# Handbook of Surgical Pathology

**Anthony S-Y. Leong** MBBS MD FRCPA FRCPath FCAP
Professor, Department of Anatomical and Cellular Pathology,
The Prince of Wales Hospital, The Chinese University of Hong Kong, Hong Kong;
Director, Division of Tissue Patholgy, Institute of Medical and Veterinary Science, Adelaide;
Clinical Professor of Pathology, University of Adelaide; Honorary Visiting Pathologist
to the Royal Adelaide Hospital, the Adelaide Women's and Children's Hospital
and the Royal Darwin Hospital, Australia

**Craig L. James** MBBS(Hons) FRCPA
Consultant Pathologist,
Gribbles Pathology, Adelaide, Australia

**Anthony C. Thomas** MBBS PhD FRCPA FRCPath
Associate Professor and Senior Consultant Pathologist,
Department of Histopathology,
Flinders Medical Centre, Bedford Park, Adelaide,
Australia

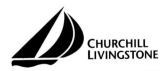

**CHURCHILL
LIVINGSTONE**

NEW YORK   EDINBURGH   LONDON   MADRID   MELBOURNE   SAN FRANCISCO   TOKYO   1996

CHURCHILL LIVINGSTONE
Medical Division of Pearson Professional Limited

Distributed in the United States of America by Churchill
Livingstone Inc., 650 Avenue of the Americas, New York, N.Y. 10011,
and by associated companies, branches and representatives
throughout the world.

First published 1996

ISBN 0443 05121 6

British Library Cataloguing in Publication Data
A catalogue record for this book is available from the British
Library.

Library of Congress Cataloging in Publication Data
A catalog record for this book is available from the Library of
Congress.

Medical knowledge is constantly changing. As new information
becomes available, changes in treatment, procedures, equipment and
the use of drugs become necessary. The authors and the publishers
have, as far as it is possible, taken care to ensure that the information
given in this text is accurate and up to date. However, readers are
strongly advised to confirm that the information, especially with regard
to drug usage, complies with latest legislation and standards of practice.

The
publisher's
policy is to use
paper manufactured
from sustainable forests

Printed in Hong Kong
NPC/01

# Contents

# Preface

The undergraduate medical curriculum is geared towards the training of a clinician so that the medical student receives exposure to a wide range of clinical disciplines. In contrast, the student sees little of the practice of surgical pathology except for brief contacts with pathologists at clinico-pathological conferences and autopsy demonstrations. The trainee or resident embarking on a career in surgical pathology carries this handicap, starting with little or no knowledge of the discipline. The first 3–6 months can be bewildering, the trainee having to learn many new practical procedures, imbibe the philosophies of the discipline, as well as assimilate massive amounts of information relevant to surgical pathology.

Much of the training in surgical pathology is an apprenticeship. The trainee receives direct instruction from the supervising pathologist or from more senior trainees. This is particularly so for the many practical aspects of the discipline. Although many excellent textbooks are available, they mostly provide instruction in pathology rather than in the practical aspects of the subject. While there are many handbooks for the clinical disciplines, there is no similar handbook for the trainee in surgical pathology. This mongraph aims to fill that hiatus, providing a comprehensive range of information required in day-to-day work with surgical biopsies.

The authors of this volume represent different chronological stages and experience in their respective careers and in the teaching of trainees, the text reflects their different perspectives. They have also worked and trained in various institutions in different continents and reflect pathology practice in different parts of the world.

In addition to the instruction and discussion of routine procedures in surgical pathology, the many other aspects of practice which are not traditionally found in textbooks are discussed. This handbook provides a brief background to the evolution of the discipline of surgical pathology and orientates the reader in the surgical pathology laboratory with emphasis on laboratory safety. The fundamentals of tissue fixation, processing and staining are elaborated in sufficient depth to allow the young pathologist to identify the causes of technical problems and artefacts, and their remedies. Besides these 'nuts and bolts' of handling surgical and cytological specimens, the reader is also instructed in the requirements and applications of many new investigative procedures including electron microscopy, immunohistochemistry, cytogenetic studies, flow cytometry, image analysis and molecular techniques which can be applied to biopsy specimens, a reflection of the rapid technological advancements in laboratory medicine. We provide lists of useful reference texts and monographs, instruction on microscopy and photography, discuss how to conduct organ and slide demonstrations, how to communicate with colleagues and clinicians, how to start a reference and slide filing system, how to use the dictaphone, and the many other aspects of day-to-day activity and function which the new trainee is exposed to but which he or she only learns through oral instruction from senior residents and pathologists.

This book does not tell you how to diagnose disease. There are many excellent textbooks on that aspect of surgical pathology. However we hope that this handbook will instruct you how to handle specimens so that they will yield the most information for diagnosis and will provide the guidance and the information necessary for a smooth, expedient and enjoyable transition from internship or other clinical disciplines into the exciting and demanding world of surgical pathology.

Anthony S-Y. Leong
Craig L. James
Anthony C. Thomas

Adelaide

# Acknowledgements

We are most grateful to Mrs Margaret Elemer who applied her considerable word processing skills to the preparation of this book.

# 1 A brief history of surgical pathology

In ancient Babylon, there was a group of important and influential individuals known as haruspices who practised the art of foretelling the future through the examination of organs of slaughtered animals. The cryptic messages derived from the examination of entrails was interpreted by the haruspex and often played an important role in the day-to-day activities of individuals living in those times. Haruspicy and histopathology share the common function of prognosticating on information obtained through the examination of tissues, but here the similarity ends. The latter is based on fact and the former on fiction. Claudius Galen (130–200 AD) was probably the first to provide detailed descriptions of the structural changes in the body associated with disease. Marco Aurelio Sevrino (1580–1656 AD) and Giovanni Battista Morgagni (1682–1771) pioneered the renaissance of morbid anatomy in Italy and Europe, and Morgagni has been regarded as the father of modern pathological anatomy. He based his work on the meticulous correlation of clinical history and autopsy findings and attempted to understand disease processes. Others assert that Marcello Malpighi (1628–1694) had stronger claims to this title, as he used the microscope more intensely, employed effective methods of fixation and also produced detailed descriptions of post-mortem examinations with clinical correlations. Matthew Baillie (1761–1823) from London, published *The Morbid Anatomy of Some of the Most Important Parts of the Human Body* in 1793, but it was only with the establishment of the microscope as a diagnostic tool in the early 1800s that information of potentially diagnostic value could be obtained from the examination of diseased tissues.

Surgical pathology probably started with the invention of the microscope. While frozen sections could be easily cut, wax embedding only became established in about 1880 and it was the advent of fixation and tissue processing that gave rise to the accelerated interest in the examination of biopsies. Bennett in Edinburgh, Scotland (1845), and Donaldson in Baltimore, Maryland (1853), were largely responsible for the use of microscopy for the diagnosis of tumours and must be regarded as contributing significantly to the birth of diagnostic histopathology and cytology.

In the 1870s, Carl Ruge and Johann Veit, at the University of Berlin, employed the surgical biopsy as a diagnostic tool, and at the German Surgical Congress in 1889, Friedrich von Esmarch, Professor of Surgery at Kiel, reinforced the need to establish a microscopic diagnosis before embarking on often extensive and mutilating surgery in cases of suspected malignant tumours. The introduction of the freezing microtome and the ability to perform frozen section examination accelerated the acceptance of this recommendation.

Rudolf Virchow (1821–1902), regarded as the 'Pope of German medicine', was responsible for the concept that each cell comes from another cell: *omnis cellula a cellula*, expounded in his book *Cellular Pathology* published in 1858. However, Virchow was a strong opponent of the use of biopsies for the diagnosis of disease, particularly cancer. This resulted from his unfortunate experience with the laryngeal carcinoma of Kaiser Frederick III. Sir Morell MacKenzie performed the biopsies which were reported as benign by Rudolf Virchow in Berlin, but a year later, at the age of 56, the Kaiser died from laryngeal cancer. This infamous case ruined McKenzie's reputation and started a wave of opposition in Europe against the technique of biopsy diagnosis, with Virchow at the forefront of this opposition. Interestingly, there is suggestion that the biopsy examined by Virchow may not have contained tumour tissue, but the material was subsequently lost and not available for review.

While interest in and the use of biopsy diagnosis stalled in Europe, it continued unabated in North America in the 1890s and quickly became an accepted procedure, with the case of the Kaiser's cancer rapidly forgotten.

In the USA, the speciality of surgical pathology was conceived and developed by surgeons and gynaecologists. Early divisions of surgical pathology were created within departments of surgery. As knowledge in pathology accumulated, the rapid advances ultimately created difficulties for physicians and surgeons who performed histopathology and cytology. With the increasing complexity coupled with the burgeoning volume of diagnostic work, surgical pathology became a fully fledged discipline with the appointment of specialists in the field of histopathology or surgical pathology.

Joseph Colt Bloodgood is regarded as the first fully fledged American surgical pathologist. Other important surgical pathologists of the past in North America include Drs Arthur Purdy Stout of Columbia-Presbyterian Hospital in New York, James Ewing and Fred Stewart of Memorial Hospital in New York, Lauren V. Ackerman of Barnes Hospital in St Louis and Pierre Masson of the University of Montreal.

Diagnostic cytology developed alongside surgical pathology. Papanicolaou, in 1928, first reported his studies on cervical cancer cytology at the Women's Hospital in New York and in the 1950s cervical cytology became an established screening procedure for cervical cancer cytology and now enjoys widespread application in many organ systems, particularly with the advent of fine needle aspiration biopsies. Today, the discipline of surgical pathology too has developed into a major branch of clinical medicine, with the surgical pathologist now completely established as an integral member of the team responsible for the care and management of the patient. While surgeons and physicians continue to be responsible for the provision of clinical services, the investigative and diagnostic backup provided by the surgical pathologist is now an indispensable component of patient management. The surgical pathologist must be able to interpret biopsies in the context of contemporary clinical practice and he/she can do this only after a solid foundation in autopsy pathology where the pathology caused by cancer and other diseases can be fully studied. Surgical pathology implies surgery, but the modern surgical pathologist is affiliated with many branches of clinical medicine including all the surgical and gynaecological specialities, internal medicine including the subspecialities of nephrology, dermatology, neurology and medical oncology, and diagnostic radiology and radiation oncology. The surgical pathologist is one of the last of a breed of true generalists who continue to examine a wide variety of tissues and retain expertise in many disease processes. However, with increasing sophistication of medical care, there is a demand for subspecialisation so that many surgical pathologists develop interest and expertise in specific organ systems and diseases.

# Further reading

King L S, Meehan M C 1973 A history of the autopsy: a review. American Journal of Pathology 73: 514–544

Lattes R 1986 Arthur Purdy Stout and his times. With a history of the laboratory of surgical pathology at the College of Physicians and Surgeons of Columbia University. American Journal of Surgical Pathology 10(suppl 1): 4–13

Ober W B 1970 The case of the Kaiser's cancer. Pathology Annual 5: 207–216

Scarani P, Salvioli G P, Eusebi V 1994 Marcello Malpighi (1628–1694). A founding father of modern anatomical pathology. American Journal of Surgical Pathology 18: 741–746

Seemayer T A 1983 The life and legacy of Professor Pierre Masson. American Journal of Surgical Pathology 7: 179–183

Tildsley G J, Lakhani S 1992 Early clinical pathologists: Rudolf Virchow (1821–1902). Journal of Clinical Pathology 45: 6–7

# 2 Laboratory layout and design

# Introduction

It is often more difficult to modify a pre-existing laboratory to comply with modern-day requirements than to design a new laboratory, and yet, the majority of pathologists concerned with laboratory layout will be faced with the former situation. Health and safety requirements demand attention to factors that are potential risks: over-crowding; ill- or over-equipped laboratories; rodent or insect infestation; poor lighting, poor ventilation or fume extraction; dangerous and inflammable chemicals; infectious material; situations which create dangerous aerosols; and unauthorised entry. Efficiency requirements demand attention to factors that influence time and motion, and documentation: geographical relationships between specimen reception and cut-up areas, and between reporting room(s) and the typing pool; the siting of filing systems for slides, blocks, photographs and reports; and the housing of departmental library books, manuals and journals. This chapter deals with the basic principles of laboratory design and its equipment, the cut-up area and its instruments and disinfectants. It should be read in conjunction with the succeeding chapter, which describes in greater detail guidelines for laboratory safety.

# Principles of laboratory layout and design

## Laboratory layout

### Routine laboratories

In some laboratories, a central area common to all branches of pathology is set aside for accessioning specimens, but in histopathology this area is usually separate from the other disciplines and forms an integral part of the surgical pathology laboratory. Ideally, it should be in close proximity to both the typing pool and the cut-up area. Within the reception area there should be facility for report storage and retrieval, to enable immediate access to previous histology on any particular case. Proximity to the cut-up area enables potentially infective material to be handled with safety. Whether accessioning is performed by clerical or technical staff, specimens should be handled with gloved hands and the request forms should be maintained free of contamination. This is largely a matter of organisation and common sense, with the exact sequence of events differing from laboratory to laboratory.

Within the proximity of the cut-up area there should be provision for specimen storage. Ideally, this should be a separate room or alcove, which, owing to formalin vapours, should be well ventilated and capable of being shut off from all other areas of the laboratory in the event of formalin spillage. Tissue processors are also best situated in a separate room which can be closed off from the remainder of the cut-up area by fire-proof doors. Embedding, sectioning, staining and mounting of sections should also be performed in close proximity to the cut-up area and tissue processors to avoid the need to transport potentially hazardous chemicals. It is this complex of reception, typing pool, cut-up area and routine laboratory that forms the nucleus of most surgical laboratories.

### Special laboratories

The provision of more specialised areas, such as small biopsy and immunohisto-chemistry laboratories, depends on the size and demand of individual departments but the same principles regarding safety and efficiency apply. An electron microscopy service, if provided, requires careful consideration in laboratory layout. The production of semi-thin and ultra-thin sections requires a dust- and draught-free environment. The area must be vibration free and the room temperature capable of being controlled within a fairly narrow range. For this reason, many such units are usually situated in the basement. Provision of a dark room in close proximity to the electron microscopy suite is essential.

## Offices

Ideally, the pathologist's office or the reporting room should be close to the typing pool, enabling reports, whether written or dictated, to be quickly and efficiently conveyed to the clerical staff and returned to the pathologist for validation. Whilst some laboratories provide for a common reporting room duly equipped with double- or multiple-headed microscopes, others have separate pathologist offices where reporting takes place. The latter requires consideration of transfer of reports to and from the typing pool. With the advent of multiple computer terminals linked to a central word processor, or central dictation facilities, the advantages of a central reporting room are reduced. Electronic validation and minor correction of reports can be made by the pathologist without the need for physical transfer of documents.

## Quiet areas

The practice of surgical pathology requires immediate access to specialised reference texts and manuals but there is often a conflict between use and accessibility. Few laboratories are fortunate enough to be able to provide a separate quiet area for reading, leading to the sequestration of books within individual offices – a practice which can be both inefficient and frustrating. A common reporting room has the advantage of doubling as a 'library' and quiet reading area, also providing a focus for consultations between pathologists. Smoking and eating should not be permitted within the work area and many institutions now ban smoking within the building confines. The provision of tea-rooms and seminar rooms is desirable, but these are luxuries which are often unaffordable; however, there should be facilities for storing outer garments and valuables.

## Interior design

### General considerations

Factors which influence the design of interior furnishing include the following:

1  Fire precautions should provide for self-closing fire-proof doors, fire extinguishers and safe handling of inflammable solvents.
2  There should be adequate exhaust systems to provide in-ward fresh air flow in all areas where solvents, formalin and other vaporising chemicals are in use.
3  Wash basins with running water should be provided in each laboratory and a dependable source of good quality water is essential. The public water system should be protected from back-flow by appropriate valves.
4  Drinking water should be provided as separate fountains outside the laboratory, for example located in the corridor. There should be no cross-connections between water for laboratory purposes and drinking water.

5   The electrical supply must be reliable and of adequate capacity, with provision of three-phase where necessary. An emergency back-up supply is desirable for the support of essential equipment. Freezers and tissue processors may be fitted with alarm systems to warn of electrical fault or breakdown.

6   First-aid facilities should be readily available and include provision of eye baths and shower facilities in the event of chemical spillage.

7   Security is of utmost importance and laboratories should not be accessible to unauthorised personnel especially outside working hours.

## Furnishings

There must be ample space and adequate lighting for conducting laboratory procedures safely. The walls, ceilings and floors should be smooth, impermeable to liquids, resistant to chemicals and easily cleanable. Floors should be slip-resistant, especially in areas subject to contamination by paraffin wax. Work tops must be stable, of suitable height and vibration free, particularly in areas where microscopes, balances and sectioning equipment are sited. Bench tops should be impervious to water, resistant to chemicals and able to withstand moderate heat. There should be adequate storage space to prevent the cluttering of benches; shelving should be of acceptable height and built-in furniture should be sturdy and easy to clean. Laboratory chairs should be stable and if fitted with castors, these should be of the locking type.

## The cut-up area

### Layout

Easy access to the reception area, the main laboratory area, tissue processors and specimen storage is essential. Photography equipment should be easily and readily available, either within a separate area adjacent to the cut-up room or through use of a portable trolley on which the camera is mounted (see Ch. 11).

### Exhaust systems

The layout of the cut-up area is often determined, to some extent, by the provision of exhaust extraction and ventilation. Direct access to the exterior where formalin fumes can be discharged negates the need for expensive ducting. There must be adequate formalin fume extraction which may be provided by enclosure in a hood or by back wall extractor fans. It should be remembered that formalin fumes are denser than air and extraction situated above the bench without enclosure will merely result in fumes being drawn past the operator. Down-draught fume extraction is more efficient and allows greater flexibility in the siting of the cut-up work bench.

### Work surfaces

Dissection benches should be of suitable height, stain resistant and able to withstand disinfectants, acids, alkalis and solvents. High quality stainless steel is a suitable material. The edges should be rounded where possible and, for ease of cleaning, there should be no awkward crevices.

### Waste disposal

Within the down-draught bench, integrated washing and flushing systems can be incorporated. Waste material can be removed by waste disposal units but care must be taken that waste is discharged in accordance with local legislation. If such units are not available, a sluice over which bowel specimens are opened can be installed.

## Emergency facilities

A wash basin should be installed, preferably at the exit of the cut-up area. This should be provided with elbow- or foot-operated taps to avoid contamination. Eye-wash facilities must be available although with the use of goggles, such injuries should not occur. A shower alcove, normally situated near the exit, should also be accessible in the event of chemical spillage.

First-aid kits must be sited in every laboratory area and regularly checked and maintained.

Fire extinguishers and fire blankets should be readily available and of the correct type to deal with either electrical or solvent-based fires.

## Chemical storage

As previously stated, wherever possible, specimen storage and tissue processors should be sited in separate areas adjacent to the cut-up area. Inflammable solvents should be stored in a fire-proof cupboard especially designed for the purpose.

## Equipment

### Infectious material and contamination

Safety cabinets must be available for examination and handling of potentially infectious tissues, such as those received for frozen section examination. Cryostats for frozen section work are best situated adjacent to the safety cabinet. Freezing of tissue is now generally performed by snap freezing in liquid nitrogen or in an isopentane slurry immersed in liquid nitrogen. This can be performed in a stainless steel thermos flask within the safety cabinet, the stock liquid nitrogen being stored in a specially manufactured refillable container.

With hand written macroscopic descriptions, care must be taken to avoid contamination of request forms and drafted reports. This often requires careful organisation. The dictation of macroscopic descriptions allows some of these problems to be overcome but then care must be taken to avoid contamination of the dictaphone equipment. Foot-operated or voice-activated recorders suitably sited over the cut-up bench are desirable.

## Protective clothing

Basic protective clothing for dissection work includes gowns, plastic aprons, rubber boots and surgical gloves. More recently, there has been greater attention given to safety within the cut-up area. The use of goggles or full face visors prevent eye splashes from formalin and tissue fluids. Face masks can be used for potentially infective specimens, whilst ventilation masks and respirators can be used in areas heavily contaminated by formalin and chemical fumes. Chemical products capable of neutralising formalin spillage are currently available. A chain-mail glove fitted over, or a protective cloth glove fitted under, the surgical glove of one hand protects against scalpel blade injury. Kevlar gloves allow greater flexibility of movement but do not protect against needle-stick and -prick injuries. These protective measures should be used by all trainees and, unless employed, many employers will not accept liability in the event of injury.

## Dissection instruments

Dissection instruments include scalpels, forceps (toothed and untoothed), scissors of different sizes, knives of varying lengths, probes and stainless steel rulers. Knives should be kept sharp at all times and this necessitates the provision of sharpening equipment. It is impossible to obtain satisfactory sections with a blunt knife. Disposable feather blades are an alternative to non-disposable knives. These come in varying sizes of blade and should be used with a blade holder. Scalpel blades should be removed from the handle with a blade remover. A sharps container must be easily accessible for used blades and needles which must not be discarded in normal waste bins. All dissection instruments should be carefully looked after. There is nothing more frustrating than forceps that do not grip properly, or scissors or knives that do not cut properly. Left-handed scissors are a scarcity and it may be necessary to have personalised instruments.

### Other cut-up equipment

Cut-up boards may be made of cork but these are sometimes difficult to clean and, more recently, polythene- or plastic-based boards similar to domestic chopping boards have come into common use. The board should be of the same height, at least, as the surrounding lip of the stainless steel work top to allow sectioning of tissues parallel to the work face without angling of the knife. Marker ink or dyes should be readily available for identifying excision margins. Stainless steel tissue cassettes are now being replaced by plastic Tissue Tek cassettes resistant to solvents. These may be used with built in plastic lids or separate, reusable stainless steel lids. Small specimens are retained by wrapping in tissue paper, then enclosure in fine mesh cassettes or with foam, although the latter can cause artefacts in tissue sections.

It is essential to maintain the utmost cleanliness in the cut-up area particularly with regard to the dissection board and instruments in order to avoid carry over from one specimen to another, one of the most serious artefacts in surgical pathology.

## Disinfectants

Although autoclaving equipment is not often available in most surgical pathology laboratories, it is generally accessible within microbiology laboratories. Equipment such as trays, cut-up instruments, gowns, staining jars, etc., can be autoclaved at 125°C for 1 hour. Instruments and work tops within the cut-up area should be disinfected daily and some laboratories place cut-up instruments in disinfectant solution in between use. Appropriate disinfectants for cleaning surfaces and for immersion of contaminated instruments and other non-disposable material which cannot be autoclaved, include Medol or other phenolic compounds, hypochlorite solution, alcoholic-iodine and Iodophor. Aldehydes such as formaldehyde and glutaraldehyde may also be used, with each disinfectant having different applications.

### Chlorine

Chlorine in the form of sodium hypochlorite is a universal disinfectant and active against all micro-organisms, although it is inactivated by protein and may not be suitable for use against mycobacteria. It is also corrosive to metals and should not be used for disinfecting items such as centrifuges and cryostats. Concentrations between 0.1% and 1% providing between 1000 and 10 000 parts per million (ppm) of available chlorine will cover most situations. Concentrations which provide between 2500 and 5000 ppm are suitable for general use and the higher concentration is recommended for decontamination of blood and body fluids.

## Phenolic compounds

Phenolic compounds are used for organic material and mycobacteria but give variable results against viruses. They are used at concentrations between 2% and 5% but may leech some plastics.

## Aldehydes

Aldehydes are effective against mycobacteria and viruses and are not inactivated by protein. Formaldehyde, either as liquid or as a vapour, is particularly useful for disinfecting cryostats and safety cabinets, whilst glutaraldehyde may be used for wiping down surfaces and for disinfecting cut-up instruments.

## Other disinfectants

Iodine has a disinfectant action similar to that of the hypochlorites and may be used in concentrations providing 75 ppm as available iodine.

Sodium hypochlorite is the most effective decontaminant known for the AIDS virus and is the disinfectant of choice for clean up of the work area, but since it corrodes metal, 95% ethanol or 10% formalin, also known to inactivate the virus, is favoured for use inside the cryostat. The older method of placing a large beaker of 40% formalin in the closed defrosting chamber overnight is less efficacious.

# 3 Laboratory safety

# General principles of laboratory safety

This chapter should be read in conjunction with the preceding chapter on laboratory layout and design which incorporates aspects of laboratory safety. All laboratory staff must be made aware of the hazards of working in a laboratory environment and the procedures required to enable them to work safely. New staff members need to be orientated to these safety practices which must be documented in a laboratory safety manual. This manual must be continually updated and brought to the attention of all staff as part of continuing education. It is also the responsibility of all trainees to ensure that they acquaint themselves with the principles of laboratory safety and their implementation.

## Laboratory code of practice

1   The laboratory should be kept neat, clean and free of articles not pertinent to laboratory work.
2   Shelves and cupboards should be kept tidy and apparatus and reagents should be put away after use.
3   Work surfaces should be decontaminated following spillage of potentially dangerous material and also on a regular basis.
4   Laboratory benches should not be used as seats.
5   Eating, drinking, smoking and the storage of food must not be permitted in the work area. Laboratory fridges must not be used for storage of food and drink.
6   Never run in the laboratory area, avoid sudden movement and always exercise care when opening and closing doors.

7   Clothing must be suited to the laboratory environment. Thongs, slippers and open-toed shoes should not be worn.
8   Long hair should be tied back.
9   Protective gowns should be properly buttoned or tied and should not be worn outside the laboratory. In particular, protective clothing must not be worn in rest room areas or canteens and contaminated clothing should be disinfected prior to laundering.
10   Safety glasses or visors must be worn, when necessary, to protect the eyes from splashes.
11   Full respiratory equipment must be available for work in rooms containing solvent or formalin vapours.
12   Protective gloves must be worn when handling all potentially infectious materials. Soiled gloves must be removed prior to handling equipment such as dictaphones, telephones, doorhandles and microscopes, and should be discarded with other laboratory waste.
13   Do not chew or place objects such as pencils and pens in the mouth and do not moisten stick-on labels and envelopes with the tongue. Never pipette fluids with the mouth; always use automatic pipettes or suction devices.
14   Regard all substances as dangerous until there is information to the contrary. Spilt materials should be cleaned up immediately, so avoiding the hazards of fumes, slipperiness, toxicity and flammability.
15   Chemical reagents must be clearly labelled and no chemical should ever be stored in containers not designed for that purpose, e.g. empty drink bottles. Labels for poisonous, infectious, corrosive and radioactive substances have been adopted by the United

Nations and examples of these are provided in Figure 3.1.

16 Broken glassware and sharps must be placed in special containers provided.

17 Always use safety carriers for glass containers of 2 litres or more. Large volume containers must be fitted with appropriate handles and managed by two people.

18 Knives should be removed from microtomes.

19 Bunsen burners should be turned off before leaving the laboratory.

20 Staff should wash their hands after handling infectious materials and when leaving the laboratory area. Wash basins must be available, preferably at the laboratory exit. Eye washes or baths must also be available in the event of eye splashes and shower alcoves should be installed near the laboratory exit for use in the event of more generalised chemical contamination.

21 Personal visitors are not allowed in the laboratory area for their own safety. Official visitors should be suitably attired and under laboratory staff supervision.

## Laboratory safety committee

It is essential that the laboratory has a safety policy and a supporting programme for its implementation. A laboratory safety committee, answerable to the management and head of the department, should be set up. The composition of the committee will vary depending on the size and nature of the laboratory but should include personnel from technical, clerical and medical staff. The committee should be responsible for providing continuing instruction in laboratory safety, for the investigation of laboratory accidents and be generally responsible

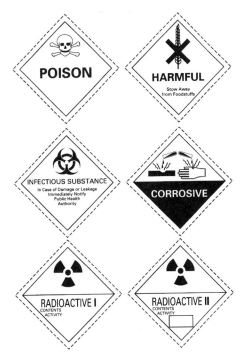

**Fig. 3.1** International hazard labels

for implementation of prescribed safety procedures.

## Immunisation and vaccination

All laboratory staff should have a Mantoux test and routine chest X-ray on commencement of employment. Vaccination against hepatitis B is also recommended and most institutions provide these immunisations routinely.

## Contingency plans and emergency procedures

The laboratory safety manual should include contingency plans in the event of emergencies. These should include procedural instructions in the event of sharps injuries, evacuation procedures and fire drills which should be practised regularly.

Following the reporting of any sharps injury, steps should be taken to ascertain the hepatitis B and C, and HIV status of the patient source of potential infection, as well as the recipient of the injury. Serological conversion over the following months must be sought and documented.

# Specific safety issues

## The handling of infectious material

### Classification of micro-organisms and infected material

Micro-organisms and infected material may be classified into four groups according to the level of hazard they present and the minimal safety conditions required for handling them.

### Category A
Category A pathogens include organisms that are extremely hazardous to laboratory staff and which may cause serious disease outbreaks. These pathogens are not normally encountered in routine laboratory work and require the most stringent conditions for their containment. If a specimen received in a clinical laboratory is suspected of being, or is subsequently shown to be, infected with a Category A pathogen, all work on that specimen must cease. The specimen must be moved to Category B1 accommodation pending transfer to a Category A laboratory. The relevant authorities must be notified and all staff who have handled such a specimen must be identified. Category A pathogens include: simian herpes (BO) virus, Lassa fever virus, Marburg virus, rabies virus, smallpox virus, Crimea (Congo) haemorrhagic fever (HF) virus, Machupo HF virus, Junin HF virus, Venezuelan equine encephalitis virus and Ebola virus.

### Category B1
Category B1 pathogens include organisms which offer special hazards to laboratory staff and for which special accommodation and conditions for containment must be provided. All specimens that contain or are suspected of containing a Category B1 pathogen must be labelled 'Danger of infection' on the specimen container and request form. Category B1 pathogens include, viruses and rickettsiae: arbovirus, *Chlamydia psittaci*, *Coxiella burnetti*, hepatitis B virus deliberately introduced into the laboratory as test materials and controls; bacteria: *Bartonella* species, *Brucella* species, *Clostridium botulinum*, *Francisella tularensis*, *Legionella* species, mycobacteria, *Pseudomonas mallei* and *pseudomallei*, *Salmonella typhi* and *paratyphi* A and *Yersinia pestis*; and fungi: all fungi isolated from pulmonary tissue (except candida), *Blastomyces dermatidis*, *Coccidiodes immitis*, *Cryptococcus neoformans*, *Histoplasma capsulatum* and *Paracoccidioides brasilliensis*. Brain and spinal cord material from patients with Creutzfeldt–Jakob disease and multiple sclerosis, and pathogenic amoebae are also included under Category B1 material and pathogens.

### Category B2
Category B2 material requires special conditions for containment but not necessarily for accommodation and includes all specimens from patients in renal units who have not been screened, all specimens from patients in risk groups such as drug addicts, all specimens other than brain and spinal cord tissue from patients suffering from Creutzfeldt–Jakob disease, all specimens from patients with defective

or altered immunological competence, all specimens known to be hepatitis B antigen positive, all specimens from patients suffering from infective, or suspected infective, diseases of the liver, e.g. hepatitis C, and all specimens known or suspected of being infected with HIV. The distinction between Categories B1 and B2 acknowledges the fact that it is not practicable to require special accommodation for biochemical and haematological tests on all specimens infected, or suspected of being infected, with some organisms such as hepatitis B, hepatitis C viruses and HIV. Whilst these specimens may be handled in routine biochemical and haematology laboratories, special precautions are required. In histopathology laboratories, tissue specimens infected with these viruses should be handled as for B1 pathogens.

## Category C

This category includes organisms, viruses and materials not listed in Categories A, B1 or B2 and which offer no potential hazards to laboratory staff provided appropriate safety codes of practice are observed.

### General principles

Portals of infection include the skin, the eye, the respiratory tract and the mouth. Methods of infection include fingers to mouth or eye, mouthing of pipettes, pencils and sticky labels, splashing of face, hands and clothing, aerosols from splashing of fluids or dried infected dust and inoculation by needle or scalpel blade. Sources of infection include blood, serum, tissues, aspirates, splattering through manipulation of tissues, grinding, sawing and homogenisation of tissues, centrifuging, leakages, spilling and overfilling.

Recently, the concept of 'universal precautions' has been adopted by many health institutions throughout the world. This concept assumes that all tissues, blood and body fluids are potentially infectious and should be handled in such a way as to minimise the risk of transferring infection. Surgical pathology is one discipline where the routine use of universal precautions is not always practicable and would introduce an unacceptable delay in the reporting of some specimens. For this reason, it is mandatory that the pathologist is made aware of the full clinical history in each case and potentially infectious material be appropriately and clearly labelled. Containers which have leaked and request forms contaminated with biological material must only be handled with gloves. Gowns should be worn and the specimen immediately transferred to a safety cabinet. The specimen should be placed in a new container, the old one being disinfected with hypochlorite and discarded in the appropriate receptacle. Contaminated paperwork should be sealed in a plastic bag, photocopied and discarded. Care should be taken to disinfect any specimen-carrying container. Specimen containers suspected of containing Category B1 pathogens must also be handled only with the gloved hand.

### Protective measures

Specimens suspected of containing hepatitis B or C virus, HIV, TB, hydatid and herpes should be adequately fixed in formalin before handling and this may take up to 24 hours or longer for large specimens. If electron microscopy is to be performed, then the tissue should be fixed in gluteraldehyde for 24 hours. Material from cases of suspected Creutzfeldt–Jakob disease (spongiform encephalopathy) should be regarded as potentially infectious even after prolonged fixation or after the application of other chemical sterilising agents. All such tissues should be placed in concentrated formalin for 14 days before phenol is added to make a 15% solution. Fixation in the formalin-phenol should proceed for a further period. A similar concentration of phenol should be used routinely in the fixatives employed in processing machines for neuropathology tissue. Specimens should only be cut up in the designated areas which have adequate fume extraction. Gloves and aprons must be used when dissecting specimens. Do not handle fixed or unfixed specimens with bare hands. Instruments and cut-up work tops must be cleaned and disinfected after use. Container lids must be properly secured on returning reserve tissue to the container. Balances should be protected through the use of disposable plastic trays and cleaned after use.

The following protective clothing should be made available: boiler suits, rubber boots, disposable plastic aprons, long sleeve gowns, full face visors, full face respirators, twin canister respirators, surgical gloves, chain-link or protective cloth gloves and protective goggles. The extent of protective clothing used should be appropriate to the situation and it should be remembered that compensation for any injury incurred is unlikely if adequate precautions are not taken.

### Safety cabinets

There are various types of safety cabinet designed for different uses. Class I open-fronted exhaust protective cabinets offer adequate protection to the worker against inhalation of aerosols and materials containing Category B1 pathogens. Class II vertical laminar flow cabinets recirculate some filtered air, exhaust some to the atmosphere and take in replacement air through the open front. They offer protection from contamination to the material handled and some protection to the worker depending upon the design. They are mainly used in tissue culture work but must not be used for handling Category A or B1 pathogens. Class III totally enclosed exhaust protective cabinets are gas tight and fitted with glove ports. They are used for handling Category A pathogens when complete isolation is required.

Any specimen that is received fresh or is suspected of containing a Category B1 pathogen should be handled in a safety cabinet. The cabinet must never be used unless the fan is switched on and the airflow indicator is in the 'safe' position. The fan should be kept on for 5 minutes after use. All work must be performed well inside the cabinet and any viewing panel that can be opened must be closed when the cabinet is in use. The ultraviolet lamp should be left on and any spills should be cleaned up, as they occur, with hypochlorite solution. The cabinet should be kept free of unnecessary equipment and reagents. Bunsen burners must not be used inside the cabinet as this can lead to distortion of air flow and may result in filters being burned. The cabinet must be frequently disinfected and there should be regular maintenance to check airflow, Hepa filters and the ultraviolet lamp.

Material received for frozen section should be handled in the safety cabinet. If it is known to be infectious, there must be good clinical reasons for proceeding with a frozen section in preference to examination after fixation. If frozen section examination is performed, double gloves, goggles, mask and gown must be worn and subsequent decontamination of safety cabinet and cryostat must be carried out. Care must be taken to limit the area of contamination and to protect staff not directly involved in the preparation of the frozen section.

Procedures with a high potential for creating hazardous aerosols must also be conducted within the safety cabinet. These include centrifugation, grinding, sawing, blending, vigorous shaking or mixing of infectious fluids or tissues.

## Exhaust hoods

There must be adequate exhaust over areas with formalin fumes, and solvent and chemical vapours. Exhaust hoods may be free standing where fumes are exhausted through a charcoal filter and the air re-circulated. With this type of system, the filter can very quickly become saturated, whereupon continued use merely redirects fumes into the laboratory area. Permanent hoods which direct fumes to the exterior are more desirable but are subject to local regulations regarding pollution and often require expensive ducting systems. When selecting or designing such a system, it should be remembered that many fumes and vapours are denser than air and an extractor hood sited over the source of the hazard will only make matters worse by drawing the fumes upward past the worker. Generally, extractors sited in the back wall of the hood offer the best protection but the draught must be sufficient to draw the vapours away from the worker. Fumes such as formalin and solvent vapours can easily be monitored and internationally accepted safe concentrations should not be exceeded.

## Cryogenic substances

Liquid nitrogen is the main cryogenic substance used in histopathology and is used in conjunction with isopentanes for snap freezing of tissues. Although it may seem relatively harmless, liquid nitrogen through extreme cold (boiling point at 1 atmosphere being −195°C) can cause injuries similar to a burn. Unprotected parts of the body will adhere to extremely cooled surfaces and flesh will tear when withdrawal is attempted. A small volume of liquid nitrogen converts to a large volume of gas which can displace oxygen from the air, and breathing of such air with lowered oxygen concentrations can result in loss of consciousness without warning symptoms. The density of the cold vapour makes this hazard greater nearer to floor level. When handling liquid nitrogen, a full face mask, loose leather gloves and closed-up footwear must be worn. The gloves should be easily removable in the event of liquid becoming trapped inside. For bulk transfer operations, there should be additional protection of a full-length leather apron. Trousers should be worn outside boots to prevent spilt liquid being trapped.

Storage must be in cryogenic containers with vented stoppers to prevent ice-plug formation. These may be filled from bulk dewars using cryogenic pumps fitted with shatter-proof silicone dispensing tubes for small quantities, and from pressurised bulk supply lines for larger quantities. With the latter, a second person should be in attendance, standing away but within visual distance. Care must be taken when transferring liquid nitrogen to a warm vessel to prevent rapid boil-off, splashing and thermal shock. Deteriorated or scratched glass vessels may explode during filling. Only long-handled tongs and instruments should be used when withdrawing objects immersed in liquid nitrogen. A blue tint indicates the presence of condensed oxygen and this may necessitate handling procedures applicable to oxygen.

Liquid nitrogen splashed onto body areas should be immediately flushed with water and affected clothing replaced as quickly as possible. Emergency first aid similar to that specified for frost bite should be sought. The affected part should not be massaged or exposed to radiant heat. Victims exhibiting signs of asphyxia should be moved to a well ventilated area. In severe cases, artificial respiration may be necessary. Solid carbon dioxide or dry ice is still used in some laboratories for freezing and transportation of tissue. Protective measures similar to those used for liquid nitrogen should be employed in the handling of dry ice.

## Chemical hazards

The most common dangers from chemicals are burns, explosions, fires and toxic fumes. Splattering from acid, caustic material and strong oxidising agents cause the greatest hazard to eyes, skin and clothing. The inhalation of excess vapours, particularly from solvents, may produce toxic effects. These may have no discernible effects on health, but can include loss of co-ordination, loss of concentration, drowsiness and increased proneness to accidents. More permanent damage to blood, lungs, liver, kidney and gastrointestinal tract may also result. Some chemicals and dyes have carcinogenic properties whilst the majority of solvents will cause skin and mucosal damage with prolonged or repeated contact. A list of reported adverse health effects of some of the more common laboratory chemicals is given in Table 3.1.

Bottle carriers should be used to carry bottles of acid or caustic material and any

**Table 3.1**   Reported adverse effects of selected laboratory chemicals

| Chemical | Acute | Chronic |
|---|---|---|
| Acetaldehyde (acetic aldehyde; ethanal) | Eye and respiratory tract irritation; narcotic effects | Bronchitis; liver damage |
| Acetic anhydride (acetyl oxide; ethanoic anhydride) | Strong eye and respiratory tract irritation, corrosive action | |
| Acetone (dimethyl ketone; 2-propanone) | Slight eye, nose and throat irritation; narcotic effects | |
| Acetonitrile (methyl cyanide) | Respiratory irritation; cyanide poisoning | |
| Acrolein | Lachrymation; respiratory irritation | |
| Aniline (aminobenzene; phenylamine) | Cyanosis due to methaemoglobinaemia; slight narcotic effects; respiratory paralysis | |
| Benzene (benzol) | Narcotic effects | Leukaemia; liver and kidney damage; aplastic anaemia |
| Carbon tetrachloride (tetrachloromethane) | Headache, nausea; slight jaundice; loss of appetite; narcosis; liver and kidney damage | Liver and kidney damage; gastrointestinal disturbances |

| Chemical | Acute | Chronic |
|---|---|---|
| Chloroform (trichloromethane) | Similar to carbon tetrachloride; liver injury; narcotic effects; nausea; loss of appetite | |
| Dioxane | Narcosis; liver and kidney damage | |
| Formalin | Respiratory and mucous membrane irritation | |
| Gluteraldehyde | Respiratory and mucous membrane irritation | |
| Methanol (methyl alcohol; wood alcohol; wood spirit) | Narcotic effects; mucous membrane irritation; damage to optic nerve possible | Damage to retina and optic nerve |
| Nitrobenzene (nitrobenzol; oil of mirbane) | Cyanosis due to methaemoglobinaemia; slight narcotic effect | Anaemia; hypotension; methaemoglobinaemia with cyanosis; bladder irritation; liver damage |
| Pyridine | Liver and kidney damage; neurotoxicity | Neurotoxicity |
| Tetrahydrofuran (diethylene oxide; tetramethylene oxide) | Narcosis; liver and kidney damage; eye and respiratory tract irritation | |
| Toluene (methyl benzene; phenyl methane; toluol) | Narcotic effects | Non-specific neurological impairment; addiction possible |
| Trichloroethylene (ethinyl trichloride) | Narcotic effects | Liver damage; non-specific neurological impairment |
| m-Xylene (1,3 dimethylbenzene) | Narcotic effects; headache, dizziness, fatigue; nausea | Non-specific neurological impairment |
| o-Xylene (1,2 dimethylbenzene) | Narcotic effects; headache, dizziness, fatigue; nausea | Non-specific neurological impairment |
| p-Xylene (1,4 dimethylbenzene) | Narcotic effects; headache dizziness, fatigue; nausea | Non-specific neurological impairment |

glass container of 2 litres or more. Bottles should be held around the body and not grasped by the neck. Exhaust hoods should be used for odoriferous, corrosive and toxic fumes and care should be taken not to contaminate hands with staining solutions and chemicals. Protective goggles should be worn when dealing with acids, caustic material and eye irritants. When diluting acids, the acid should always be added slowly to water; water should never be added to acid. All chemicals should be dispensed with automatic pipettes and never by mouth pipette. All reagents must be properly labelled and preferably with the date of preparation and expiration or dye batch number if applicable. Spillage of hazardous chemicals must be dealt with immediately and spill kits should be readily available within all laboratory areas. Splashes to the eyes should be flushed immediately with water and proper medical assistance sought. Many chemicals commonly found in the laboratory undergo dangerous reactions if allowed to come into contact with each other. A list of some incompatible chemicals is given in Table 3.2.

Table 3.2    Incompatible chemicals. Many chemicals commonly found in the laboratory undergo dangerous reactions if allowed to come into contact with certain other chemicals. Some incompatible chemicals are listed below

| | | | |
|---|---|---|---|
| Acetic acid | With chromic acid, nitric acid, hydroxyl-containing compounds, ethylene glycol, perchloric acid, peroxides and permanganates | | finely divided organics or combustibles, carbon |
| Acetone | With concentrated sulphuric and nitric acid mixtures | Chlorine | With ammonia, acetylene, butadiene, benzine and other petroleum fractions, hydrogen, sodium carbide, turpentine, and finely divided powdered metals |
| Acetylene | With copper (tubing), fluorine, bromine, chlorine, iodine, silver, mercury, and their compounds | Chlorine dioxide | With ammonia, methane, phosphine, hydrogen sulphide |
| Alkali metals | With water, carbon dioxide, carbon tetrachloride, and other chlorinated hydrocarbons | Chromic acid | With acetic acid, naphthalene, camphor, alcohol, glycerol, turpentine, and other flammable liquids |
| Ammonia, anhydrous | With mercury, halogens, calcium, hypochlorite, hydrogen fluoride | Copper | With acetylene, hydrogen peroxide |
| Ammonium nitrate | With acids, metal powders, flammable liquids, chlorates, nitrates, sulphur, and finely divided organics or combustibles | Cyanides | With acids and alkalis |
| | | Flammable liquids | With ammonium nitrate, chromic acid, hydrogen peroxide, nitric acid, sodium peroxide, halogens |
| Aniline | With nitric acid, hydrogen peroxide | Hydrocarbons | With fluorine, chlorine, formine, chromic acid, sodium peroxide |
| Bromine | With ammonia, acetylene, butadiene, butane, hydrogen, sodium carbide, turpentine, and finely divided metals | Hydrogen peroxide | With copper, chromium, iron, most metals or their respective salts, flammable fluids and other combustible materials, aniline, nitromethane |
| Carbon, activated | With all oxidising agents | Hydrogen sulphide | With fuming nitric acid, oxidising gases |
| Chlorates | With ammonium salts, acids, metal powders, sulphur, | Iodine | With acetylene, ammonia |

| | | | | |
|---|---|---|---|---|
| Mercury | With acetylene, fulminic acid, hydrogen | | Sodium | With carbon tetrachloride, carbon dioxide, water |
| Nitric acid | With acetic, chromic and hydrocyanic acids, aniline, carbon, hydrogen sulphide, fluids or gases, and substances that are readily nitrated | | Silver | With acetylene, oxalic acid, tartaric acid, ammonium compounds |
| Oxalic acid | With silver, mercury | | Sodium azide | Commonly used as a preservative, it forms unstable explosive compounds with lead, copper and other metals. If flushed into sinks, the trap can explode when worked on by a plumber |
| Oxygen | With oils, grease, hydrogen, flammable liquids, solids and gases | | | |
| Perchloric acid | With acetic anhydride, bismuth and its alloys, alcohol, paper, wood and other organic materials | | Sodium peroxide | With any oxidisable substance e.g. methanol, glacial acetic acid, acetic anhydride, benzaldehyde, carbon disulphide, glycerol, ethylene glycol, ethyl acetate, furfural |
| Phosphorus pentoxide | With water | | | |
| Potassium permanganate | With glycerol, ethylene glycol, benzaldehyde, sulphuric acid | | Sulphuric acid | With chlorates, perchlorates, permanganates, water |

All compressed and liquefied gas cylinders should be clearly marked with the name of the contents and gas cylinders should be regularly examined and tested for worthiness. Cylinders must not be left free standing but should be secured so that they cannot fall. Pressure-relief devices and regulators must be fitted and protection caps must be in place when not in use.

## Fire hazards

Many chemicals and reagents used in histopathology are flammable and a potential fire hazard. Containers in which these chemicals are kept should be clearly labelled as to contents and stored in cabinets with the appropriate fire rating for storing of flammable liquids. Only restricted quantities should be allowed in the laboratory workplace outside designated storage areas. Volatile flammable solvents should only be handled in exhausted areas. Although it is desirable that these solvents should be stored at low temperatures, they should not be kept in domestic fridges to avoid thermostat spark-generated explosions. Highly corrosive or oxidising agents such as nitric acid must never be stored with solvents such as acetone. Fires have been caused by the build up of pressure and subsequent explosion of acid bottles igniting the solvent.

It is desirable for tissue processing machines, in which flammable solvents are in continual use, to be located separately from the rest of the laboratory area, preferably with intervening fire-proof doors. Bunsen burners and gas taps should be regularly checked for gas leaks and deteriorated hoses immediately replaced.

Joiners and T-pieces, and plastic tubing should not be used. Gas supplies must be turned off after use and gas taps must be accessible at all times.

Fire extinguishers and blankets must be located at strategic points throughout the laboratory; the number, maintenance and location are subject to local fire regulations and these must be adhered to. Smoke detectors must be installed and fire alarm systems regularly checked. Escape routes in the event of fire must be clearly designated, so that visitors and regular staff alike can safely evacuate the building. Water extinguishers are used for fires of ordinary combustibles such as paper, cloth and wood. Carbon dioxide and dry chemical extinguishers are used for fires of flammable liquids such as alcohol or xylene and for fires involving electrical motors and wiring. Never use water extinguishers for these types of fire. Other types of extinguisher include foam, soda acid and BCF. These should all be used in accordance with local fire regulations.

## Radiation hazards

The increasing use of radioimmunoassays in clinical laboratories makes it necessary for staff to be aware of radiation hazards and related safety precautions. The amount of radiation is small but certain rules should be followed. Radioactive material must be properly labelled and stored in specific designated areas. Gloves, a long-sleeved gown and plastic apron should be worn and appropriate shields used for protection against direct rays. Spills should be contained and contaminated surfaces washed with alkali reagents. This should be repeated until the radioactivity count is below 300 counts per minute. Radioactive waste should be disposed of in properly designated containers and never

down the sink. Staff routinely working with these reagents should wear film badges and these should be regularly monitored.

Occasionally, radioactive specimens such as tumours and thyroid glands will be received by the laboratory. Any tumour in which 'needles' are embedded should be suspected of being radioactive. Most health institutions have strict regulations controlling the use of radioactive substances, and advice from the radiation safety officer must be obtained when dealing with these specimens.

X-ray cabinets used for X-raying bony specimens and for angiographic procedures should be under the control of the radiation safety officer and regularly inspected for leaks.

## Electrical and mechanical hazards

With the increasing use of electrical equipment in laboratory areas, there is an increasing danger of electrical shock and malfunction. All electrical installation must be carried out by qualified electricians but laboratory staff must be aware of certain safety precautions: do not overload circuits; do not attempt to operate equipment requiring three phase wiring on single phase circuits; do not use multiple plugs with the one socket, as this can lead to overloading and fire risk. Similar situations can occur with portable power boards. Worn or damaged wiring must be replaced before further use. Electrical equipment, plugs or sockets should not be touched with wet hands. If reagents are inadvertently spilled on electrical equipment, the equipment should be immediately turned off at the socket. Similarly, unplug all equipment before maintenance or adjustment. Equipment should not obstruct power outlets. In the event of an electrical fire, the equipment should be turned off, unplugged and the fire extinguished using a carbon dioxide extinguisher.

Microwave ovens should be regularly checked for leakage of electromagnetic energy. Drying ovens should be fitted with a safety cut-out switch. Centrifuges are a common source of potential injury. They should always be balanced before use and the maximum speed rating must not be exceeded. The lid must not be opened until the rotor has stopped and on no account should the rotor be stopped by hand. Keep hands and any articles of clothing or jewellery, e.g. necklaces, away from moving parts. Centrifuges must be regularly checked for corrosion, wear and tear. Band saws, slicing machines and grinders are used from time to time in the histopathology laboratory. These appliances must be switched off at the socket when not in use. They must never be used without the appropriate factory fitted guards. Goggles must be worn but long loose sleeved gowns should not be worn for fear of becoming caught up in the moving parts. Operation of this equipment requires the utmost concentration and the operator must not be distracted or bumped. If there is danger of an aerosol being created, full-face visors, masks or respirators should be worn. Microtome knives must not be left unattended in the microtome. Disposable blades must be discarded in the appropriate sharps container. Microtome knife sharpeners must have the protective hood in place when in operation. Autoclaves should be operated correctly and regularly checked for damage and corrosion. The results of a build up of pressure could be disastrous.

## Waste management

### Sharps

Hypodermic needles and used scalpel blades must be placed in commercially available, clearly identified containers having rigid and impenetrable walls. When full, these should be placed in 'infected waste containers' and incinerated. Disposable syringes should be discarded in a similar manner.

All broken glass must be placed in clearly identified impermeable containers. If the glass is thought to be infective, it must be autoclaved before disposal even though it may have been placed in disinfectant.

### Solvents, chemicals and fluids

Waste immiscible solvents used in tissue processing and section staining should be decanted into fire- and explosion-proof containers.

Chlorinated waste should be kept separate from non-chlorinated waste. Containers must be clearly labelled as to contents. The burning of such wastes causes atmospheric pollution and is no longer acceptable practice. In many countries, commercial agencies are licensed to carry out bulk chemical waste disposal.

The disposal of chemical waste down the sink is subject to local legislation. Large amounts of water to flush the reagents should be used and particularly between disposal of different reagents. It should be remembered that all such waste drains into the sewage system and remains in the environment as pollutants. Chemicals which are explosive when dry should never be poured down the sink. Mercury-based fixatives are particularly difficult to dispose of and require special precautions. They, too, should never be discarded down the sink as they are toxic. Indeed, there is little justification for their continued use as a fixative.

After overnight contact with infected material, disinfectants must be emptied down the sink through a sieve, the solid matter being autoclaved and disposed of as non-infected waste or placed in 'infected waste containers' and incinerated.

### Body fluids and tissues

Non-infective body fluids and tissue waste can be disposed of via a sluice or waste disposal unit but there must be adherence to local health regulations. Infected tissue may be autoclaved and incinerated, or bagged in 'infected waste containers' and incinerated. Fixed specimens requiring disposal should be similarly bagged and incinerated.

Incinerators must be effectively commissioned and fitted with an after burner to prevent the dispersal of infected particles into the atmosphere.

### Transport of specimens

Special trays or boxes must be provided for the internal transport of specimens between wards and laboratories. These must be able to withstand repeated autoclaving and disinfection procedures. They must be fitted with bottle or tube racks and must be maintained in the upright position. For external transport, similar boxes must be fitted with a lid that can be fastened and clearly labelled. When infected material is sent to another laboratory, a record must be kept of its nature, destination, method of transport and the person authorising dispatch. Transport by air freight must meet the requirements laid down by the International Air Transport Association (Restricted Articles Regulations). Packing

for dispatch by post must be in accordance with local post office regulations and those of the recipient country in the case of specimens sent overseas. Specimens must be sealed in plastic bags and surrounded by sufficient absorbent material to prevent leakage in the event of tear or breakage. They should be placed in containers or canisters specifically designed for the purpose and these should be clearly labelled. There should be no glass-to-glass or plastic-to-plastic contact.

Slides and tissue blocks sent for consultation may also be subject to similar controls depending on local legislation. Slides must be properly packaged in slide boxes and placed in padded envelopes for dispatch. Slides and blocks may be sent by registered mail, recorded delivery or special courier. It is sometimes prudent to inform the intended recipient that the material has been despatched.

## Accident report procedure

All accidents, however minor, must be reported immediately to the appropriate supervisor and documented on incident report forms. It is advisable for all injuries to be seen by appropriately qualified medical staff. Worker's compensation is unlikely to be considered unless these basic protocols are followed. All injuries should be brought to the attention of the laboratory safety committee and institution safety officer. Regular feedback on the incidence of accidents has been found to be very helpful for maintaining staff safety awareness.

All institutions must formulate written protocols to be followed when staff have suffered injury or have been exposed to blood or body fluid. The protocol should include immediate first-aid advice and deal with issues of patient consent in the event of a comatose patient. If a staff member has parenteral or mucous membrane exposure to blood or body fluid, the source should be identified and tested for HIV, and hepatitis B and C. If the source material is positive for HIV antibody/virus/antigen or hepatitis antigens, the worker should be counselled regarding the risk of infection and should be evaluated clinically and serologically for HIV, and hepatitis B and C infection. Immediate therapy (within 24 hours) with azidothymidine (AZT) should be considered when the infecting source is HIV positive. The prophylactic efficacy of AZT has not yet been proven but it is the only agent so far that has been shown to prevent infection in experimental animals. Any illness within 3 months of exposure should be reported and the worker's serum should be retested at 3 months and if negative, again at 6 months. If the source material is negative for HIV, no follow up is necessary unless there is a high risk of HIV infection when the worker should be retested at 3 months.

If the staff member responded effectively to vaccination and less than 5 years has elapsed since vaccination, then neither source nor staff member need be tested further for hepatitis B. If the staff member did not respond effectively to vaccination then anti-hepatitis B immunoglobulin should be given as soon as practical and repeated 1 month later if the source material is hepatitis B positive. Vaccination should be commenced if this has not yet been done. If the source material is negative for hepatitis B, no further investigation is necessary but vaccination should commence if this has not yet been performed.

As yet, no immunisation programmes, either passive or active, are available for the prevention of hepatitis C. However, it is becoming more widely appreciated that, although often having a prolonged time course, hepatitis C infection may be just as serious as hepatitis B infection, with as many as 50% of post-transfusion hepatitis C cases progressing ultimately to cirrhosis. Although hepatitis E appears to be more like hepatitis A in its epidemiology, the new discoveries of other viruses responsible for hepatitis highlights the need for universal precautions whenever possible and for appropriate documentation of all needlestick injuries no matter how slight.

## Further reading

Coghill G 1995 Safety in the histopathology laboratory. In: Bancroft JD, Stevens A (eds) Theory and practice of histological techniques, 4th edn. Churchill Livingstone, Edinburgh

CSIRO 1975 Laboratory safety. Code of practice for safe handling of cryogenic fluids. CSIRO safety booklet, Australia

DHSS 1987 Code of practice for the prevention of infection in clinical laboratories and post mortem rooms. HMSO, London

Guidelines for transportation of specimens as regular commercial freight 1987 National Pathology Accreditation Advisory Council publication, Woden, Australia

Leong AS-Y 1995 Principles and practice of medical laboratory science: Basic histotechnology, Churchill Livingstone, London

Marcus R, the CDC Cooperative Needlestick Surveillance Group 1988 Surveillance of health care workers exposed to blood from patients infected with the human immunodeficiency virus. New England Journal of Medicine 319: 1118–1123

US DHSS: PHS, CDC and NIH 1988 Biosafety in microbiological and bio-

medical laboratories. US Government
Printing Office, Washington
WHO 1983 WHO laboratory biosafety
manual. WHO, Geneva

# 4 Using the dictaphone

## Using the dictaphone

Your work can be considerably expedited with the proper use of a dictaphone. Macroscopic descriptions as well as microscopic descriptions can be dictated and in order that they be accurately transcribed, your dictation must be clear, concise and understandable.

While dictaphones come in many different forms with varied facilities, they can be divided into those which are hand-held and hand-operated, and those which are operated by a foot pedal. Whatever the type of machine used, it should be remembered that frequent stop-starts disrupt a smooth dictation and make transcription difficult. Furthermore, it should be remembered that with each stop-start, it takes the machine a short time to attain the optimal recording speed, adding further to the unevenness of the dictation. It is, therefore, desirable that you formulate your sentence before commencing dictation and stops should occur only at the end of sentences.

Identify yourself at the commencement of dictation and state the date and time. Also provide special instructions, if any. Similarly, say 'this is the end of the dictation' when you conclude and state the time. Dictate punctuations and capital letters, where appropriate. Avoid introducing distracting sounds, such as 'um' and 'eh', and background noises from running water, and clanging containers. Before and during dictation, think about the specimen, possible diagnoses, and anticipated pathological changes. With gross descriptions, examine the entire specimen before beginning dictation. Proceed in an orderly, organised, and generally standardised or reproducible, manner. Do not jump from area to area but rather organise your approach anatomically from external to internal appearances of the specimen. With all descriptions, avoid

pathological diagnoses, assumptions or conclusions. However, do not be circumlocutory – there is no harm in 'calling a spade a spade', i.e. an intramural leiomyoma is quite distinctive and may be called so rather than described in full.

Another major disruption to the smooth transcription of dictation is extraneous noise. While modern dictaphones tend to cut out background noise during dictation, earlier models record both the dictation as well as distracting extraneous noise.

For the smooth and even flow of dictation, speak directly into the microphone at a constant distance as well as at a uniform pace, and a sufficiently loud and even tone of voice. Always spell difficult or uncommon words, or words which may not come across well in your dictation or pronunciation.

It is a useful exercise to listen to your own dictation as this will provide an insight into how you are heard by others.

During dictation avoid playing back too often. This disrupts the even flow of the dictation. With practise, it is possible to remember what has been dictated and to avoid doing this. Frequent playbacks are not necessary and reflect insecurity or lack of concentration. However, it is prudent to ensure that your dictation is recorded and this can be done by noting that the 'recording light' is on while dictating or by playing back for a short distance immediately after each case. It can be a disappointing experience to find, after dictating for 10 or 15 minutes, that the dictation button was not depressed or, more commonly, the recording tape was malaligned and failed to record a single word!

It is possible, with practise, to adopt a standard approach to most specimens so that the macroscopic and even microscopic descriptions can be done smoothly. In exceptional cases, the nature of the specimen may require a non-standard approach, e.g. a mass of adherent large bowel due to multiple adhesions and peritonitis will require a different format from the more usual segment of large bowel which lends itself to a standard macroscopic description. Avoid using jargon or superfluous phrases, such as: 50 g 'in weight'; blue 'in colour'; 'measures' $10 \times 10 \times 15$ mm; square 'in shape'; 'total' three 'in number'; and small 'in size'. It is also redundant to state 'is of small size, measuring 1 mm in diameter', as the size is provided and the judgement can be made by the reader. Do not use 'approximately' to describe dimensions. If you have actually measured the parameters, then the values are not 'approximate'. Other examples of redundancy include: 'a majority of' for 'most'; 'reducing in width' for 'narrowing'; 'for the most part' for 'mainly'; 'shows congestion' for 'is congested'; 'posterior aspect of' for 'posterior'; and 'focal areas' for foci.

Words ending with 'ish' often add to uncertainty and ambiguity, e.g. 'round', not 'roundish'; 'dark', not 'darkish'; and 'blue', not 'bluish'. Do not use analogies to vegetables, fruits and other foods, such as 'prune-like' for wrinkled and 'jelly-like' for soft. Use only primary, secondary or other common colours, avoiding descriptors such as 'mauve' and 'teal'. Beginning sentences with phrases like 'there is', 'sections show' and 'the slides show' is boring and redundant. Another grammatically incorrect phrase is 'skin is present' or 'epithelium is present' for 'there is skin (or epithelium) present'.

Dictation is an important skill for the surgical pathologist as it will greatly expedite his/her work. It is a skill which is worth mastering well. The following summarizes the tips to good dictation:

1 Identify yourself and state the date and time at commencement of dictation. Also indicate the termination of dictation and the time.
2 Dictate at an even pace and in a loud and uniform tone of voice, directly into the microphone.
3 Pause only at the end of sentences and indicate punctuation marks.
4 Avoid frequent playbacks.
5 Check that the dictaphone is on 'dictate' mode before commencing.
6 Be simple and direct, concise and clear. Avoid long words, long phrases and lengthy sentences. Do not use jargon.
7 Describe precisely, avoid making diagnoses and conclusions in macroscopic descriptions.
8 Minimise words and maximise information, avoiding needless words and adjectives.
9 Describe in present and active tense.

## Glossary of descriptive terms

The ultimate goal in gross and microscopic pathological descriptions is an accurate and concise documentation devoid of controversy and confusion. It should create in the mind of the physician reader a vivid mental picture of the pathology present. Accomplishment of this goal is difficult and requires both language and communication skills which come only with maximum mental discipline. This skill is separate from the ability to dissect specimens for examination and sampling for microscopy.

The following is a glossary of descriptive terms which are useful in gross pathology:

### Words describing shape

| | |
|---|---|
| Acuminated | sharp; tapering to a point |
| Angulated | bent; forked |
| Arciform | arched, arcuate, bow-shaped |
| Circular | round |

| | |
|---|---|
| Concave | depressed, hollowed surface; opposed to convex |
| Conical | cone-shaped |
| Convex | bulging, rounded surface; opposed to concave |
| Cordate | heart-shaped |
| Cuboidal | cube-shaped; with equal square sides |
| Cuneiform | wedge-shaped |
| Cylindrical | shape of a cylinder |
| Elliptical | oval; ellipsoid |
| Filamentous | fibre-like; string-like |
| Fimbriated | fringed; filamentous; ciliated |
| Fusiform | with tapered ends |
| Lanceolate | lance-shaped |
| Lenticular | lens-shaped |
| Linear | like a line |
| Multifaceted | many small flat surfaces |
| Oblong | rectangular, longer than broad |
| Oval | egg-shaped |
| Polygonal | many sided |
| Polypoid | a rounded mass on a stalk |
| Pyramidal | pyramid-shaped solid |
| Rectangular | four sided with all angles at right angles |
| Reniform | kidney-shaped |
| Ribbon | narrow and long band |
| Stellate | star-shaped |
| Spherical | round body |
| Trapezoid | four sided with two sides parallel |
| Triangular | three sided |
| Wedge | a body which slopes to a thin edge at one end |

## Words describing outlines and margins

| | |
|---|---|
| Angulated | many angles |
| Arciform | arcuate; arched |

| | |
|---|---|
| Circumscribed | limited; restricted |
| Clefted | fissured; creviced |
| Curvilinear | curved lines |
| Dentate, sawtooth, serrate | toothed; like the edge of a saw |
| Indistinct | poorly demarcated; ill-defined |
| Infiltrating | penetrating |
| Interdigitated | interlocking finger-like processes |
| Lobate | with lobes or rounded divisions |
| Macerated | soften; broken up |
| Papillary | small elevation; nipple-like |
| Pushing | generally rounded; expansive |
| Semilunar | crescentric; half moon-shaped |
| Serpentine | tortuous; serpiginous |
| Serpiginous | tortuous; serpentine |
| Sinuate | winding |
| Smooth | even |
| Undulating | rising and falling like waves |
| Villous | with numerous frond-like or finger-like projections |

## Words describing surfaces

| | |
|---|---|
| Arcuate | arc-shaped; curved |
| Bulging | distended; rounded |
| Bosselated | numerous protuberances or nodules |
| Centrifugal | tending away from the centre |
| Centripetal | tending toward the centre |
| Clear | translucent |
| Cobblestone | numerous rounded raised projections |
| Concentric | having a common centre |
| Contused | bruised but with intact surface |

| | |
|---|---|
| Crinkled | corrugated |
| Cystic | hollow; bag-like |
| Dull | not bright |
| Eroded | superficial ulceration or destruction |
| Furrowed | grooved |
| Geographic | many different interlocking shapes; map-like |
| Glistening | sparkling; bright; reflective |
| Honeycombed | numerous even holes |
| Homogeneous | uniform |
| Indurated | firm; hard |
| Mosaic | pattern-like interlocking shapes |
| Notched | clefted; scored |
| Opaque | dull; not translucent |
| Perforated | penetrated; a through-and-through hole |
| Petechial | small; pin-point |
| Punctate | dotted; punctured |
| Radial | radiating from a point from the centre |
| Scored | notched |
| Septated | divided; partitioned |
| Serpentine | winding; snake-like |
| Serpiginous | creeping |
| Serrated | jagged; nicked |
| Shiny | bright; reflective |
| Solid | resisting pressure; not hollow, liquid or gaseous |
| Stellate | star-shaped |
| Stippled | filled in with dots |
| Streaked | striped; striated |
| Striated | streaked |
| Translucent | clear; transmits light |
| Transparent | can see through, translucent |
| Ulcerated | localised loss of epithelium |
| Undulating | wavy |
| Wrinkled | creased; furrowed |

## Useful words to describe consistency, texture and contour

| | |
|---|---|
| boggy | pedunculated |
| bosselated | plastic |
| clayey | pliable |
| coarse | polypoid |
| cobblestone | puckered |
| compressible | pulpaceous |
| depressed | putty-like |
| dimpled | raised |
| dry | resilient |
| elastic | resistant |
| elevated | rough |
| fine | rubbery |
| firm | sessile |
| flat | sharp |
| flocculant | smooth |
| granular | soft |
| gritty/sandy | spongy |
| grumous | stony |
| hard | thick |
| indurated | umbilicated |
| invaginated | vegetation |
| leathery | velvety |
| lobulated | villiform |
| lush | viscid |
| malleable | viscous |
| moist | wet |
| nodular | |

# 5 Principles of macroscopic examination and sampling

The aim of tissue sampling is to obtain representative tissue blocks for microscopic examination, and to document, by description and photographs, the macroscopic abnormalities present. Specimens arriving in the laboratory, therefore, need to be correctly identified and accessioned, dissected and described, and finally, sampled for processing and microscopic examination. This sequence may be modified by the additional requirements of an ever-increasing array of ancillary techniques which can be applied to the biopsy to aid in diagnosis and prognosis. The correct handling, macroscopic description and sampling of specimens is an important area in pathology training and it is clear that many diagnostic problems are a direct result of failure to handle the specimen correctly in its early stages.

## Specimen identification and accessioning

Before any specimen is sampled, it is essential to ensure that the material received was indeed that removed from the designated patient and a mix-up of specimens has not occurred. The checking of specimens cannot be over-emphasised, as mix-ups can result in dire consequences and represent unmitigated negligence. It is the laboratory's responsibility and ultimately the pathologist's responsibility to ensure that the specimen received with the patient's name corresponds to the patient demographics on the surgical pathology request form. Specimens are sent to pathology laboratories from operating theatres, various clinics and consultation rooms which can sometimes be located a long distance from the laboratory. On removal, these biopsies are placed into containers of appropriate size which should contain sufficient quantities of 10% buffered formalin to immerse the specimen completely. The container is then labelled with the patient's name, age and sex, hospital registration number and other pertinent data such as the referring doctor's name, date of biopsy and, importantly, the nature of the specimen. The specimen should be accompanied by a laboratory-provided request form which is completed with similar patient information and should be duly signed by the requesting clinician. As this matching of specimen, patient's name and request form is done before receipt in the accessioning laboratory and by someone other than the laboratory staff, it is essential that both specimen and request form be matched again on receipt in the laboratory, just prior to macroscopic examination and cut-up, as they may be separated during transportation. The specimen is next assigned an accession number which can be done simply by sticking printed labels with the same accession number to both the specimen container and to the request form, and entering the patient's demographics in a log book. Modern technology permits entry of such accessioning data by bar code scanning, but whatever the method, the purpose of the procedure is to match the request form and the specimen, record its receipt in the laboratory, and assign a laboratory accession number before macroscopic examination and tissue sampling. Although there is no accurate means for the pathologist to ensure or check that the specimen in the container indeed came from the patient whose name is on the container, the information provided by the requesting clinician allows another means of checking as it should also identify the nature of the specimen which can then be matched against its macroscopic appearance. For example, specimens designated 'skin' can be readily recognized as such macroscopically, thus allowing one method of checking that the specimen is correctly matched with the patient's demographics. Immunohistochemical staining for blood group antigens and molecular DNA fingerprinting techniques are more sophisticated methods which can be employed to determine the source of specimens in mix-ups.

In the case of multiple biopsies from the same patient, these should be retained under the same accession number and be clearly identified as separate parts of the same specimen, e.g. parts 1, 2, 3, etc.

## Clinical history

Histopathological examination is a consultative procedure and the diagnosis rendered by the surgical pathologist is a distillate of his/her experience and knowledge which is integrated into the clinical setting of the individual patient. To provide an opinion which is of optimal benefit to the patient, the pathologist must be given the relevant clinical information which also enables immediate orientation to the problem at hand. This consultative process between clinician and surgical pathologist is discussed in detail in Chapter 16.

Infectious specimens, especially if received fresh, must be labelled or identified appropriately by the requesting clinician and safety precautions should be adopted. Do not hesitate to contact the responsible clinician if a specimen requires orientation or if other clinical information is required. Do not hesitate to request the surgeon or his/her assistant to orientate the specimen in relation to resection margins and other important anatomical landmarks.

## Macroscopic examination

Pathological examination of all tissues removed from patients should be mandatory, although this is not so in every medical centre. However, whether microscopic examination is necessary in each instance is left to the pathologist's discretion. Ingrowing toenails, bunions and hard or metallic foreign-bodies are examples of specimens which do not require routine microscopic examination, although the routine paraffin embedding and sectioning of all tissues forms a convenient method of storing representative tissue from all specimens. In such circumstances, a gross description and macroscopic diagnosis is made with the notation that no microscopic sections were taken.

Proper gross examination and description is based upon a systematised and orderly approach to the specimen according to its anatomy. Tips on concise, clear and accurate description are provided in the preceding chapter. In general, the gross or macroscopic description should consist of the following parts in order of importance:

1 Record the designation of the specimen as found on the specimen container and the name of the patient and accession number. Also note the state in which the specimen is received – whether it is fixed or fresh, previously opened, etc.
2 Describe the specimen including its dimensions and weight, and describe the pathological changes including the location of the lesion in reference to a fixed structure such as the surgical margin or an anatomical landmark.
3 Describe other tissues and adjacent structures according to their anatomy.
4 Provide a block key of the tissue blocks sampled for microscopy.

In examining solid organs, make parallel slices at 5–10 mm intervals so that the largest surface area is exposed by your slices. For hollow viscera, open the organ longitudinally with scissors, gently washing off its contents with running water before examination. Hollow viscera can be dissected fresh or pinned out on a cork board and fixed in 10% buffered formalin overnight, or hardened by immersion in normal saline and by multiple exposures to microwaves to allow easy dissection.

While it is useful to fix some specimens before dissection, it should be remembered that the situation may vary. It may be necessary to separate the various components of a specimen while still in the fresh state, such as in a radical neck dissection, or it may be necessary to remove only some components such as regional lymph nodes and leave the rest of the specimen as a single piece for fixation. Some specimens can be satisfactorily injected, such as injecting the bronchial tree of a lobectomy specimen with a syringe or catheter, and in the case of cystic lesions, the cavity can be packed with cotton impregnated with formalin.

## Special situations

### Lymph node dissection

The dissection of lymph nodes is one of the most important steps in the examination of a radical operation for cancer. While in the fresh state, it is easy to separate the adipose tissue containing lymph nodes from the main specimen. This can be done with sharp scissors and in the case of the gastrointestinal tract and other sites, the nodes are mostly found in very close proximity to the bowel so that the removal of the fat or mesentery should be done in such a way that the fat and serosa are stripped and the muscular bowel wall is

exposed. This can similarly be done with the greater and lesser omentum for gastrectomy specimens. In the case of axillary dissections accompanying mastectomies, the axillary fat should be removed from the mastectomy specimen to allow easier dissection of lymph nodes. Lymph nodes are pink in colour in the fresh state and can be dissected by careful palpation and by making 1–2 mm slices through the fat with a sharp scalpel. Alternatively, the fatty tissue containing the nodes can be fixed by immersion in normal saline and irradiated with microwaves. This produces enhancement of the pink colour of the nodes which contrasts against the yellow fat, allowing easier identification. Clearance of fat by fixing for 16 hours in Carnoy's solution (ethanol 60%, chloroform 30%, glacial acetic acid 10%) provides a higher yield of lymph nodes but the specimen becomes greasy and offensive smelling, and there is no good evidence that the higher yield of lymph nodes provides better prognostic information. All lymph nodes dissected should be submitted for histological examination. Large nodes are sliced at 1–2 mm intervals and placed in individual cassettes, while small nodes, less than 2 mm diameter, may be placed collectively in one cassette.

### Specimens with bone and soft tissues

The handling of specimens which contain both bone and soft tissues will vary according to the nature of the specimen and the pathology present. One method is to freeze the entire fresh specimen to enable slicing with a bandsaw while the specimen is still frozen hard. Washing of the slices with water results in good demonstration of the pathology, particularly when present within bone. It is useful to dissect away the soft tissue before specimens are subjected to slicing in the bandsaw. When there is pathology in the soft tissue, these can be submitted directly for fixation and processing without being subjected to decalcification which not only delays the histological examination, but also results in suboptimal cytomorphology.

## Resection margins and marking inks

The assessment of surgical margins is an important part of the examination of radical resections for neoplasm. The margins should be sampled before the specimen is destroyed by dissection. Macroscopic examination provides the best guide as to which margins require sampling and the extent of microscopic examination. Obviously, it is not practically possible to sample all margins. Margins closest to the tumour require the most extensive sampling. The pathologist's judgement and experience dictate the appropriateness and extent of sampling margins and he/she must determine if more pertinent information is to be gained by taking parallel or perpendicular sections, if quadrants should be sampled, if only one area needs to be studied or if the entire margins should be evaluated. Theoretically, blocks including the margin of resection, whether on a parallel or perpendicular axis, could be entirely sectioned to provide complete information regarding tumour at the margin and distance of tumour to the margin. Each technique of margin evaluation has inherent disadvantages. Sections parallel or circumferential to the lesion will evaluate the line of resection, but will not give information about the distance of the tumour to the margin. Conversely, sections perpendicular to the line of resection will determine the distance of the tumour to the margin, but will not evaluate the surgical margin in its entirety. Conventionally, in

the majority of excisional biopsy specimens, the margins are sampled as sections perpendicular to the margin and in larger specimens, one section perpendicular to the closest margin and the remainder of the margins are examined by sections parallel to the margin.

In all instances, the margins should be inked before any sections are taken. India ink is the most common pigment used to paint the margin and this can be done by gently wiping the surgical margins with gauze before carefully covering the entire surgical surface with the ink, using a cotton swab stick. Smearing of the ink should be prevented by carefully blotting the surfaces with gauze or paper towel. Dipping the inked surface in Bouin's solution is another method to stop spreading of the ink. Other indelible inks, including tattoo pigments and alcohol-insoluble marking pens, can be used to paint margins and surfaces. Separate colours may be employed to identify different margins and surfaces. Alternatively, the margin can be identified by notching with a scalpel but it is not always easy to distinguish these cuts and notches from artificial clefts in the tissue.

Apart from the examination of specimens containing tumour, the pathologist is also required to examine specimens in which the primary lesion may be ischaemic or vascular, infectious, inflammatory or metabolic or degenerative. In the case of ischaemic or vascular lesions, an assessment of the location of the lesion and their exact nature and the organ or tissue consequences need to be assessed including the viability of resection margins. Transverse sections of visible vascular obstruction or narrowing should be sampled and the entire vascular bundle should be examined by transverse cuts at close intervals. Obviously inflamed and potentially infectious tissues, when received fresh, should be sampled under sterile conditions in a biological safety cabinet, for microbiological culture and sensitivity. In the case of metabolic diseases, the tissues mostly show diffuse involvement making representative sampling easy; however, fresh tissue may need to be submitted for biochemical investigations.

## Tissue sampling

The general principles of macroscopic examination and sampling are: (1) all pathology present should be assessed; (2) features of prognostic and therapeutic relevance should be noted; and (3) there should be as little distortion and destruction to the specimen as possible during dissection, to allow it to be demonstrated to clinicians and pathologists, if necessary, and to enable further sampling of specific areas if required. For the correct sampling of a specimen, the pathologist must be aware of the desired clinical objectives of the examination. These may be to confirm a clinical diagnosis, to make a diagnosis, determine the degree of tumour spread, examine the resection margins, determine the presence of pre-cancerous lesions, and exclude some important clinical differential diagnoses. Biopsies may be diagnostic and/or therapeutic and it should be the aim to minimise sampling errors by taking tissue for microscopic examination which are representative of the pathology present. The difficulty lies in the heterogeneous and focal nature of many disease processes and the magnitude of the error is inversely proportional to the relative sample size, i.e. the error is small at the gross macroscopic level and increases with magnification so that it becomes very great in the small tissue sample selected for electron microscopy.

It is difficult to generalise on the number of blocks required in any given case as the number is determined by the size and complexity of the specimen, research interests, possible legal ramifications, costs and importantly, common sense and the experience of the pathologist. Ideally, the entire specimen should be examined microscopically but this is obviously not a cost-effective exercise. All small biopsies which can be contained within three to five cassettes should be processed in their entirety, whereas all larger specimens should be examined by representative sampling. Careful and good dissection techniques are important prerequisites for macroscopic sampling and ultimately for the histological diagnosis. For example, the chance of detecting a solitary 5 mm incidental metastasis in a large piece of liver removed for another reason would be very small if the specimen was examined with a single knife cut; whereas if the specimen was finely sliced at less than 1 cm intervals, the odds of detecting the metastasis increase significantly. Careful gross examination with the naked eye serves as a low power microscopy and reduces the number of blocks taken in a given case. In some situations, statistical analyses have been performed to assess the optimal number of blocks for examination. For example, with prostatic chips removed during transurethral resections, it has been shown that six cassettes provide the optimal diagnostic returns. It is impractical and probably not justified to process all the prostatic fragments received regardless of the total amount. As a general rule, specimens which can be submitted entirely in one or two cassettes are examined in their entirety, e.g. diagnostic endometrial curettage. However, if the curettage was performed for incomplete abortion and gross examination shows obvious products of conception, one representative block is usually adequate.

One important function of specimen sampling is the provision of material for special investigations such as immunohisto-chemistry, electron microscopy, tissue culture, cytogenetics and molecular diagnostic procedures. The actual investigative procedure employed will be dependent on the state in which the biopsy is received. The trainee must be familiar with the list of special procedures that can be performed on fresh tissue and should be able to assess the need for such techniques in each case. For example, it would be incomplete to examine a lymph node removed fresh for possible malignant lymphoma by routine H & E examination only. A complete lymphoma work-up includes imprints, fresh frozen tissue for immunohistochemistry, fresh tissue in transport/culture media for lymphocyte surface markers or flow cytometry studies, tissue in glutaraldehyde for possible ultrastructural examination, and consideration of possible cytogenetics and other molecular studies. These ancillary investigative procedures are discussed further in Chapter 7.

## Block size

Tissue blocks taken from solid specimens should be in blocks of no more than 2–3 mm in thickness and $15 \times 20$ mm in area. Adipose tissue does not process well and this should be no more than 2 mm for the best results. Tissues will not process well if the cassettes are over-filled. Bone and other calcified material should be removed unless the tissue is subjected to decalcification, and sutures, metal clips and other foreign material should be excluded to avoid microtome blade damage. Partially calcified

tissues can be processed routinely following short decalcification.

If one side of a tissue block needs to be sectioned, the opposite surface can be indicated with India ink. Some specimens require to be embedded on edge, such as in the case of pieces of mucosa and membranes. For smaller specimens orientation is more difficult but may be just as important. Such specimens are embedded uncut, in toto, and are sectioned as multiple levels. Other methods, such as surrounding a small specimen with a solution of 3% agar in distilled water or embedding in paraffin by the pathologist him/herself, are more time-consuming procedures. Correct tissue sampling and orientation requires a close working relationship between the pathologist and medical technologist. Regular or square tissue blocks of solid tissue are embedded flat, and it should be remembered that the surface of the block which is facing down in the cassette will be cut. If it is imperative that one surface should be cut, the opposite surface should be marked with India ink or grooved or notched with the scalpel.

Multiple microscopic sections or levels provide a better sampling of small specimens such as endoscopic biopsies of the bronchus, gastrointestinal tract and bladder, needle and punch biopsies, and fragmented specimens of less than 3–4 mm. For example, as a generous needle biopsy of the liver is estimated to contain one-fifth millionth of the liver volume, sampling error is a real possibility, particularly if the lesion is focal and the biopsy was not radiologically directed to the lesion.

Tubular structures such as vas deferens need to be embedded on end to allow a complete transverse section and hollow visceral organs such as bowel and cyst walls are usually embedded on edge, as are sections of skin. With organs such as bowel which are covered by a folded mucosa, better sections are taken perpendicular rather than parallel to the mucosal folds and cord-like structures such as nerves are often embedded as a combination of longitudinal and cross-sections, the latter from either end.

## Block key

The sampling of larger specimens may entail multiple tissue blocks, and unless an accurate block key is provided to indicate the sites of each of these blocks it is almost impossible to identify their location in the specimen. For example, the distal and proximal margins of a segment of colon may be histologically similar and a special area of a lesion may be sampled but, unless specifically identified, cannot be distinguished from the other 25 blocks taken from the specimen. An accurate block key describing the location of each sample is essential if another pathologist, other than the prosector, is to understand the sections. This block key can be greatly enhanced by a line diagram, photograph or specimen photocopy on which the sites of all, or only the important samples, can be indicated.

## Photographs, line diagrams and specimen photocopies

The adage that 'a picture or photograph is worth a thousand words' is very true in descriptions of pathological findings. Black-and-white photographs serve well as objective illustrations and their liberal use is only limited by cost considerations. Besides recording the pathological changes, these prints can also be used to indicate the sites of sampling which can also be done with line diagrams. One method of producing rapid images of the specimen surface is with a photocopying machine. By

placing the specimen on a transparent plastic sheet to avoid contamination and soiling of the photocopier, a true-to-size image of the specimen surface can be produced. This is a particularly cheap and effective method for cut surfaces and specimens with flat external surfaces.

## Cleanliness

The need for a clean cut-up bench during tissue examination and sampling is important to avoid contaminant tissue crossing in between cases. It is important to wash the cutting board or surface with clean water and to sponge or wipe the board in between cases. Instruments employed in cut-up should also be washed in running water between cases. Certain specimens such as products of conception, uterine curettings and friable bowel and bladder tumours are notorious for producing 'visitors' and contaminants and can be avoided with clean techniques. Examination of the paraffin block may give an indication of the nature of such pick-ups. Floaters, on the other hand, are picked-up in the water-bath during sectioning and these are more readily identified as they do not appear in deeper levels from the block.

## Further reading

Leong AS-Y, Duncis CG 1986 A method of rapid fixation of large biopsy specimens using microwave irradiation. Pathology 18: 222–225

Olson DR 1978 Specimen photocopying for surgical pathology reports. American Journal of Clinical Pathology 70: 94–95

# 6 Examination, description and sampling of specimens

## Introduction

Specimens from a wide variety of body sites arrive in the pathology laboratory for examination and diagnosis. The trainee must be familiar with the handling and processing of these different specimens, acquire a knowledge of the likely pathology from the macroscopic examination, and judge when and what ancillary studies will be helpful or essential for diagnosis and yielding information of therapeutic relevance. This chapter outlines the range of specimens by organ system (arranged alphabetically) seen in a diagnostic laboratory and provides guidelines on the examination, dissection, sampling and gross description of such specimens. It does not portend to be an exhaustive list and rarer specimen types are omitted. Biopsies requiring special investigative procedures are also discussed in Chapter 7. An in-depth discourse of each type of specimen is beyond the scope of this book and only principles will be discussed.

## Principles of gross examination and dissection

Diagnostic specimens may take a variety of sizes and shapes and range from small needle cores and fragments through to radical resections and exenteration where several adjacent structures and organs are removed.

The general principles of specimen documentation, examination and sampling are discussed in Chapter 5 and summarised below:

### 1 Take photographs and draw diagrams

'A picture is worth a thousand words' – this statement is very true for the macro-scopic documentation of surgical specimens. With developments in digitisation of images it may be possible to have the macroscopic appearances of all specimens stored as numerous images, but until such time, accurate descriptions can be supplemented by photographs, line diagrams and photocopies of the specimens. These ancillaries should be employed as often as possible, especially for complex specimens and those that are of sufficient interest to be shown at clinicopathological conferences or be used for teaching or publication.

### 2 Provide an accurate and clear description of the specimen

Until adequate numbers of images of the specimen can be readily stored and reproduced inexpensively in the pathology report, it will be necessary to provide clear and accurate descriptions of the specimen.

Describe the pathological lesion, giving its size, shape, texture and colour, with measurement of its dimensions and relationship to adjacent structures and anatomical landmarks in the specimen, measuring these distances if appropriate. Use descriptive terms which are clearly understandable. Do not employ unusual terms or abbreviations.

### 3 Small specimens of 1–3 mm are difficult to orientate

These specimens are best embedded intact and in toto. Levels may be cut to ensure adequate examination.

### 4 Sample the lesion and take representative non-lesional tissue

As a general principle, all pathological tissue should be sampled, including both primary pathology as well as secondary changes. In addition, tissue blocks representative of the different histological types of non-lesional tissue in the specimen should also be taken for microscopic examination. The purpose of gross and microscopic examination of any pathological specimen is to identify the nature of the lesion, document its extent, study any complications or consequences of the primary pathology and note any accompanying, contributory or aetiological changes in the specimen. A more recent aspect of such histological examination includes the prediction of the biological behaviour of the lesion, particularly in the case of neoplasms.

The detailed documentation and examination of biopsies and excisions are primarily for the purpose of diagnosis, management and prognosis of the patient, with additional aims of educating through the medium of the written report and through photographs used at clinicopathological conferences, in publications, for medico-legal and record purposes, and in research.

## 5 Identify and sample margins

Sample all surgical margins, particularly in radical resections for tumours, marking the margins in an identifiable manner if necessary.

## 6 Lymph node dissection

Dissection of lymph nodes, particularly in radical resections, can be aided by first clearing adipose tissue in Carnoy's solution.

## 7 Provide a block key

Provide an accurate block key of all samples taken, if necessary, indicate sites of sampling in a line drawing of the specimen or on photographs or specimen photocopy.

## 8 Perform ancillary investigations where appropriate

In all unfixed specimens, particularly of tumours, and other relevant lesions, perform ancillary investigations including the preparation of cellular imprints for cytology, snap freeze tissue samples for frozen section immunohistochemistry and biochemical assays, fix tissue in 2.5% glutaraldehyde for electron microscopy, submit tissue in culture medium (e.g. RPMI 1640) for flow cytometry, lymphocyte surface marker studies and cytogenetics. Submit infectious material for culture and sensitivity studies. Details of these special ancillary techniques are provided in Chapter 7. As a general rule, priority should be given to obtaining adequate representative tissue for histological diagnosis and samples taken for ancillary studies only after this requirement is satisfied. In exceptional circumstances where histological diagnosis is already established, the biopsy may be performed solely to obtain tissue for special investigations.

## 9 Request immunohistochemical and special stains where appropriate

It is also expedient to anticipate the requirement for multiple or deeper levels and for special histochemical stains in appropriate cases and to request these at the time of dissection and cut-up. Additional stains may be required after microscopic examination.

# Breast

Needle biopsy, lumpectomy, micro/macrodochectomy, subareolar wedge resection, segmental resection, mastectomy and silicone prostheses capsule

## Clinical indications

Biopsies are taken from the breast to investigate the nature of palpable breast lumps (fibroadenoma, fibrocystic change, fat necrosis, papilloma, carcinoma, etc.), nipple bleeding, and ever increasingly from regions of mammographic abnormalities such as mass lesions and microcalcifications. These biopsies are often preceded by breast fine needle aspiration. Micro/macrodochectomy is utilised to remove papillomas in major ducts and duct ectasia. Segmental breast resection is indicated for smaller peripheral unifocal breast tumours, possible local residual neoplasm post lumpectomy or for mammographic abnormalities with positive cytology. Mastectomies are, in the majority of instances, performed for malignant tumours not suitable for removal by segmental resection. Subcutaneous mastectomy preserves the nipple and/or skin. It can be used to resect some types of primary breast tumours. Smaller resections of breast tissue may be received for ductal papillomas, cosmetic breast reduction and gynaecomastia. Silicone breast prostheses may rupture and leak into the surrounding breast tissue where painful fibrosis and distortion necessitate removal. Prostheses are also removed because of a possible association between silicone and a number of conditions, particularly autoimmune disease.

*Lumpectomy (tylectomy)* specimens are measured and the resection margins inked.

Orientating clips and sutures are noted. Margins can be differentially inked with coloured dyes, notched or scored for orientation. If a lesion is palpable, the specimen is cut at 3–4 mm intervals and the slices kept in sequence. If suspicious for carcinoma, tumour tissue should be submitted for oestrogen/progesterone receptors by biochemical cytosolic assays or immunostaining. Many laboratories can now perform hormone receptor immunostaining in paraffin sections, allowing the examination of small tumours detected by mammography and, importantly, allowing correlation of morphology with hormone receptor expression.

The sampling of mammographic-detected breast lesions requires special precautions to ensure that areas of mammographic abnormality are completely sampled and their relationship to the closest resection margins determined. The specimen may be received with a hook wire placed into the area of interest or carbon may have been injected into the lesion to direct the surgeon. Occasionally, the breast tissue is stapled to cardboard with a V-shape of staples whose apex indicates the nipple end. Specimens submitted compressed between acrylic grids enable accurate localisation of the lesion but tend to obscure specimen radiography, are bulky and require cleaning, so that they have fallen from favour. A specimen X-ray should be provided to indicate the areas of interest (microcalcifications and mass lesions), or, alternatively, the specimen may be received either fresh or in formalin previously sliced at 3–5 mm intervals with orientation to the superior, superficial and medial surfaces. Rapid freezing of fresh tissue to –20°C in a cryostat enables easy slicing of the fresh breast tissue with either a feather blade or meat slicer and does not produce freezing artefact. The slices are then laid on X-ray film and covered by moistened towelling paper. The X-ray film can be marked with a permanent marking pen to indicate the sequence of slices and margin orientation. Radiography of the slices enables accurate selection of blocks with microcalcification and soft tissue for histological sampling. This allows the selection of appropriate blocks to be step sectioned for further examination. Calcifications may not be associated with a grossly visible lesion in the tissue. Description of the radiological abnormality should form part of the macroscopic description, and the area of interest is best identified by the radiologist or surgeon who should also confirm that the mammographic lesion of concern is contained in the specimen, i.e. it has been removed. Representative tumour tissue can be retrieved after histological identification for hormone receptor immunostaining. If a specimen radiograph is not available, the breast specimen should be sliced at 3–5 mm intervals, retaining the slices in sequence, with orientation of the margins. Any visible lesion and all breast tissue around the hook wire, particularly non-adipose fibrous connective tissue, should be sampled.

*Micro/macrodochectomy* and *subareolar wedge resections* may be received fresh or in formalin. Microdochectomy removes only one or two ducts while macrodochectomy clears all the subareolar ducts with a disc of surrounding breast tissue. Often, the main duct in the specimen is marked with a suture or stent and the nipple end identified. For smaller specimens containing non-palpable tumours, the margins should be inked before removal of the stent. Serially slice the specimen perpendicular to the duct. For larger specimens with palpable lesions, the duct may be opened longitudinally with a pair of fine scissors, exposing

the typically papillary tumour and pinning out the specimen on corkboard for fixation.

*Breast segmental resections* may be received with sutures or radio-opaque clips to mark the margins. The segmental resection may contain a skin ellipse with a central carbon track injection site. Hook wires, if used, have a tendency to move after placement. Segmental resection is often performed for carcinoma or multiple localised mammographic calcifications. The tumour may be palpable or impalpable and may require specimen radiography, in which case it is handled as described above. Axillary contents are treated as for mastectomy specimens described below.

The *mastectomy* for carcinoma is often received fresh to enable sampling for hormone receptor analysis, although this is no longer necessary with the advent of immunohistochemical staining in paraffin sections. The specimen is weighed, palpated from the deep aspect, and the margin closest to the tumour is inked. The weight is especially helpful in cosmetic breast reduction as it provides a guide to symmetry. Specimen radiographs may be required in the case of multiple impalpable mammographic abnormalities. Parallel cuts in a sagittal plane at approximately 1 cm intervals are made through the deep aspect, leaving the slices connected by the overlying skin. Alternatively, complete slices can be made and laid out in sequence. If fresh tumour is required for hormone receptors, a sample is taken without compromising histology. A section of the deep margin over the tumour should be taken at this stage before specimen distortion occurs. Photograph the specimen if appropriate. The sliced specimen is fixed in a large bucket of formalin for several hours or overnight. Any attached axillary tissue should be removed from the main mastectomy prior to formalin immersion and placed into Carnoy's fixative for easier lymph node dissection. Alternatively, lymph nodes can be dissected in the fresh state by either slicing the fat with a scalpel and inspecting the cut surface or with a combined dissection and palpation technique (see 'Radical neck dissection', p. 80). Between 17 and 20 lymph nodes should be retrieved from an extended axillary dissection and a minimum of eight nodes should be present in a good axillary sampling specimen. The attached axillary tail, if present, is a guide to the lateral edge of the specimen and the surgeon may separately mark the superior and lateral skin edges and the apex of the axillary tail. The Patey modified radical mastectomy includes the pectoralis minor muscle and level I and II nodes whilst the Halsted mastectomy includes additional level III nodes (see below). Supraradical mastectomies are extended to include the pectoral muscles, internal mammary nodes and, sometimes, supraclavicular node, but it is now a rare operation.

The fat and nodes of the axillary contents course across the posterior surface of the pectoralis minor muscle which was used to divide the nodes into three levels: Level I (low, inferior to muscle), Level II (middle, between upper and lower borders of pectoralis minor muscle) and Level III (high, superior to muscle), but such a division of nodes has no bearing on prognosis. Prognosis is determined by the number of nodes involved by tumour, provided the sampling is adequate. Tumour invasion of the pectoralis major muscle should be noted.

The nipple and areola are examined with parallel sections at 3 mm intervals perpendicular to the skin surface. Alternatively, the nipple can be sampled by horizontal or vertical sections and the areola with radial sections.

If a *silicone prosthesis capsule* is received it should be weighed, measured and examined for rupture and leakage or contracture. Photograph the specimen if ruptured and retain indefinitely in case of litigation.

# Cardiovascular system

## Endomyocardial and pericardial biopsies, and valve cusps

### Clinical indications

Endomyocardial biopsies are rarely performed outside of cardiac transplant centres. Such biopsies are done for the investigation of transplant rejection and they have a role in the investigation of restrictive type cardiomyopathy and to rule out conditions such as haemochromatosis, sarcoidosis, amyloid, glycogen storage disease and hypertrophic cardiomyopathy. Endomyocardial biopsies are also used to diagnose drug-induced cardiotoxicity, myocarditis and to assess idiopathic chest pain or arrhythmias. The vast majority of biopsies sample the right interventricular septum. Pericardial biopsies may be performed in cases of chronic restrictive pericarditis due to tuberculosis and malignancy such as mesothelioma and metastatic carcinoma. Pericardial samples may also arrive as multiple strips and fragments obtained at pericardectomy performed for the relief of tamponade. Cardiac myxomas are round or ovoid gelatinous masses usually removed from the atrium. Complete or partial removal of mitral or aortic valves are performed for stenoses or incompetence, either congenital or acquired. The latter may be degenerative, as in senile calcific aortic stenosis or myxomatous floppy mitral valve disease, or be post-inflammatory in nature.

## Examination and dissection technique

Small biopsies usually defy accurate orientation although the endocardial surface may be apparent in some endomyocardial biopsies. They generally range from 1 to 3 mm in diameter and are embedded uncut. In some instances, separate fresh biopsies will be taken for viral cultures, iron quantitation, lymphocyte subtyping, or snap frozen in liquid nitrogen for biochemical analysis. In suspected anthracycline toxicity, a portion should be placed into glutaraldehyde for ultrastructural analysis. Larger pericardiectomy specimens are measured and transversely sliced at 5 mm intervals, and examined for focal lesions. If infection, including tuberculosis and fungi, are suspected, a portion should be removed under sterile conditions and submitted for culture, and fixed for at least 24 hours prior to examination and sampling.

With biopsies of *cardiac myxomas* it is usually difficult to identify the point of attachment of the tumour to the endocardium. The specimen is photographed and after fixation cut in parallel 5 mm slices and embedded.

The macroscopic examination of *cardiac valves* often yields more information than microscopy. Accurate measurements and photographs of both sides of the valve cusps are essential and if there is cusp calcification, X-ray and decalcification will be needed prior to sectioning. Valve cusps are sectioned transversely, and if intact, obtain a section across commissures which are fused. When vegetations are present and if unfixed, a portion should be taken for culture. Examine for ballooning and myxoid change and check chordae tendinae,

if present, for fibrosis and shortening or stretching. Rounded ends suggest previous rupture. With semilunar valves note the number of cusps and their symmetry and examine for a ridge which would suggest an inflammatory aetiology for a bicuspid valve.

## Aneurysm sacs

### Clinical indications

Aneurysm sacs may be from the aorta or iliac vessels and obtained at the time of repair. Although aneurysms of cerebral vessels are common, they are rarely excised for histopathological assessment. Infective mycotic or vasculitic aneurysms are occasionally received.

### Examination and dissection technique

The specimen is cut using parallel sections from the intima to the adventitial surface. With unfixed mycotic aneurysm, a portion should be cultured.

Record the dimensions of the aneurysm sac and examine for the presence of thrombus, atheroma, intimal thickening, plaque disruption, calcification, thinning of wall, dissection, thrombotic occlusion of ostia of smaller vessels, rupture, and other complications. In the case of berry aneurysms, examine for rupture and 'daughter' aneurysms. Elastic stains are useful in the examination of vascular lesions.

## Arteries and veins

### Clinical indications

Segments of small or medium sized arteries are excised to diagnose arteritis, the temporal artery being the commonest specimen. Parts of larger arteries may be removed during reconstructive surgery for atheroma or quiescent arteritis and usually form part of an aneurysm wall. Thrombosed varicose veins and haemorrhoids may be submitted for histological examination.

### Examination and dissection technique

Small muscular artery segments are cut transversely with a fine scalpel blade at 3 mm intervals and embedded on end. Veins are also cut via serial transverse sections. In the examination of blood vessels, particularly the temporal artery, the entire segment of excised vessel should be submitted for histological examination as the changes may be very localised.

Haemorrhoidal tissue is difficult to orientate and is either embedded uncut or the larger fragments bisected.

Elastic stains are useful in the microscopic examination of blood vessels.

## Limb amputation

Amputations include below knee and above knee amputation, forefoot amputation and arm amputation. The following comments pertain to lower limb amputation as an example.

### Clinical indications

Extremities, typically legs, may be amputated in severe occlusive peripheral vascular disease, gangrene, trauma and chronic osteomyelitis. Amputation for soft tissue or osseous tumours, including pelvic and shoulder girdle disarticulation, is described under 'Osteoarticular system and soft tissues' (see p. 86).

### Examination and dissection technique

Confirm that the amputated specimen corresponds with the specimen label, the nature and side of the body, and the clinical history. Many of these specimens arrive fresh, labelled 'for disposal'. It is the pathologist's responsibility to determine the extent of dissection required and the need for microscopic examination. In most cases of peripheral vascular disease, with or without gangrene, expose and dissect the major vessels and nerves proximal to the ankle and examine for stenosis and thrombosis by making serial parallel transverse sections or by opening the vessels longitudinally with a fine pair of blunt-ended scissors.

A more detailed examination of the femoral, popliteal, posterior tibial, anterior tibial and peroneal vessels and associated nerves may occasionally be necessary. This may be done by incising the skin longitudinally in the midline posteriorly from the popliteal fossa to the lower third of the leg down to the level of the superficial fascia. Extend the incision obliquely to about 2 cm below the posterior body of the medial malleolus. Using blunt and sharp dissection with scissors and scalpel, separate the semitendinous, semimembranous and medial head of the gastrocnemius muscle from the biceps femoris and lateral head of the gastrocnemius to expose the femoral and popliteal vessels as well as the sciatic and posterior tibial nerves. The posterior tibial neurovascular bundle lies deep to the intermuscular fascia. The sciatic and posterior tibial nerves can be dissected free down to the level of the popliteal vessels. Starting proximally, excise the femoral and popliteal vessels down to the level of the posterior tibial nerve. The posterior tibial neurovascular bundle is then excised down to the medial malleolus and the peroneal vessels are next removed with surrounding muscle. These vessels lie posterior to the fibula and the interosseous membrane and within the flexor hallucis longus. To remove the anterior tibial neurovascular bundle, turn the limb over and incise the skin anteriorly commencing between the head of fibula and tibial tuberosity and down distally to the midpoint between both malleoli. The incision extends into the superficial fascia and in the mid-portion through the tibialis anterior muscle down to the interosseous membrane exposing the anterior tibial vessels and nerves. Further dissection of muscle proximally and tendons distally reveals the rest of the vessel and nerve which can be removed with adjacent muscle and interosseous membrane. The dorsalis pedis vessels can be removed by outlining a 4 cm wide rectangle on the dorsum of the foot between the lower part of the previous anterior tibial incision and the first interosseous space. The overlying skin and tissue down to the deep fascia and dorsum of underlying bones are removed exposing the vessels deep in this region. Finally, the medial and lateral plantar vessels are removed. With the sole of the foot uppermost, trace out a rectangle over the proximal 60% of the foot between the posterior border of the medial malleolus, medial side of the foot, base of the metatarsals and lateral side of foot. The outlined skin and subcutaneous tissue are removed with the incision extending through the plantar aponeurosis, fascia, muscle and tendon to bone. The removed block is divided into medial and lateral halves and each contains the respective plantar vessels.

In suspected osteomyelitis, X-ray the limb, remove the bone in question and decalcify prior to sampling. With unfixed specimens, take a swab or a piece of tissue for culture.

With traumatised limbs, particularly in medico-legal cases, X-ray the specimen and photograph the injuries present. Make a determination of possible causes of trauma (flailing, degloving injury, patterned abrasions, stabbing, crushing, burns).

Many pathologists do not routinely take sections from limbs amputated for peripheral vascular disease or gangrene, particularly if labelled 'for disposal'.

If microscopic examination is deemed desirable, the following are sampled: arteries showing high grade stenosis, thrombosis or dissection, skin ulceration, or gangrene, major nerves and veins and one to two blocks of the proximal resection margin to assess viability. Bone and joints are sampled when relevant, e.g. osteomyelitis.

Macroscopic documentation of the injuries is usually adequate for cases of trauma and microscopic examination is only required when there is infection, osteomyelitis, fracture or if injuries require dating.

## Central and peripheral nervous system

### Brain, meninges and spinal cord

#### Clinical indications

Most intracranial biopsies are of space occupying lesions including primary and secondary neoplasms, abscesses and, less often, haematomas, all of which are detected radiologically or found incidentally at craniotomy for another condition. Biopsies are taken to confirm, type and grade brain neoplasms as a guide to treatment and prognosis. Frozen section examination is often performed in the first instance for diagnosis and the procedure may be followed by tumour debulking. Post-treatment biopsies to assess tumour response may also be performed. Less commonly, brain biopsies are taken to confirm or exclude a herpetic or other viral encephalitis or to investigate early onset dementia.

Meningeal biopsies are usually performed to confirm and subtype meningioma, and separate from cerebellopontine angle tumours such as acoustic nerve schwannoma and other tumour types including metastatic deposits and astrocytoma. The wall of chronic subdural haematomas may be submitted for examination, as may the contents of evacuated cerebral haematomas.

### Examination and dissection technique

Biopsies from *brain and meninges* often arrive fresh for initial frozen section examination and to confirm adequacy of the sample for paraffin section diagnosis. It is essential to know the patient's age, biopsy site and radiological diagnosis. In unusual tumours, such as childhood primitive neuroepithelial tumours, further tissue may be required for deep freezing, electron microscopy and cytogenetic studies. A portion of tumour should be submitted for lymphocyte surface markers/flow cytometry in suspected lymphoma. Touch, or squash preparations or smears of unfixed brain tumours form an important adjunctive method of diagnosis. Toluidine blue or a rapid H & E stain can be used on the smears. Typing and grading of the tumour at frozen section will determine the extent of attempted surgical debulking. Fresh material may be used for rapid immunofluorescence, culture and/or negative staining rapid transmission electron microscopy in cases of suspected viral encephalitis, and there may be special processing requirements for the investigation of dementia and storage disease.

*Brain* biopsies are typically small irregular fragments which are difficult to orien-

tate. Occasionally, a larger specimen may be received from the cerebellum where the grey matter is recognisable and the tissue can be cut perpendicular to the surface before blocking.

*Meningeal* biopsies vary from multiple small fragments, through rubbery round masses of tumour tissue to excisions taken in continuity with part of the inner table of the skull and/or brain cortex. Mark the margins of larger specimens. The skull bone will need to be dissected from the tumour and decalcified prior to sectioning. Some tumours with heavy calcification may also need decalcification.

If a length of nerve is identified, sample blocks both longitudinally and transversely to assess the tumour/nerve relationship.

*Spinal cord* specimens may be from primary and secondary neoplasms, abscesses, vascular malformations, haematomas, prolapsing intervertebral discs or osteophytes. The lesions may be extradural or subdural, the latter comprising intramedullary and extramedullary lesions. These specimens are handled similarly to brain and meningeal biopsies. For intervertebral discs see 'Osteoarticular system and soft tissues' (see p. 86).

### Peripheral nerve

### Clinical indications

Peripheral nerve biopsies are performed to confirm vagotomy or for the investigation of peripheral neuropathy. For the latter, the sural nerve is typically chosen. Peripheral nerve sheath tumours such as neurofibroma are often accompanied by a portion of nerve whilst schwannomas can often be removed without the nerve of origin (see 'Soft tissue including skeletal muscle biopsy' p. 88). Ganglia are occasionally received to confirm the adequacy of sympathectomy. Tumours such as ganglioneuroma may be removed from the mediastinum or retroperitoneum (see 'Adrenals' p. 57).

## Examination and dissection technique

As with all linear or tubular structures, peripheral nerve bundles are best sampled as longitudinal and cross sections, the latter taken from the centre or the ends.

Peripheral nerves removed for the investigation of neuropathy require specialised handling for optimal assessment and to reduce artefacts. The nerve is best received fresh and unfixed and handled only by its ends to minimise crushing and stretching as myelin sheaths are almost liquid in the unfixed state. The surgeon should avoid the use of diathermy and not dab the nerve with gauze. Most peripheral nerve biopsies range between 10 and 60 mm in length. Cut the nerve on dental wax as it is less adhesive than cork. If a 60 mm segment is received it is divided as follows: a 2 mm length is snap frozen in isopentane/liquid nitrogen for immunofluorescence in cases of suspected vasculitis; a 5 mm segment is placed into formal calcium; a 20 mm length is tied at each end with cotton string, one of which is attached to a 3 g lead sinker. The weighted nerve is suspended in a container of Fleming's fixative (Na/K dichromate, glacial acetic acid and osmium tetroxide) for 24–48 hours with the string at the opposite end secured under the lid. This procedure reduces contraction. Another 35 mm segment is handled in the same way and placed into glutaraldehyde for 3 hours and transferred to buffer for teased nerve preparations and electron microscopy. The weight can be cut away after 3 hours fixation.

Peripheral nerve biopsies for peripheral neuropathy can be examined as follows:

one frozen section block for immunofluorescence; one block fixed in formal calcium, embedded in paraffin and stained with haematoxylin and eosin, Congo red, Masson's trichrome, and Glees and Marsland for myelin; two blocks in Fleming's fixative, one embedded transverse and one longitudinal and stained with Kulchitsky Pal for myelin; and a glutaraldehyde-fixed block osmicated to blacken the myelin. A portion of nerve is teased with fine forceps under the dissecting microscope after immersion in 66% glycerine in water for 12 hours. A length of at least five nodes of Ranvier should be obtained. Approximately five nerve fibres per slide and 60 fibres per case should be examined. The other portion is placed into resin, embedded transversely and longitudinally for both light and electron microscopy.

# Ear, nose, oral cavity and larynx

## Ear

### Clinical indications

Biopsies and excisions are performed for congenital malformations, inflammatory lesions, some metabolic diseases, and epithelial, soft tissue and osseous neoplasms. Fragments of cholesterol granulomas and cholesteatomas are also not uncommon.

Stapedectomy is used to remove foci of otosclerosis and congenital footplate fixation.

Partial or total temporal bone resection is indicated for some carcinomas and other rare malignant neoplasms of the deep external auditory canal, middle ear or mastoid.

Grommet tubes may be submitted for microbiological culture, but histological examination is not performed on them.

*Examination and dissection technique*

Most biopsies from the *external auditory canal* or middle ear or mastoid air cells are small and are submitted in toto. Those with bone will require decalcification. A hand lens or dissecting microscope may be needed at the time of embedding to ensure that cutting is perpendicular to the epithelial surface. Ink the margins of larger excision biopsies which are cut in parallel transverse sections and perpendicular to the epithelium.

The *stapes* is the most commonly received ossicle and requires decalcification before sectioning. The bone is embedded longitudinally so the shape of the whole ossicle is revealed in the section. Otosclerosis may present as a pink swelling of the footplate.

For *ear-temporal bone* resection, a specimen X-ray is essential and comparisons should be made with pre-operative films. Orientate the specimen into antero-posterior, supero-inferior and medio-lateral edges and mark the edges. There are two methods of sectioning, either hemisected with the auditory canal longitudinal or cut in a series of transverse sections using either a hand-held saw or band saw. The choice will depend on the location and size of tumour. Portions of bone require decalcification. This can take several days as the temporal bone is extremely dense. Decalcified bone immediately adjacent to the tumour needs to be assessed for osseous spread.

## Nose and nasopharynx

### Clinical indications

Mucosal biopsies are taken from the nasal vestibule, cavity, mastoid antrum, sinuses and post-nasal space to investigate inflammatory, infective and neoplastic processes.

Nasal polyps, typically inflammatory and bilateral, are commonly removed and need to be distinguished from neoplastic polyps such as Schneiderian papilloma and carcinoma. Adenoids are removed for chronic inflammation, and often accompany tonsils.

### Examination and dissection technique

The biopsies are generally embedded uncut in toto but larger biopsies may need to be bisected. Some biopsies, such as those for suspected fungal infection of the sinuses, may arrive fresh whereupon a portion should be removed under sterile conditions and submitted for culture.

*Nasal polyps* may be quite large and all should be bisected and inspected closely. Many have cystic foci and myxoid cores. Fragments of incorporated bone and calcification are common and, if prominent, may necessitate decalcification prior to sampling. Polyps comprising dense grey/white tissue may be neoplastic and if the resected base is intact and identifiable, ink the margin.

*Tonsils and adenoids* are examined for sulphur granules of actinomyces and for focal lesions.

## Oral cavity

### Clinical indications

A vast array of inflammatory, developmental and neoplastic disorders occur in the oral cavity mucosa, soft tissue and jaws. Common entities such as papillomas, inflammatory papillary hyperplasia, pyogenic granuloma and leukoplakia/erythroplakia patches are commonly biopsied or excised, the latter to exclude squamous dysplasia and carcinoma. Jaw cysts are divided into odontogenic and fissural (developmental) subtypes. Various dermatoses such as lichen planus and pemphigus commonly involve the mouth. The jaws are also a site of primary neoplasms, or may be involved by direct spread from adjacent soft tissue or metastases. Radical curative resections of oral cavity soft tissue and bone in continuity are occasionally received.

## Examination and dissection technique

Biopsies of *oral cavity* bullous lesions or suspected lichen planus should be received fresh, in saline or transport media, for immunofluorescence. Excision biopsies, particularly of larger lesions of the tongue, buccal mucosa or floor of mouth, may be orientated by the surgeon and should have their margins inked and a block key diagram or specimen photocopy made. The tissue must be well fixed before sectioning as the edges of these specimens may be irregular and the oral mucosa may fold due to the loose submucosal tissue. Pinning out larger specimens on corkboard and fixation for a few hours is helpful. Some specimens will be attached to bone or teeth. The mucosa and soft tissue is dissected from the bone which needs decalcification. Mark the bone resection margins in the event of bone involvement by tumour.

*Radical resections* from this region may include the alveolar ridge, floor of mouth, part of the tongue and cervical lymph nodes plus attached tissues from the neck. They can be quite daunting and present an apparently bewildering array of possible surgical margins and lack of clearly recognisable anatomical structures in some cases. Orientating sutures placed by the surgeon may be helpful but if there is uncertainty of specimen orientation, the attending surgeon must be called to assist. The trainee must be familiar with the anatomy in this region and should not hesitate to consult an anatomy atlas. For floor of mouth specimens, the location of the tumour is identified, the lingual and mandibular mucosal edges located and the following structures should be identified if included in the specimen: mylohyoid muscle, major nerves and vessels, sublingual/submandibular glands and mandible. The tongue is anatomically divided into an anterior two-thirds distal to the V-shaped line of circumvallate papillae and a posterior third which ends at the tonsillar pillars. This division is important as the lymphatic drainage is different for the two areas. Lymphatics of the tongue, particularly more dorsally and in the posterior one-third, can cross the midline.

All radical resection specimens must be well fixed before sampling. Some specimens are best fixed pinned to corkboards. The resection margins should be inked, photographed and a block key diagram or specimen photocopy is necessary. The tumour (especially floor of mouth tumours) relationship to upper cervical soft tissue margins should be carefully examined. Dissection of lymph nodes included in a radical neck resection are described under 'Radical neck dissection' (see p. 80). The tumour and soft tissue are dissected from attached bone (e.g. mandible) which is decalcified, clearly marking resection margins.

*Teeth* may be received as a separate specimen, with an attached cyst or in situ as radical resections of the mandible or maxilla. Jaw cysts should be well fixed before sectioning. Larger cysts can be opened to aid fixation. The identification of a tooth as an incisor, canine, premolar and molar is possible by external examination. The full human dentition comprises 32 permanent teeth, some individuals retaining deciduous childhood precursors.

Each tooth has a contact or occlusal surface, crown, neck and root. Classification of dental cysts requires accurate identification of the tooth/cyst relationship. Teeth can be decalcified for histological examination but this is a prolonged procedure and fillings need prior removal.

## Larynx

### Clinical indications

Endoscopic biopsies are used to evaluate tumours, nodules and ulcerated areas in the larynx. The larynx is removed in part or in toto for laryngeal tumours, most commonly carcinoma. Hemilaryngectomy involves resection of one half of the thyroid cartilage plus the true and false vocal cords, and the ventricle on the same side. Supraglottic laryngectomy excises the proximal part of the larynx horizontally through the ventricle. Total laryngectomy specimens comprise the entire larynx, lower pharynx, epiglottis and upper tracheal rings, and often include an epsilateral hemithyroidectomy, hyoid bone, anterior strap muscles and occasionally the overlying skin if involved by tumour. The latter is usually seen around tracheostomy stoma.

### Examination and dissection technique

The larynx may be accompanied by attached epsilateral or bilateral radical neck dissection, which should be dissected off the main specimen and handled in the manner described in the lymphoreticular system (see 'Radical neck dissection' p. 80). Total and supraglottic laryngectomies are opened along the posterior midline and either pinned to a corkboard or splinted open with cotton-tipped sticks during formalin fixation. The specimen should then be photographed and a block key diagram or photocopy constructed. The pharyngeal, lingual and tracheal resection margins should be marked. Longitudinal sections through the midline between the left and right true and false cords, and ventricle and to the level of cartilage should be taken, as well as blocks of the soft tissue resection margins. Laryngeal carcinoma has a tendency to spread between the thyroid, cricoid and arytenoid cartilages, and it is essential to examine deep sections of the anterior margin. The remaining intact laryngectomy specimen can be subjected to parallel longitudinal sections after decalcification, allowing the relationship of tumour to cartilage to be assessed. Very large sagittal blocks can be made to assess tumour spread, enabling correlation with radiology (Fig. 6.1). Alternatively, by careful sampling the blocks can be submitted in several cassettes and the sections reconstructed to show the

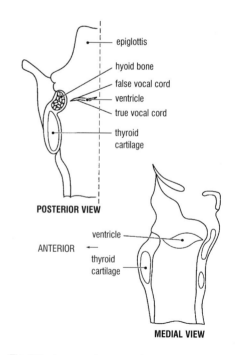

Fig. 6.1   Laryngectomy specimen

entire sagittal block, including the surgical margin. The laryngeal cartilage calcifies with increasing age. An alternative method is to slice the fixed laryngectomy specimen transversely at 4–5 mm intervals with a bandsaw. Slices generated in this way should be kept oriented and photographed. Some blocks will need decalcification prior to processing. The hyoid bone, if present, should be dissected free and sampled after decalcification.

If the thyroid gland has been resected, search for parathyroid glands as well as perithyroid and prelaryngeal (delphian) lymph nodes and examine microscopically for tumour deposits.

# Endocrine system

## Pituitary gland

### Clinical indications

Pituitary gland removal is indicated primarily for tumours, mainly adenomas, which may be hormonally functioning or non-functioning.

### Examination and dissection technique

All dissected fragments or curetted specimens including blood clot are submitted uncut for processing. Aspirated material should have formalin added immediately (preferably in theatre) and is strained to retrieve the fragments. Many suspected pituitary tumours are submitted to frozen section diagnosis to ensure that abnormal pituitary tissue is removed. A 1 mm or greater fragment should be fixed for ultrastructural study. If more tissue is available, a portion can be frozen for biochemical hormone assays although immunohistochemical staining for pituitary

hormones can be performed on fixed paraffin-embedded tissues.

## Adrenals

### Clinical indications

Core biopsies of adrenal gland are uncommonly performed for assessment of adrenal mass lesions, typically metastasis, and have largely been superseded by fine needle aspiration. Primary adrenal cortical tumours (adenoma, carcinoma) and medullary tumours (phaeochromocytoma, neuroblastoma, ganglioneuroblastoma/neuroma) apart from adenoma are uncommon, and if resectable, are removed with the whole adrenal gland. The adrenal gland may be included as part of a radical nephrectomy for renal adenocarcinoma or pelvic transitional cell carcinoma. Bilateral adrenalectomy has been employed to palliate the effects of ectopic ACTH producing tumours when the primary site remains elusive and was previously performed in association with oophorectomy to palliate breast carcinoma. Ectopic adrenal cortical tissue may be removed incidentally at laparoscopy/laparotomy or herniorrhaphy.

### Examination and dissection technique

The specimen is weighed and the dimensions recorded, as cortical tumours over 100 g and 5 cm diameter may behave in a malignant fashion irrespective of their histological features. The specimen may be submitted fresh and if phaeochromocytoma is suspected, the entire specimen or a selected block can be immersed in potassium dichromate fixative. The presence of catecholamines in the tumour will result in the chromaffin reaction, revealed as brown granules in the cytoplasm of tumour cells microscopically and as a brown colouration macroscopically. This procedure is now not necessary, as immunostaining allows clear distinction between cortical and medullary tumours. Prior formalin fixation renders the reaction unreliable. Tumours containing aromatic amine-rich granules such as the catecholamines will also exhibit formaldehyde-induced fluorescence and this can be demonstrated by exposing a cryostat section to formalin vapour generated by flame heating. The catecholamine type expressed by the tumour is more reliably determined from fresh tumour extracts, or by immunostaining for noradrenaline and adrenaline, or electron microscopy. If possible, a portion of tumour tissue should be frozen and in childhood adrenal tumours, a fresh sterile piece for cytogenetics is mandatory and often yields important diagnostic and prognostic information. Ultrastructural examination can be very helpful in the separation of cortical from medullary tumours, as well as for the diagnosis of malignant small round tumours of childhood such as neuroblastoma, rhabdomyosarcoma, lymphoma, Wilm's tumour and most metastatic tumours. If the tumour is large and is accompanied by attached organs such as kidney and liver, the specimen margins should be inked. A careful search should be made for the adrenal hilar vessels and periadrenal lymph nodes which are often involved by cortical carcinoma. The separated adrenal gland is sliced at parallel 2–3 mm intervals and sampled for microscopy. Radiography of paediatric adrenal/periadrenal tumours may reveal calcification which is common in ganglioneuroma/blastoma.

Adenomas associated with Cushing's syndrome often have a variegated, marbled or uncommonly yellow colour with haemorrhagic degeneration. They tend to be greater than 3 cm in size and the extratumoral cortex is atrophic. The finding of a thin layer of peritumoral adrenal gland suggests a functioning glucocorticoid-producing cortical tumour, as atrophy is not seen with tumours which are non-secreting, or produce sex steroids or aldosterone. The adenomas of primary aldosteronism are typically less than 3 cm, yellow, or less commonly brown. Non-functioning adenomas are often greater than 3 cm, yellow, uncommonly black and frequently show haemorrhagic degeneration. Neuroblastomas are classically large, soft and grey-pink, with extensive necrosis and frequent haemorrhage, whilst ganglioneuromas are white/grey firm and homogeneous with focal calcification. Phaeochromocytomas are soft, haemorrhagic tumours, red-brown, yellow or grey on cut section.

## Thyroid

### Clinical indications

The use of thyroid core biopsies to investigate nodules has markedly declined with the advent of fine needle aspiration cytology. 'Cold' thyroid nodules which may be removed include adenomas, carcinomas, dominant nodules in multinodular goitres or even Hashimoto's disease. Subtotal thyroidectomy is performed for multinodular goitre and toxic goitre following failure of medical suppressant therapy. Total thyroidectomy is generally reserved for malignancy.

### Examination and dissection technique

Weigh, measure and orientate the specimen. Accompanying lymph nodes or parathyroid glands (on the posterior surface) should be identified and sampled.

Parathyroid glands are typically 2–3 mm in size and brown or tan in colour. Lymph nodes are often a darker pink or black/grey from accumulation of carbon pigment but distinction from parathyroid glands is not always easy. Ink the margins of resection if malignancy is suspected. To enhance fixation, cut parallel slices at 4–5 mm intervals, keeping the slices ordered as to lobe side and position. These cuts can either be in the transverse or sagittal plane. Many nodules in the thyroid are soft and friable and their contents easily extruded when slicing. The use of a long feather blade knife in a sawing motion rather than a conventional scalpel blade produces less trauma to the specimen. Alternatively, the whole specimen can be fixed prior to slicing. If the specimen arrives unfixed, imprints can be obtained and a sterile portion obtained for cytogenetics, and samples fixed for electron microscopy (in medullary carcinoma) and frozen for hormone assays and immunohistochemistry. If the trachea is attached, it is opened posteriorly to expose its relationship to the tumour. Decalcification may be needed on the separated trachea before sectioning. Neck dissections are dissected as described under 'Lymphoreticular system' (see p. 79). Specimen photographs may enhance the macroscopic description.

For diffuse and inflammatory processes take two to three blocks from each lobe and one block of isthmus. For solitary well-circumscribed nodules of less than 5 cm, block the entire lesion with most sections to include the capsule and/or adjacent thyroid gland. Capsule sections are essential in follicular lesions to assess the presence of capsular and vascular invasion. For larger nodules take one additional block per centimetre diameter. With multinodular glands, generally take one block from each nodule up to a maximum

of eight blocks. Take care to sample the periphery of the nodules with inclusion of the adjacent gland and any solid white or grey areas. In the case of suspected papillary carcinoma ideally block the entire thyroid gland in view of the high incidence of multifocality, alternatively, slice the gland at 1 mm intervals and sample any opaque areas. For invasive tumours other than papillary carcinoma take three to six blocks of tumour including a section of any capsular permeation, three blocks of each thyroid lobe away from tumour, one block of isthmus resection margin in hemithyroidectomy specimens. Submit all lymph nodes or parathyroid glands in toto.

## Parathyroids

### Clinical indications

Parathyroid glands are usually excised for hyperparathyroidism, primary, secondary and tertiary. Hyperparathyroidism may be due to adenoma or hyperplasia. Generally, three and a half glands are excised in cases of hyperfunction, as the ability to reliably distinguish adenoma from hyperplasia requires histological examination of all four glands. Removal of only one gland, even if clearly enlarged, should be discouraged. The remaining half gland may be left in situ, or transplanted subcutaneously or intramuscularly in the forearm to enable easy removal in the event of recurrent hyperfunction. A fifth parathyroid gland may be present in up to 3% of patients. Rarely, six glands may be found and glands may be ectopically located deep in the neck, mediastinum or even in the thyroid gland. In many instances, parathyroids are submitted for frozen section examination where the principle role of the pathologist is to identify parathyroid tissue and exclude lymph nodes, fat and small nodules of thyroid gland. Parathyroid carcinoma is very rare, may be palpable, and typically infiltrates surrounding tissue.

## Examination and dissection technique

Suspected parathyroid glands should have surrounding fat removed before weighing each gland on an accurate, preferably digital, balance. This must precede sampling of tissue for frozen section examination and the location of each gland should be documented. Each parathyroid gland weighs approximately 30 mg, the combined weight of four parathyroid glands in the adult male being $120 \pm 3.5$ mg and in females being $142 \pm 5.2$ mg. A gland of more than 60 mg is generally considered abnormal (provided the surgeon has identified three other normal glands).

Generally, all the parathyroid glands are submitted in toto for examination, unless they are very large when they require bisection. The periphery of large glands should be sampled to identify any residual compressed normal parathyroid gland.

## Endocrine pancreas

### Clinical indications

Islet cell tumours of the pancreas may be single or multiple, benign or malignant, and tend to be preferentially located in the tail and body of the pancreas where the density of islets is greatest. They account for less than 1% of pancreatic tumours. Other endocrine tumours such as carcinoids are extremely rare.

### Examination and dissection technique

The resection margins of the distal pancreatectomy are inked before slicing the pancreas at 5 mm intervals perpendicular to the direction of the pancreatic duct. As islet cell tumours are often small, the cut surfaces must be inspected carefully. If the spleen is included, it is removed and handled as described in the 'Spleen' (see p. 81). Complete pancreatectomies are dissected as described under 'Exocrine pancreas' (see p. 79). The external surface should be inspected for lymph nodes. If the specimen is submitted fresh and there is clearly identifiable tumour, freeze away a portion and submit tissue for ultrastructural examination.

Take three to six blocks of the tumour, at least one block of each tumour if multiple. The blocks should include the relationship of the tumour(s) to the resection margins and main pancreatic duct. Also sample two to three blocks of uninvolved pancreas and take sections of any other focal lesions such as cysts. Sample the proximal excision margin in excisions of the distal pancreas.

## Paraganglia

These extra-adrenal neuroendocrine organs are widely distributed through the body and may be affected by hyperplasia or neoplasms, which, on occasion, are functional or may be difficult to locate. Paraganglia tend to follow vessels and include the parasympathetic tympanic, jugular, intravagal, intercarotid, superior laryngeal and inferior laryngeal nerves in the neck, and the subclavian, aortico-pulmonary and coronary vessels, and around the aortic arch. The sympathetic system includes the superior cervical ganglion in the neck, the sympathetic trunk in the posterior mediastinum and retroperitoneum, the organ of Zuckerkandl around the origin of the inferior mesenteric artery in the abdominal aorta, and within the bladder wall. Rare sites include the gallbladder, prostate, uterus and the spermatic cord.

The term phaeochromocytoma is best restricted to a tumour of the adrenal medullary paraganglioma.

### Examination and dissection technique

If tumour tissue is received fresh, a portion can be stored for frozen section immuno-histochemistry and 1 mm fragments may be fixed for ultrastructural examination, both useful examinations in the difficult case. DNA ploidy and static image cytometry are less helpful.

Biopsies of paraganglioma can be quite small and be composed predominantly of tumour or be included with other associated viscera such as the urinary bladder. As a general rule, the resection margins should be inked and larger specimens opened or sliced to enhance fixation. Fresh tumour specimens should have a cut surface imprinted. Chromaffin paragangliomas can be placed into potassium dichromate fixative for the chromaffin reaction. Formaldehyde-induced fluorescence can be used to demonstrate catecholamines. Argyrophil and argentaffin stains are useful in the study of paragangliomas.

## Eye and eyelids

### Eyelids, conjunctiva and lacrimal gland

#### Clinical indications

Biopsies from the eyelids, conjunctiva and lacrimal gland are removed for a variety of inflammatory and degenerative disorders which are often actinic-related conditions such as pinguecula and pterygia. In addition, cysts, benign and malignant tumours, congenital abnormalities and systemic metabolic disorders may manifest in these sites.

### Examination and dissection technique

Most specimens from these sites are small and represent biopsies for diagnosis or curative excision. The eyelid specimens with skin are handled like other small specimens, while biopsies from the lacrimal gland and conjunctiva are generally so small that they are embedded uncut. If sufficiently large, lacrimal gland biopsies should be cut into transverse sections. Biopsies of the bulbar conjunctiva, particularly for pterygium, should be cut longitudinally to show the transition between conjunctiva and corneal limbus. The tissue can be laid on filter paper to stop curling. If infection is suspected, fresh tissue should be sent for culture. Calculi (dacryoliths) may sometimes be received and these generally do not require microscopic examination.

### Cornea

#### Clinical indications

Full thickness corneal buttons are removed at the time of corneal transplant for corneal endothelial decompensation (bullous keratopathy), keratoconus, some corneal dystrophies, failed corneal grafts, corneal scarring and chronic herpetic keratitis. Rarely corneal transplants may fail and be removed. Partial thickness or small biopsies may be received in the above conditions and for diagnosis of tumour masses.

#### Examination and dissection technique

Most cornea specimens arrive in formalin as buttons of about 8 mm diameter. The diagnosis of some corneal dystrophies such as the lipid keratopathies will need fresh tissue frozen sections or special fixatives, whilst others such as Meesman's corneal dystrophy show diagnostic ultrastructural features and require fixation in glutaraldehyde. Careful handling of corneal biopsies is essential, as the posterior corneal endothelium is easily denuded. Examine the cornea for opacities, ulcers and vesicles, and cut the biopsy at 2 mm intervals. Three levels ordered at the time of cut-up and special stains including PAS, Hale's colloidal iron, Alcian blue, von Kossa, Masson's trichrome and Congo red may be helpful in the study of dystrophies.

## Intraocular biopsies (lens, choroid, retina, iris, trabecular meshwork)

### Clinical indications

Cataractous lenses are now rarely received as many centres use high frequency sound waves to emulsify the lens before aspiration. Prosthetic lenses composed of polymethylmethacrylate may be removed if they are loose, as they can mechanically damage the iris, cornea (pseudophakic bullous keratopathy) or induce intraocular inflammation. The trabecular meshwork (trabeculectomy) can be excised in glaucoma to improve the drainage of aqueous. Intraocular biopsies of other parts of the eye may be taken from intraocular tumours and some forms of chorioretinitis. Fragments of ocular tissue may be removed following trauma.

### Examination and dissection technique

The biopsy specimens are usually small and are embedded in toto. Specimens which are slightly larger and display a recognisable epithelial surface should be cut perpendicular to the surface or across the junction between normal and abnormal tissue. In

cases of suspected infection, particularly in immunosuppressed patients, a portion of fresh tissue should be submitted for microbiological culture. Prosthetic lenses have a central optical zone and peripheral extensions. They are flat and can be placed on glass slides for surface inspection. Trabeculectomy specimens are ideally inspected with a dissecting microscope to ensure correct orientation.

## Periorbital soft tissue

### Clinical indications

Developmental abnormalities such as teratomas and meningocoeles, primary and metastatic neoplasms, thyroid ophthalmopathy and inflammatory masses including mucocoeles which present as proptosis may be biopsied or excised.

### Examination and dissection technique

The resection margins of excision specimens should be inked, and if unfixed, portions of tumour should be snap frozen for immunohistochemistry and 1 mm cubes fixed for electron microscopy. Fresh tissue should be kept for lymphocyte surface marker studies by flow cytometry or frozen section immunohistochemistry in lymphoid tumours. Imprints of the freshly cut tumour surface aid in diagnosis, especially of lymphoid tumours. Larger specimens are sliced at 5 mm parallel intervals and small biopsies are submitted uncut in toto.

## Eye enucleation

### Clinical indications

Enucleation removes the eye globe, leaving in situ the eyelids and retrobulbar tissues. It is performed for trauma, to reduce the risk of sympathetic ophthalmitis in the contralateral eye, painful blind eyes (phthisis bulbi), intractable glaucoma, severe intraocular inflammation and intraocular tumours (typically melanoma). Evisceration is performed for severe intraocular infections; to decrease the risk of post-operative meningitis, the globe contents are removed, leaving the sclera intact and the dura around the optic nerve.

## Examination and dissection technique

The intact globe needs to be fixed for a minimum of 24–48 hours in formalin before sectioning. The temptation to open the sclera, cut widows or inject formalin into the vitreous should be resisted unless there is a pressing need for fresh tissue such as for molecular analysis and cytogenetics in retinoblastoma. Before cutting, the eye should be washed well in running water. The clinical reason for enucleation should be reviewed. To establish the side of eye, view from the posterior aspect. The optic nerve is on the medial or nasal side of the globe relative to the tendinous insertion of the superior oblique muscle and the muscular insertion of the inferior oblique muscle. The long posterior ciliary vein and nerves are on the extreme nasal aspect of the globe (Fig. 6.2). Callipers are used to measure the antero-posterior, horizontal and vertical dimensions of the globe, the length of the optic nerve and the diameter of the cornea are noted. Any surgical injuries should be documented. Examine the eye by transilluminating with a strong light beam in a darkened room. If there is a clinical history of intraocular foreign bodies or retinoblastoma, X-ray the globe in a faxitron before cutting the specimen. The eye is best cut horizontally with a new, sharp, single-edged razor blade rather than a scalpel, with the blade held between the

thumb and middle or ring finger of the pathologist's dominant hand. The eye is cut into three pieces, the central cross-section containing the important structures including the cornea, lens and optic nerve. By resting the globe on a soft surface such as cotton wool, cornea downwards, the first cut should be made vertically through the globe about 2 mm to one side of the optic nerve down to just above the superior edge of the cornea. By lying the cut surface on a hard surface, the second cut is made parallel to the first to pass to the opposite edge of the cornea. The cuts should be as smooth as possible, but in practice, an element of sawing is almost inevitable. This first cut may be modified slightly depending on the location of any lesion established by transillumination. The interior of the globe is then examined systematically with the aid of a hand lens or dissection microscope and photographs are taken. The two asymmetric calottes of globe are placed into an alcohol-containing jar and fixed for 2 days. Artificial lenses may be left in situ as they dissolve during processing.

Examine each structure of the eye systematically particularly for retinal

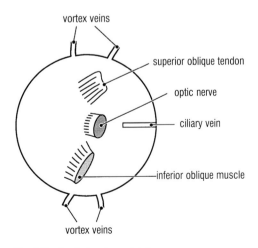

**Fig. 6.2** Posterior view of left eye

detachment, haemorrhage and necrosis, and trans-scleral spread or optic nerve infiltration by tumour. Cut levels of the whole block mounts, especially of the central portion, so that some levels include the optic disk and macula. Routine Masson's trichrome and PAS stains are useful. For tumours, especially retinoblastoma and malignant melanoma, a cross-section of the optic nerve margin, and samples of vortex veins from each eye quadrant respectively should be taken. In cases of early trans-scleral extension, the resection margin should be assessed.

## Orbital exenteration

### Clinical indications

This uncommon operation removes, in addition to the globe, the retrobulbar soft tissues and muscle, the lacrimal gland and the eyelids. It is occasionally performed for large cutaneous eyelid or conjunctival neoplasms, and aggressive intraocular tumours manifesting trans-scleral extra ocular spread.

### Examination and dissection technique

The elliptical eyelid skin is pinned open and the specimen fixed well before sectioning. The surgical margins are painted with ink. The eyeglobe is cut horizontally as described for eye enucleation, and the eyelids and soft tissues are left attached.

In addition to blocks to assess the depth of tumour invasion and involvement of globe, sample other anatomical structures in the specimen (lacrimal gland, eyelids, conjunctiva, palpebral fissure, periorbital soft tissues). Also sample the margins of the soft tissue, globe, optic nerve and skin.

# Female genital system

## Vulva

### Clinical indications

Inflammatory dermatoses, dystrophy, cysts, abscesses, condylomas, dysplasia (vulvular intraepithelial neoplasia – VIN) and neoplasms are lesions subjected to biopsy or excision. Vulvectomy is indicated for some neoplasms and occasionally is employed for symptomatic relief of some chronic inflammatory conditions such as lichen sclerosus. Unilateral labium majus and skin may be excised, or a radical excision of the entire vulva, perineum and inguinal nodes may be performed.

### Examination and dissection technique

The butterfly-shaped vulvectomy specimen is pinned on a corkboard for fixation in formalin. The specimen should be photographed and a photocopy or drawing made for a block key diagram. Ink the resection margins. Focal lesions are cut transversely to demonstrate the deep and lateral extension of the tumour. Bilateral inguinal lymph node dissection may be present either in continuity with the vulvectomy or separately in cases of radical vulvectomy. Separate the node-containing fat and clear in Carnoy's fixative before dissecting for nodes as described in 'Inguinal dissection' (see p. 81).

Indicate the type of vulvectomy and whether there is attached or separate inguinal node dissection. Record the specimen dimensions (labia minus and majus, clitoris, diameter of introitus and length of distal vagina) and describe focal lesions, noting their distance to margins of excision and if the tumour crosses the midline or spreads into the perineal/perianal skin.

## Vagina

### Clinical indications

Vaginal biopsies are rare compared to biopsies from the cervix and vulva. They are performed to investigate inflammatory disorders, dysplasia, cysts, polyps, adenosis post-diethylstilboesterol exposure, human papilloma virus infection and tumours. Vaginectomy is very rarely performed for malignancy, although partial vaginectomy often forms part of a vaginal repair operation for prolapse and a vaginal cuff is often included with a radical hysterectomy for cervical carcinoma (see 'Cervix' and 'Uterine corpus' pp. 65, 67).

### Examination and dissection technique

Many specimens are blocked uncut but cysts, polyps and condylomas may be of a size requiring bisection or further parallel sections before embedding. If a well defined lesion has been excised, ink the margins for identification.

The vaginectomy specimen may be accompanied by vulva, uterus, tubes, ovaries, bladder and rectum in continuity. The other organs are handled as described elsewhere in this chapter. If the tumour has not directly extended onto the cervix, the vagina is separated from the uterus and cervix before being opened along the wall opposite to the tumour mass or the bulkiest part of a circumferential lesion. It is pinned flat on a corkboard. Attached organs such as bladder and rectum are opened and their mucosal surfaces, in the region of the tumour, inspected closely for infiltration and fistula formation. Photocopies or a block key diagram of the specimen helps orientation. Ink the resection margins and photograph specimens with tumours. Inspect the perivaginal soft tissue for lymph nodes using serial cuts at 5 mm intervals. The upper half of the vagina drains to the external iliac nodes whilst the lower half drains to the hypogastric nodes. Some lymphatics may drain to the vulva or cervix. These nodal groups may be resected in cases of vaginal malignancy and can be placed into Carnoy's solution to facilitate fat clearance. Carefully evaluate any attached vulval or cervical tissue, as vaginal carcinoma is associated with a second primary neoplasm in 10–20% of women.

## Cervix

### Clinical indications

Biopsies of the cervix are often guided by colposcopy following identification of abnormal cervical cytology and are used to assess conditions such as cervicitis, human papilloma virus infection, dysplasia, both squamous and glandular, and carcinoma. Endocervical curettage is a technique used to sample the endocervical canal and is sometimes used in conjunction with endometrial curettage (fractional curettage) as a staging procedure in endometrial carcinoma. Polyps are common, may cause bleeding and are easily removed. Cone, large loop excision of transformation zone (LLETZ) and loop electrosurgical excision procedure (LEEP) biopsies are employed as curative resection of dysplasia and for microinvasive carcinoma. The latter two procedures employ a thin wire loop and low voltage diathermy. Cervical amputation with preservation of the uterine corpus is rarely employed in the treatment of prolapse.

### Examination and dissection technique

Biopsies and curettings are often difficult to orientate and are usually embedded uncut.

Larger cervical biopsies (> 5 mm) can be bisected at right angles to the epithelial surface in the long axis. The long axis can be identified by longitudinal endocervical grooves. Small cervical polyps are embedded uncut whilst larger polyps can be bisected.

The ideal cone biopsy is received intact with identification of the 12 o'clock position. Most specimens are received in formalin and the surgical margins should be inked. The anterior margin can be marked with a second marking material or scored transversely with a scalpel. Many cone biopsies are now removed by laser rather than scalpel (cold knife). They are smaller and have burnt margins and orientation can be difficult because of distortion and charring. With deep cone biopsies, take a transverse section of the apex and cut 3 mm thick parallel sagittal sections in the 12–6 o'clock plane, from 3 o'clock to 9 o'clock (Fig. 6.3a). The transverse apical block is not taken in small

cone biopsies as it makes resection margin epithelium more difficult to assess. An alternative method involves opening the cone biopsy longitudinally at 12 o'clock using scissors placed in the endocervical canal. The opened cone biopsy is pinned to a corkboard with the mucosal surface up and fixed in formalin for several hours. The entire cervix is then cut into 3 mm serial radial sections moving clockwise from 12 o'clock and keeping the pieces oriented. Blocks need to be taken so that each includes the squamo-columnar junction but it is difficult to consistently get epithelium in all sections and the stroma of the wedge-shaped blocks has to be trimmed to achieve this (Fig. 6.3b).

LLETZ and LEEP biopsies may be received as one piece or as multiple charred fragments. In the latter situation, the larger pieces (> 5 mm) are cut as parallel longitudinal sections and embedded in toto. Intact LLETZ and LEEP specimens are handled as

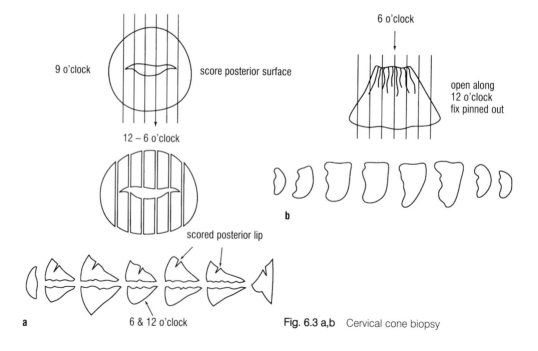

**Fig. 6.3 a,b**   Cervical cone biopsy

with cone biopsies, although orientation can be more difficult. The margins of such biopsies are often readily identified by diathermy changes.

The amputated cervix from a vaginal repair usually has attached triangular cuffs of anterior and posterior vaginal wall. The cervix can be opened longitudinally through the os to aid fixation.

With small and fragmented biopsies of cervix, three levels of each block should be examined.

## Uterine corpus

### Clinical indications

Specimens from this part of the female genital tract are very common. The commonest indication is the investigation of abnormal per-vaginal bleeding which may be dysfunctional and related to hormonal imbalance, or due to endometritis, polyps, adenomyosis, submucosal leiomyomas, endometriosis, hyperplasia, malignancy and pregnancy (intra- or extra-uterine). Curettage and pipette biopsy is usually an initial examination. Myomectomy of uterine leiomyomas with preservation of the uterus is helpful in younger women who wish to retain fertility. Endomyometrial ablation is a more recent alternative to hysterectomy for the treatment of persistent dysfunctional uterine bleeding. Hysterectomy is indicated for the reasons listed above as well as for prolapse. The uterus may be removed with attached vagina, fallopian tubes, ovaries and parametria, and in the case of malignancy of the cervix or endometrium, pelvic lymphadenectomy may also be performed.

### Examination and dissection technique

All tissue received is strained through a sieve or alcohol-soaked foam and blocked in toto. Bulky curettings which fill more than one cassette generally indicate late secretory phase endometrium, hyperplasia, malignancy or pregnancy. Yellowish friable tissue is suggestive of carcinoma. In the case of abortion, inspect closely for fetal parts, membranes and chorionic villi. Spongy tissue often represents chorionic villi whilst haemorrhagic membranous tissue with a shiny surface on one side and a rough surface on the other is suggestive of decidua. If the specimen is received fresh or in saline for investigation of recurrent abortion, submit a sample of chorionic villi for cytogenetic analysis. In incomplete abortions, embed pale solid areas which may represent decidua and chorionic villi. If fat is seen, warn the clinician of a possible uterine perforation. Because of the friable nature of products of conception it is easy to contaminate the cut-up area. Be careful to wipe clean the area and rinse all instruments used. If possible, do not follow the case with another uterine curettage.

Endomyometrial resections are handled in a similar manner to curettings and are embedded in toto. Some large pieces may need bisection. Diathermy artefact is often pronounced. Leiomyomas resected during myomectomy are cut in parallel slices at 1 cm intervals.

For simple hysterectomy performed for cervical in situ or microinvasive carcinoma, endometrial hyperplasia or carcinoma, the uterus is weighed and the following dimensions recorded: length, intercornuate and antero-posterior diameter, dimensions of the cervical os and the sounded depth of the uterine cavity. There is a broad range of normal uterine weights. The nulliparous uterus of a premenopausal woman weighs approximately 30–40 g whilst a parous uterus is usually between 75 and 100 g. Uterine weight generally increases with parity. Many uteri are received opened to enhance fixation of the endometrium which otherwise undergoes autolysis quickly. The peritoneal reflection extends more inferiorly over the posterior surface of the uterus and the insertion of the fallopian tubes is posterior to that of the round ligaments.

The cervix is amputated from the uterine corpus 2.5 cm above the external os and the external resection margins are inked. In cases with cervical cancer, the cervix is treated like a cone biopsy. It is either cut in serial sagittal sections or opened at the 12 o'clock position and pinned out on a corkboard. If bulky tumour is present or a previous biopsy suggests an unusual neoplasm, fresh tumour tissue may be frozen for ancillary investigations and 1 mm cubes fixed in glutaraldehyde. The uterine corpus is dissected separately from the tubes and ovaries which are transected. The uterus may be examined by parallel horizontal slices at 5 mm intervals (Fig. 6.4) or by parallel sagittal slices. If leiomyomas are received separately, they are

examined by 5 mm slices. If a portion of vagina has been resected in continuity with the cervix, it may need to be removed to fit into the tissue blocks. In these circumstances, it is important to orientate the true resection margin and mark it. Following sampling of the myometrium and endometrium, the entire uterine cavity can be scraped with a scalpel to provide an almost complete sampling of the endometrium.

In Wertheim's hysterectomy, lymph node resection will be received as separately identified groups which should be blocked in toto. Photograph interesting specimens.

Gestational trophoblastic disease requires cytogenetic and possibly DNA ploidy studies. Ovaries and fallopian tubes are examined as described below.

## Fallopian tube

### Clinical indications

Segments of fallopian tubes are often submitted to confirm sterilisation whilst salpingectomy is performed for ectopic pregnancy, severe endometriosis, pyo/hydrosalpinx and other inflammatory conditions, and very rarely for carcinoma of fallopian tube.

### Examination and dissection technique

The tube is cut into 3–5 mm parallel transverse sections. If there is a pyosalpinx and the tube is received fresh, submit some of the luminal contents for microbiological examination. In tubal pregnancy, sample the contents of any vesicle or grey tissue found within the intraluminal clot, as they represent chorionic villi or fetal parts. If such tissue is not apparent macroscopically, take several blocks of the intraluminal clot where chorionic villi may reside. Additional

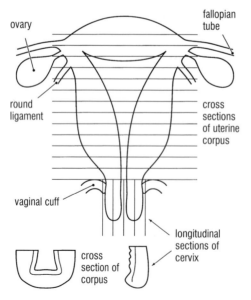

Fig. 6.4　Hysterectomy specimen

blocks may be required if products of conception are not identified in the initial sections. Examine for pre-existing pathology that may have lead to the ectopic pregnancy, e.g. strictures, endometriosis.

## Ovary

### Clinical indications

The ovary may be biopsied to investigate infertility, premature menopause and endometriosis. Wedge biopsies are employed in both the diagnosis and treatment of polycystic ovary syndrome. Unilateral oophorectomy is performed for benign ovarian neoplasms, torsion, severe endometriosis and envelopment in dense adhesions. Bilateral oophorectomy is undertaken for malignant tumours of the ovary, endometrium and cervix in combination with hysterectomy, salpingectomy and omentectomy, the latter in ovarian carcinoma. Oophorectomy is now rarely performed for palliation of breast carcinoma. Ovaries are often removed together with the uterus for dysfunctional uterine bleeding, in patients over the age of 40 years.

### Examination and dissection technique

Small ovarian biopsies are embedded uncut, whilst larger wedge biopsies should be bisected perpendicular to the capsule in the long axis.

Most cystectomies are less than a few centimetres in size. The cysts should be measured and weighed if intact. Simple cysts are opened and allowed to fix further, whilst more complex solid and cystic lesions are examined as described for tumours below. Collapsed cysts are measured and submitted as multiple cross-sections of the cyst wall and adjacent ovarian parenchyma.

The ovary should be measured and weighed if enlarged. If removed for ovarian malignancy and received fresh, a portion of tumour can be snap frozen for immunohistochemistry and 1 mm fragments fixed for ultrastructural examination. With both cystic and solid tumours, several parallel cuts should be made to enhance formalin permeation. Neoplasms filled with hair and sebaceous material indicate a teratoma. As much of the contents should be removed as possible to enhance formalin permeation. The sebaceous material adheres readily to dissection instruments and warm water is helpful in its removal. In the benign cystic teratoma, solid areas are often present and such areas should be sampled as they display the broadest array of tissue types in such tumours. Similarly, all other cystic lesions should be carefully examined for solid and papillary areas which must be sampled for microscopy. Fallopian tubes and the uterus are examined as described earlier. The omentum, removed in cases of ovarian malignancy, is inspected for surface tumour deposits and dissected for tumour deposits and lymph nodes.

Tumour infiltration of the serosal surfaces should be carefully searched for in ovarian malignancy and in hormone-secreting ovarian tumours; the endometrium should be examined for hyperplasia or neoplasia.

## Placenta

### Clinical indications

Small fragments of placental tissue may be received as part of a spontaneous or therapeutic abortion or from retained postpartum products (see 'Fetus' and 'Uterine corpus' pp. 67, 71). Normal term or pre/post-term placentas are not routinely received but those from multiple births, stillbirths, growth-retarded babies, intrauterine infection, maternal disease and fetal malformations may be submitted for examination.

## Examination and dissection technique

Placentas are best examined in the fresh state where microbiological cultures or a portion of fetal membranes for cytogenetic studies can be obtained and, if the placenta is incomplete, the obstetrician can be informed. Cotyledons or the succenturiate lobe may be missing and the only indication may be the presence of precipitate-ending membranous fetal vessels. Examine the container for detached pieces of placenta and estimate the amount of blood and clots present. The grape-like appearance of the grossly swollen and cystic chorionic villi of hydatidiform mole are usually readily recognised. The placenta is measured and its singleton, twin or multiple state determined.

With the *singleton placenta*, the following examination sequence is adopted for membranes, umbilical cord, fetal surface and maternal surface. The membranes are examined for completeness, meconium staining, colour, opacity, retromembranous haemorrhage, oedema, decidual necrosis, cord insertion and extra-amniotic pregnancy. A 2 cm wide section of membranes is taken from the point of rupture to include the nearest placental edge. This strip can be rolled with the amnion inward around a pair of forceps, prised off and fixed before cross-sections are taken from the centre as described for the Swiss roll technique for the ureters. The length of the umbilical cord and the distance from the cord insertion to the placental margin are measured. Other features examined for include: membranous versus non-membranous insertion, velamentous, fetal vessel

damage, number of cord vessels on cross-section, colour, strictures, haemorrhage, thrombosis, atresia, twists and true knots. The cord should be removed from the placenta 3 cm proximal to the insertion and sectioned. The fetal surface is examined for amnion nodosum, squamous metaplasia, thrombosis of fetal vessels, colour, subchorionic fibrin, cysts (number, size, contents) and chorangioma. The maternal surface is examined for completeness, fissures and lacerations, depressed white areas of old infarction, and retroplacental haemorrhage (estimated volume, distance from edge). The placenta is then placed fetal side down on a cutting board and incomplete parallel sections are made at 1–2 cm intervals with a long bladed knife, leaving the slices attached by the fetal surface. A transverse section of the mid-maternal surface should be taken to assess the maternal vessels.

*Twin placentas* may be dichorionic-diamniotic (separate), dichorionic-diamniotic (fused), monochorionic-diamniotic and monochorionic-monoamniotic (Fig. 6.5). The latter two appearances reflect monozygotic twins whilst the former two may be monozygotic or dizygotic twins. Histological examination of the membranous septa between the twins allows the distinction of mono- from di-chorionic placentation. In the monochorionic-diamniotic placenta the dividing membrane is transparent, thin, easily stripped and has a smooth continuous attachment to the fetal surface. Numerous twin-to-twin vascular anastomoses are present. Fused dichorionic-diamniotic placentas have thick, opaque dividing membranes which are difficult to strip and attach to the fetal surface with a ridge. Separate twin placentas are both examined as singleton placentas. The absence of a dividing membrane suggests the very rare monochorionic-monoamniotic placenta. A 2–3 cm strip of dividing membrane is made into a Swiss roll by rolling around a pair of forceps, prised off and fixed before a 3 mm cross-section is taken of the mid-portion for histology. The vascular anastomoses in monochorionic-diamniotic placentas occur as artery to artery, vein to vein or artery to vein anastomosis. They can be studied by injecting one twin's artery along the fusion point with 30–50 ml of dye and determining whether the dye exits from the lobular veins of the other twin. Arteries run superficial to veins. The twin placentation in a case with vascular anastomoses will show pallor and oedema in one placenta and deep congestion of the other. The fused twin placenta is best divided along

the vascular pole rather than the base of the dividing membrane and each half is then examined as a singleton placenta.

Take blocks of membranes, cord and placenta, the latter from the central and peripheral areas of both maternal and fetal aspects and any gross lesions. In addition to these, the dividing membrane in twin placentas is sampled with the Swiss roll procedure.

## Fetus

### Clinical indications

Fetuses may be received intact in a gestational sac, or in fragments with placental tissue and endometrium, as part of a miscarriage or therapeutic termination of pregnancy. Larger fetuses from mid-trimester miscarriages may also be sent for examination but the specialised investigation of these deaths requires a detailed and complete necropsy with analysis of congenital defects by dissection, histology and radiology, exclusion of transplacental infection and retention of tissue for possible metabolic studies and cytogenetics. Malformed fetuses should be photographed.

### Examination and dissection technique

The dissection method varies with the gestational age and preservation of the fetus. Small fetuses can be embedded uncut whilst larger fetuses are cut sagittally. Fetuses less than 10 cm in crown–heel length are inspected externally and can be cut into three transverse sections through the head, thorax and abdomen. The gross sections generated can be inspected with a hand lens or dissecting microscope to

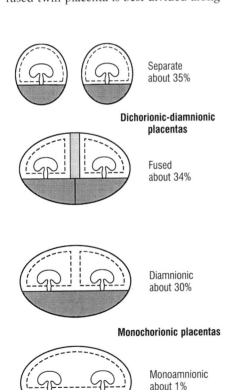

Separate
about 35%

**Dichorionic-diamnionic placentas**

Fused
about 34%

Diamnionic
about 30%

**Monochorionic placentas**

Monoamnionic
about 1%

Fig. 6.5   Twin placentas

evaluate the positioning of internal organs and for congenital malformations.

In the case of fragmented fetal parts, try and establish whether there is one or more fetuses and examine for gross external morphological abnormalities. Record the foot length or crown–rump length if possible to give an estimation of gestational age (Table 6.1).

**Table 6.1** Approximate gestational age guide as indicated by measurement of foot length and crown–rump length

| Foot length (mm) | Crown–rump length (mm) | Gestational age (weeks) |
| --- | --- | --- |
|  | 2 | 5 |
|  | 5 | 6 |
|  | 8 | 7 |
|  | 12 | 8 |
| 2 |  | 8.5 |
| 3 | 17 | 9 |
| 4 |  | 9.5 |
| 5 | 25 | 10 |
| 6 |  | 10.5 |
| 7 | 50 | 11 |
| 8 and 9 |  | 11.5 |
| 10 | 56 | 12 |
| 11 |  | 12.5 |
| 12 |  | 13 |
| 13 and 14 |  | 13.5 |
| 15 and 16 | 87 | 14 |
| 17 |  | 14.5 |
| 18 and 19 |  | 15 |
| 20 and 21 |  | 15.5 |
| 22 | 112 | 18 |
| 39 | 160 | 22 |
| 50 | 203 | 26 |
| 59 | 242 | 30 |
| 68 | 277 | 34 |
| 79 | 313 | 38 |
| 83 | 350 | 40 |

These measurements and the crown–heel length should also be recorded in intact

fetuses, which should also be assessed for gross external and internal malformations. The state of preservation should be noted. The normal umbilical cord has two arteries and one vein. The umbilical cord and placenta (if present) should be sampled and representative samples of internal organs be taken for microscopic examination.

# Gastrointestinal system

## Oesophagus

### Clinical indications

Endoscopic biopsies are typically performed to diagnose oesophagitis resulting from a variety of causes such as reflux, candida or viruses; to confirm Barrett's columnar lined oesophagus and monitor any transition to dysplasia, and to examine polyps and tumour masses.

Oesophagectomy and oesophagogastrectomy are executed mainly for malignant and, rarely, intractable benign strictures. A partial pharyngectomy is occasionally included with the specimen excised for tumours of the upper oesophagus.

### Examination and dissection technique

The oesophagus is opened longitudinally along the wall opposite the tumour if it is eccentrically located. If the stomach is included, the cut is extended along the greater curve and the specimen pinned out, mucosal side up, on a corkboard for further fixation. The specimen should be photographed and a block key diagram drawn. The perioesophageal soft tissue surgical margins around the tumour are inked and the same done for the proximal or distal margins if close to the tumour. A search for lymph nodes is undertaken in the perioesophageal fat, particularly around the cardia in the case of lower oesophageal tumours. The lymph nodes may be divided into peritumoral, proximal and distal groups. Alternatively, the proximal and distal ends of the unopened specimen can be ligated after sampling of the margins and the specimen fixed by inflating with formalin introduced by injection or by stuffing the lumen with gauze or cotton permeated with formalin.

## Stomach

### Clinical indications

Endoscopic biopsies are primarily performed in the investigation of gastritis, ulcers, polyps and tumour masses.

Gastrectomies are performed for malignant disease, intractable peptic ulceration and for life-threatening haemorrhage where the site of bleeding is not identifiable. The gastric antrum with or without part of the gastric body is removed to reduce the acid output of the stomach in peptic ulceration. The specimen often does not include the ulcer which may be in the duodenum and not excised, or may form part of the distal margin of the gastrectomy. Local gastric wall resections are uncommonly performed for benign polypoid tumours such as leiomyomas or localised vascular lesions responsible for recurrent upper gastrointestinal tract haemorrhage such as in Dieulafoy's disease. The stomach may also be removed as part of radical surgery for malignancy in adjacent sites such as the oesophagus (oesophago-gastrectomy) or pancreas (Whipple's procedure).

### Examination and dissection technique

The stomach is usually opened along the greater curve unless there is a tumour or ulcer in this location, whereupon the specimen is opened along the lesser curve. If attached, the duodenum and oesophagus are opened longitudinally and in continuity. In the case of tumour, the lymph nodes are dissected out in groups (cardiac, lesser curve, greater curve, pyloric, omental and perisplenic) and the omentum is detached. The spleen may be excised in resections for gastric carcinoma. After dissecting out the hilar nodes, the spleen is weighed, measured, sliced at 1 cm intervals and placed in formalin. The detached omentum and perigastric fat are cleared in Carnoy's fixative to aid lymph node dissection. The opened stomach is pinned on a corkboard, mucosal surface up and fixed in formalin, preferably overnight. Photograph the specimen and draw a block key diagram. An alternative method involves clamping or tying the ends of the gastrectomy specimen after sampling the margins. The specimen is then injected with formalin or the stomach can be distended with formalin-soaked gauze or cotton. Total sampling of the mucosa for multifocal lesions and detailed mapping can be done with the Swiss roll method described in the section on 'Bladder' (see p. 96). This method is preferable to multiple separate blocks of mucosa. Sections of stomach are best taken perpendicular to the mucosal folds. Angiography is helpful to outline vascular lesions in unfixed stomach resections (see Ch. 7).

PASD, Alcian Blue and Giemsa stains (for helicobacter) are useful in the assessment of gastritis and can be ordered at the time of cut-up.

### Duodenum

Endoscopic biopsies for duodenal ulcers and duodenitis are occasionally performed and the distal duodenum instead of the jejunum may be sampled to investigate malabsorption. Resections of duodenum may be included with gastrectomies for peptic ulcer disease or may form part of a Whipple's resection for head of pancreas carcinoma.

## Small intestine

### Clinical indications

Endoscopic biopsies of the proximal jejunum or fourth part of the duodenum are taken to investigate malabsorption. The Crosby capsule is sometimes used to biopsy the jejunum and produces larger biopsy fragments. Ulcerated lesions are occasionally biopsied. Segmental resections are typically performed for small bowel obstruction due to adhesions or following entrapment in hernial sacs or, more rarely, for tumours such as carcinoids, lymphoma or adenocarcinoma. A portion of the terminal ileum is often included with right-sided colonic resection for carcinoma or inflammatory bowel disease.

### Examination and dissection technique

The duodenal and jejunal biopsies may be submitted free-floating in formalin but are best adhered to a stiff support such as filter paper, foam or millipore filter with the mucosa uppermost. The biopsy should be evaluated with a dissecting microscope to establish the mucosal pattern (normal finger-like villi, leaf-like, cerebriform or the flat mucosa of villous atrophy). Keep the specimen moist with normal saline. In immunosuppressed patients and Whipple's disease, a separate portion should be fixed for ultrastructural examination. The biopsy should be embedded at right angles to the mucosal surface and levels should be cut into the centre of the biopsy. A PASD stain and other special stains, including Ziehl–Neelsen, Warthin–Starry and Giemsa stains, are needed for the assessment of

infective organisms in immunosuppressed patients. *Giardia lamblia* are visible as motile organisms in aspirates and wet imprints of bowel fluid.

Segments of small bowel are opened along the anti-mesenteric border unless there is focal pathology such as a Meckel's diverticulum along this edge. Luminal contents are gently washed off with a slow stream of water or with a saline-filled 50 ml syringe. The opened bowel is pinned to corkboard and fixed in a formalin tank before sampling.

## Appendix and Meckel's diverticulum

### Clinical indications

The appendix is a common surgical specimen removed in cases of clinical appendicitis which may, on rare occasions, be the presenting symptom of carcinoid tumour, mucinous neoplasm, Crohn's disease or endometriosis of the appendix. Appendectomy may be performed as a prophylactic measure at the time of abdominal surgery for other conditions.

Meckel's diverticulum is present in 1–2% of the population and may be a source of abdominal pain due to ectopic acid-secreting gastric mucosa.

### Examination and dissection technique

The specimen should be sampled after fixation. The appendix is sampled as a 2 cm longitudinal section of the tip and the rest of the appendix is examined by serial 3 mm transverse sections, taking samples from the base and mid-body.

The Meckel's diverticulum is removed typically with a short segment of attached ileum and can be handled similarly to the appendix. Alternatively, the ileum and diverticulum can be opened in a T-shape incision.

## Large intestine

### Clinical indications

Colonoscopic biopsies are performed to investigate proctocolitis found at colonoscopy, and ulcerated foci, and evaluate evolving dysplasia in chronic ulcerative colitis. In the patient with diarrhoea, biopsies are taken from the mucosa, even if macroscopically normal, to exclude microscopic colitis. Biopsies via the endoscope are very useful in the assessment of polyps and malignancy to enable planning of definitive surgical treatment. The colonoscope enables resection of smaller polypoid lesions whilst larger villous adenomas and small carcinomas may be amenable to local submucosal resections. Colectomy is performed to remove large adenomas not resectable through the colonoscope, carcinoma and other neoplasms, and for non-neoplastic conditions such as ischaemic or radiation stricture, diverticular disease especially complicated by haemorrhage, stricture, perforation, and pericolic abscess, volvulus, chronic inflammatory bowel disease and angiodysplasia. Panproctocolectomy is usually reserved for longstanding ulcerative colitis with dysplasia and for carcinoma, and involves removal of the terminal ileum, large bowel, appendix, anus and perianal skin.

Suction biopsies of the rectum include the submucosa and are used to identify ganglion cells in colonic dysmotility disorders such as Hirschsprung's disease.

### Examination and dissection technique

If multiple, separately labelled biopsies from different parts of the large bowel or terminal ileum are received, it is important to identify these biopsies separately. The biopsies can be adhered to millipore filters which are processed, embedded and sectioned with the biopsies, minimising tissue distortion and allowing orientation. Up to eight biopsies can be orientated and laid in a straight line on the filter.

Polyps may be sessile or pedunculated and be of a variety of types such as inflammatory, prolapse, hamartomatous, juvenile, hyperplastic, adenomatous and malignant. Microscopic examination determines the type and, for neoplastic polyps, adequacy of excision. Small polyps are embedded uncut whilst larger sessile polyps are bisected and embedded with the cut surface down. The cut should divide the polyp into two asymmetrical pieces, leaving the intact stalk in one piece to allow its examination by trimming into the block. This is particularly important in polyps with narrow stalks. A cross section of the base of polyps with long stalks can be taken.

Submucosal resections for villous adenomas and small polypoid carcinomas are often accompanied by a thin layer of mucosa which retracts and wrinkles easily. These are best fixed pinned out with the margins inked.

Colectomy specimens need to be opened prior to fixation to ensure adequate formalin penetration. Occasionally, the large bowel may have attached organs or tissues such as the coccyx, uterus, vagina and bladder which need to be identified prior to dissection. Typically, these large specimens are removed for neoplasia with spread into contiguous viscera. The purpose of the dissection is to demonstrate the primary site of tumour, assess involvement of adjacent organs, nerve plexuses, vessels and metastasis to regional nodes, and appraise the surgical resection margins for each organ. Delays in specimen handling should be avoided, as digestive enzymes and intestinal flora induce rapid mucosal autolysis. The colon should be received fresh with extramural vessels clearly marked in cases of suspected angiodysplasia to enable angiography with an injected barium/gelatin mixture prior to opening the bowel (described in Ch. 7). This enables localisation of lesions that may otherwise be imperceptible on inspection of the mucosal surface.

Colons received for other conditions are palpated to localise focal lesions before opening longitudinally along the antime-senteric aspect with blunt-ended scissors. The sigmoid colon and rectum are general-ly opened along the peritoneum-covered anterior wall, unless this is the site of a localised lesion. Wash away faecal material with a slow running stream of cold water. Vigorous washing should be avoided as the mucosal surface damages readily. Do not attempt to remove adherent mucin. Formalin may be employed to wash out the colon but the risks of splashing and fume generation outweigh the alleged benefits. Pin out opened colons on cork-board and immerse in formalin tanks. Instillation of formalin into the bowel lumen as described elsewhere allows the demonstration of strictured areas in diverticulosis and Crohn's disease, but this may be difficult to accomplish if the stenosis is very tight.

The sequence of dissection will vary with the pathology. For malignant tumours, it is convenient to first remove the pericolic fat and mesentery from the opened bowel before taking representative blocks from the colon. The fat can be cleared in Carnoy's fixative before lymph node dissection, or may be immediately dissected in the fresh or partly fixed state. The dissected nodes can be separated into caecal, ascending colon, transverse colon, descending colon, sigmoid colon and perirectal groups. The

adipose tissue is sliced with a scalpel or feather blade, at parallel 5 mm intervals, and the cut surface visualised and palpated for tan/white nodes which are firmer than the surrounding fat. Nodes found in the most proximal mesocolon or around the vascular pedicle can be separately identified. An average of 13 lymph nodes may be found in a hemicolectomy. A block should be taken to include the site of deepest penetration by tumour. In rectal and sigmoid resections, it is important to ink and sample the subserosal or posterior margin which is shaved off the sacrum, as this area is not bound by peritoneum and is a common site of recurrence in penetrat-ing tumours. Carcinoma complicating ulcerative colitis may be diffusely infiltrat-ing and difficult to identify macroscopically. While extensive lymph node sampling is not necessary in inflammatory bowel disease, if carcinoma is found, it will be necessary to re-examine the specimen for lymph nodes.

The thickened colonic wall of diverticular bowel disease often precludes pinning out of the specimen which should be opened before placement in formalin. The fixed segment of colon can be sliced longitudinal-ly with a long bladed knife in parallel 1 cm slices, from the proximal to the distal margin, leaving the mesocolon to hold the slices in together. The diverticula are exposed in an ideal plane for sectioning and small foci of perforation, serosal inflamma-tion and fistula can be demonstrated.

Photographs of colonic resections for unusual tumours and inflammatory bowel disease are recommended and block key diagrams or photocopies of the specimen are invaluable.

Sections of colon are best taken perpen-dicular to the direction of the mucosal folds. Diverticula are sectioned as longitu-dinal and cross-sections. Doughnuts of the proximal and distal resection margins may arrive separately with the two apposed pieces of colon held together by sutures or staples. The sutures and staples are removed before blocking as bisected halves.

The diagnostic biopsy for investigation of neuronal dysplasia must include a series of mucosal/submucosal biopsies from high enough in the rectum to clear the normal hypoganglionic zone which extends up to 1 cm from the pectinate line, but not too high to miss a short aganglionic segment. The biopsies should be labelled as to their exact site and multiple levels should be examined. Agangliosis can often be identified on fixed H & E stained tissue but fresh tissue enables acetylcholinesterase staining, a proliferation of lamina propria nerves being observed in aganglionic segments.

Immunohistochemical staining for neurofilaments is an alternative which allows ready identification of ganglion cells. A rapid non-specific esterase method for adrenergic nerves can be used on frozen sections and formalin-induced fluorescence has been utilised. A diagnosis of agangliosis rendered on the initial submucosal biopsies is often followed by frozen section examination to assess bowel wall innervation at the level where colostomy is planned. Hypoganglis or hyperganglis requires multiple full wall thickness biopsies for evaluation, including acetylcholinesterase staining.

# Hepatobiliary system and pancreas (exocrine)

## Liver

### Clinical indications

Liver core biopsies are used to investigate diffuse liver disease, commonly due to chronic viral hepatitis or alcohol, and to determine the nature of focal lesions such as adenoma, focal nodular hyperplasia and tumours, commonly metastatic carcinoma. Core biopsies may also be submitted for the evaluation of impaired hepatic function in liver transplants (conditioning treatment effect, rejection, graft-versus-host disease, recurrence of native disease, infection and surgical complication). Wedge biopsies may be taken at the time of laparotomy for any of these reasons.

Partial hepatectomy and hemihepatectomy are performed for traumatic rupture, hydatid or other cysts, and tumours such as adenoma, fibrolamellar carcinoma, small hepatocellular carcinomas and, rarely, for solitary metastatic deposits.

### Examination and dissection technique

Core biopsies are embedded uncut whilst wedge biopsies may be sliced at right angles to the capsule into smaller pieces. In infections, separate core biopsies may be submitted fresh for culture and in haemochromatosis or Wilson's disease, a separate biopsy may be taken for iron and copper quantitation respectively, and is submitted unfixed wrapped in foil. Liver transplant biopsies are usually received in formalin unless there is infection, whereupon fresh tissue is submitted for culture (bacterial including mycobacteria, fungi and viral). Fresh tissue may be submitted for lymphocyte subset typing. In unusual tumours and metabolic diseases, electron microscopic examination may be performed.

In cases of trauma, specimen photographs are recommended, particularly when there is anticipated medico-legal or forensic implications. The tissue received from trauma cases is often in the form of multiple ragged pieces which are difficult to orientate but should be weighed.

The dimensions and weight of partial hepatectomy and hemihepatectomy specimens should be recorded and, if containing tumour, the resected surface is inked. Parallel slices through the liver at 1 cm intervals at right angles to the excision margin aid formalin fixation. Hydatid cysts and other infections should be fixed for at least 24 hours prior to handling. Imprints of fresh tumour tissue can be prepared, portions of tumour tissue snap frozen and 1 mm cubes of tumour fixed in glutaraldehyde. Photographs are recommended, and in complex cases a block key diagram is helpful.

Special stains for liver biopsies are requested routinely at the time of cut-up (PAS for glycogen, PASD for alpha-1-antitrypsin globules, Gordon and Sweet's reticulin, Sirius red to assess architecture, Fouchet's stain for bile, Perls' stain for iron, rhodamine stain for copper and orcein stain for copper binding protein and hepatitis B surface antigen). Immunostaining for hepatitis B surface and core antigens, hepatitis C, cytomegalovirus and herpes is also available and can be included for liver transplant biopsies.

## Gallbladder

### Clinical indications

Gallbladders are common specimens. They are removed for recurrent biliary colic from calculi, cholecystitis and rarely for carcinoma. The latter is typically seen in gallbladders with calculi and is unsuspected prior to surgery. The gallbladder is often removed incidentally at the time of surgery for neoplasms in adjacent organs (partial hepatectomy, Whipple's procedure).

### Examination and dissection technique

Gallbladders are generally received partially opened by the surgeon so that calculi may have been removed. If intact, the gallbladder should be opened longitudinally from the fundus to the neck. The cystic duct is left intact to enable a transverse section of the resection margin. Calculi are transected to inspect their core and can be submitted for chemical analysis. Calculi can be large pure yellow cholesterol stones or small black calcium bilirubinate pigment stones. Mixed calculi show a variable composition of cholesterol, calcium bilirubinate and calcium carbonate or a combination of pure and mixed stones. Flat surfaces form between calculi and are a feature indicating the presence of more than one calculus. In cases of neoplasms, the resection margin over the tumour is inked and in gallbladder tumours, the cystic duct lymph node should be sampled.

## Bile ducts

### Clinical indications

The extrahepatic bile ducts include the left and right hepatic ducts, the common bile duct and the ampulla of Vater. The cystic duct is considered to be part of the gallbladder. Mainly small biopsies are received from this region to investigate benign and malignant duct strictures. They are often submitted for frozen section diagnosis.

### Examination and dissection technique

The duct may be identified by a suture or stent but many specimens are difficult to orientate. The proximal or distal end of larger specimens is often identified. Sections should be made perpendicular to the duct at 3 mm intervals.

## Exocrine pancreas

### Clinical indications

The Whipple's procedure for tumours of the head of pancreas involves block excision of the proximal pancreas, distal stomach and duodenum, and the common bile duct. Total pancreatectomy involves excision of the entire pancreas, partial gastrectomy, duodenectomy and splenectomy. Distal pancreatectomy comprises resection of the body and tail of the pancreas with the spleen. There are various modifications to these procedures which may include transverse colon, mesenteric vessels and even segments of inferior vena cava.

Needle biopsies of the pancreas are typically performed to investigate radiologically detected pancreatic masses. The biopsies may be performed intraoperatively or be guided by CT scan or ultrasound, but the use of fine needle aspiration cytology has reduced the frequency of the core biopsy.

Pancreatectomy is executed for resectable pancreatic or bile duct neoplasms, and is occasionally used for painful chronic pancreatitis.

### Examination and dissection technique

Correct orientation of the anatomical structures is the key to handling pancreatectomy specimens. In the case of a Whipple's procedure, the proximal gastric and distal duodenal margins, the distal pancreatic margin and the common bile duct margin are identified and sections taken of these margins. Lymph nodes from different sites are separately identified and blocked. The peripancreatic soft tissue margins closest to the tumour are inked and the stomach and duodenum are opened with scissors along the greater curve and free border respectively, and the ampulla of Vater defined. The pancreatic and common bile ducts can be probed to assess patency. The pancreas is cut longitudinally into anterior and posterior halves with a sharp knife, using a probe in the pancreatic duct as a guide. The probe can be passed into the pancreatic duct via the ampulla. If the duct is blocked by tumour or calculi, the pancreas is examined by serial sagittal slices parallel to the distal excision margin. An effort should be made to distinguish the primary site of the tumour, although in a number of cases, with extensive infiltration, this will not be possible. If not involved by tumour, the stomach can be transected at the pylorus and examined separately. Photograph the specimen and draw a block key diagram.

## Lymphoreticular system

### Lymph nodes

### Clinical indications

Lymph nodes are examined in the investigation of lymphadenopathy (reactive, specific infections, lymphoma and metastatic carcinoma/melanoma). Needle biopsies are used in some cases of suspected metastatic carcinoma, particularly when the patient is old, or too ill for lymphadenectomy and fine needle aspiration biopsy has been unsuccessful. In the investigation of lymphoproliferative disorders, the lymph node should be removed with capsule intact and submitted unfixed. Core biopsies should be avoided. Regional node dissections are performed for carcinoma and melanoma which do not show clinical evidence of distant metastatic disease.

## Examination and dissection technique

If the lymph node is received fresh, in cases of infection, it should be examined under sterile conditions in a biological safety cabinet. Submit a portion for culture. On occasion, the need for culture may only become apparent after routine examination, such as when caseous necrosis is seen on the cut surface. In such circumstances, the node should immediately be transferred into a sterile Petri dish and material taken for culture before overnight fixation. Contaminated instruments and cut-up area should be appropriately decontaminated. In non-infectious cases, imprints should be made of freshly cut surfaces. In necrotic or bloody specimens, gentle dabbing of a clean glass slide on the node surface reduces blood on the slide. Smears fixed in alcohol or 10% formalin can be stained with Gram, ZN, PASD, GMS, and Warthin–Starry and Giemsa to show infective organisms. When the node is thinly sliced at 1–2 mm intervals, fixation in 10% formalin produces good cytomorphological preservation so that mercury-based reagents, which are environmental pollutants, need not be used. H & E sections of well-fixed lymph nodes remain the mainstay of diagnosis. While it is still useful to keep a portion of node frozen for immunostaining of the more labile lymphocyte markers, many antigens can now be studied in well-fixed, paraffin-embedded tissue. Frozen tissue can be employed for molecular studies, cytogenetics or cell culture. Fresh tissue may be sent for lymphocyte surface marker studies or flow cytometry. If adequate tissue is available, material may be submitted for electron microscopy, especially for the diagnosis of metastatic tumours such as carcinoma and melanoma.

Two options are available for the handling of radical lymph node dissections. The fresh specimen can be examined by palpation and dissection or by a combination of palpation and a series of close parallel cuts through the fat with a sharp knife or feather blade to expose the pink-tan nodes. Alternatively, the specimen is first fixed in formalin prior to examination or placed in clearing agents such as Carnoy's fixative for a few hours to dissolve the fat, rendering nodes visible as white masses.

### Radical neck dissection

The standard neck dissection removes cervical nodes, sternomastoid muscle, internal jugular vein, spinal accessory nerve, submandibular gland, the deep portion of the platysma and sometimes part of the parotid. The modified radical neck dissection (Bocca functional neck dissection) spares the internal jugular vein, spinal accessory nerve and sternomastoid. Regional node dissection removes only the sentinel nodes considered to be the first point of lymphatic drainage from the primary tumour. Extended radical neck dissection removes, in addition to the standard excision, nodes from some or all of the following groups: paratracheal, parotid, retropharyngeal, suboccipital and upper mediastinal nodes. An orientating diagram, photocopy or photograph is very helpful in these dissections. Anatomical landmarks are lost in modified or regional node dissections unless orientated by the surgeon. The cervical nodes can be divided into six groups – superior anterior, superior jugular, superior posterior, inferior posterior, inferior jugular and inferior anterior. More commonly, the nodes are divided into five groups, the superior, middle and inferior jugular, posterior and anterior triangle groups (Fig. 6.6). The resection margins overlying nodes with palpable tumour can be inked. The internal jugular vein should be opened longitudinally to assess tumour involvement. A minimum of 30 lymph nodes should be retrieved.

### Inguinal dissection
The specimen is usually received as a single mass of fat with nodes, but occasionally the superficial and deep node groups may be separated. The internal saphenous vein is opened longitudinally to examine for tumour involvement. The resection margins over obvious palpable tumour deposits should be inked. A minimum of 12 lymph nodes should be retrieved.

### Retroperitoneal dissection
The different lymph node groups should be received in separately labelled containers as common iliac, periaortic, pericaval, inferior interaortocaval, superior aortocaval and suprahilar (above renal artery) nodes. A minimum of 25 lymph nodes should be retrieved.

With regional node dissections, all retrieved lymph nodes should be sampled. If the lymph node is less than 3 mm, embed whole. Several nodes may be embedded in the one block. Larger nodes may need bisection and both halves should be embedded in the same block. Adherence to this method allows accurate lymph node counts, which provides important prognostic information in some tumours such as breast carcinoma.

## Spleen

### Clinical indications

Splenectomy is usually performed for lymphoproliferative/myeloproliferative diseases, traumatic laceration, rupture, spontaneous rupture, e.g. in infectious mononucleosis, hypersplenism. It may be received together with a gastrectomy for gastric carcinoma or as part of a staging laparotomy for lymphoma, which will include abdominal lymph nodes, wedge biopsies of left and right liver lobes and an open iliac crest bone marrow biopsy. The spleen may also be removed when involved by pancreatic or colonic carcinoma.

### Examination and dissection technique

The spleen is separated from attached structures such as stomach, measured and

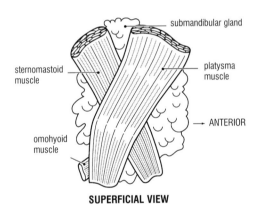

**SUPERFICIAL VIEW**

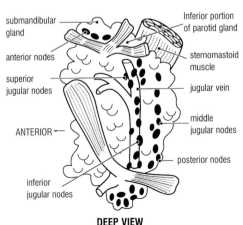

**DEEP VIEW**

Fig. 6.6   Right radical neck dissection

weighed. If it is received fresh and there is a possibility of infection, submit a portion for culture by searing the surface with a flame-heated scalpel and removing a sample into a biological safety cabinet. A 1 cm cube of fresh tissue is placed into culture medium for lymphocyte surface marker studies in cases of suspected lymphoma and fresh samples may be sent for cytogenetics or cell culture. With a sharp long-bladed knife, the spleen is cut into 5–10 mm parallel slices and imprints are obtained of the fresh cut surfaces. In suspected sickle cell anaemia, a deep section should be taken and fixed immediately in formalin. Examine for hilar lymph nodes, splenunculi and pancreatic tail tissue.

## Bone marrow

### Clinical indications

Bone marrow biopsies are taken for the investigation of haematological disorders, both neoplastic and non-neoplastic, and metastatic tumour.

### Examination and dissection technique

Needle cores are immediately fixed in either formalin or Zenker's fixative and, when well fixed, are washed and decalcified for a short period to enable sectioning. Aspirates are allowed to clot before fixation. Bilateral iliac biopsies should be separately designated.

Deep levels, reticulin and Giemsa stains can be ordered routinely at time of cut-up. If the methyl green pyronin is required, decalcification should be with EDTA rather than acids. The latter, particularly strong acids, also adversely affect the preservation of cellular antigens.

## Thymus

### Clinical indications

The thymus is removed for cysts and neoplasms such as thymoma, germ cell tumours or lymphoma and as treatment of myasthenia gravis.

### Examination and dissection technique

The thymus is weighed and cut into 5 mm parallel slices after inking the relevant resection margins. Imprints may be helpful and freeze away a portion. If lymphoma is suspected, obtain tissue for the various procedures described for lymph nodes.

## Tonsil

### Clinical indications

Tonsils are removed for inflammation and neoplasms such as carcinoma, and lymphoma.

### Examination and dissection technique

Tonsillectomy for lymphoma should be submitted fresh. The tonsil can be cut into 3–4 mm parallel slices. If fresh, make imprints and treat as with lymph nodes for lymphoma.

# Male genital system

## Testes

### Clinical indications

The testis is removed or biopsied for a variety of clinical conditions, which include the investigation of infertility, chronic epididymo-orchitis, infarction following torsion, maldescent, tumours, palliation for prostatic adenocarcinoma and, occasionally, at herniorrhaphy.

*Examination and dissection technique*

Biopsies for investigation of infertility should be submitted in Bouin's fixative which produces optimal cellular detail. Fixation in Bouin's solution should not be prolonged and if the biopsy cannot be processed immediately, it should be transferred to formalin after 1 hour to prevent tissue brittleness. As biochemical assays for luteinising hormone and follicle stimulating hormone, and sperm counts provide useful diagnostic information in the assessment of male infertility, the need for histological examination of testicular tissue is much reduced.

The testicular tissue removed for other purposes is usually received in formalin. If infection is suspected, fresh tissue should be sent for microbiological culture. The tunica vaginalis is opened and examined for hydrocoele. The volume of the intact testis can be measured by volume displacement by immersing in a measuring cylinder (normal range 15–25 ml). Photograph and draw block key diagrams if appropriate. Cut serial 5 mm slices perpendicular to the original cut through both halves, leaving the tunica albuginea intact to keep the slices together. Cut the epididymis longitudinally and make cross-sections of the spermatic cord. Sample lesional and non-lesional testicular tissue including the overlying tunica in cases of tumour. Also sample the epididymis, spermatic cord and the surgical margin of the spermatic cord.

## Epididymis and vas deferens

*Clinical indications*

Biopsies are performed for chronic epididymitis, obstruction, sterilisation and, rarely, neoplasms such as adenomatoid tumour.

*Examination and dissection technique*

The epididymal tissue received is often small and not always easy to orientate. The specimen is best sectioned transversely. Vasa deferentia are often separately labelled as to side. They should be cut into parallel transverse sections and submitted in their entirety.

## Prostate

*Clinical indications*

Prostatic tissue is removed for microscopic examination in chronic prostatitis, hyperplasia and tumours.

Needle cores, transurethral resections and retropubic prostatectomy were common procedures, but there has been a return to total prostatectomy and the ultrasound-guided transrectal biopsy is a newer procedure.

*Examination and dissection technique*

Prostatic chippings should be weighed. Chippings which are very hard or yellow should be preferentially selected for histological examination as they are more likely to contain neoplastic tissue. Smaller pieces are more likely to represent tissue from the periphery of the prostate, a more common location for neoplasia.

The retropubic prostatectomy specimen is serially sliced at 3–4 mm intervals, either fresh or after formalin fixation. Areas that are hard, very soft or yellow should be sampled. With prostatic chippings, fill five or six cassettes regardless of weight (approximately 10 g = 5 blocks). Estimate the percentage of chippings submitted for histology. It has been shown that embedding 12 g of random chippings will detect 92% of Stage A tumours. Controversy persists as to whether all remaining tissue should be embedded if high grade prostatic intraepithelial neoplasia (PIN III) or adenocarcinoma is found in the chippings.

The radical prostectomy specimen requires special attention. It is orientated as to anterior/posterior/superior/inferior edges, and the urethral, bladder base and vas deferens margins identified. It should be well fixed prior to sampling and the margins, especially at the base of the prostate, inked. Serial transverse slices are generally made from the urethral margin to the bladder base at 3–4 mm intervals. The McNeal prostate model emphasises the oblique course of the urethra through the prostate and oblique sectioning of the prostate may provide information which can be better correlated with the anatomical segments of the prostate (Fig. 6.7). Photocopy the prostatic slices or draw a diagram of the slices to orientate the exact location of sections taken. Transillumination of thin slices may aid identification of foci of carcinoma which are opaque.

Sample the seminal vesicles, vas deferens, bladder and all lymph nodes in radical prostatectomy specimens. Several options are available in sampling of the radical prostatectomy specimen. At one extreme, the entire gland can be blocked as whole mounts of cross-sections, or selected sections can be taken. Whatever the method, it is essential to keep the tissue slices in sequence to enable further sampling, if required, after initial microscopic examination. It is difficult

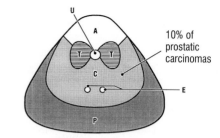

**TRANSVERSE SECTION**

10% of prostatic carcinomas

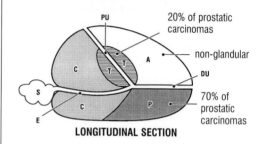

**LONGITUDINAL SECTION**

20% of prostatic carcinomas

non-glandular

70% of prostatic carcinomas

**Fig. 6.7**   Diagrammatic representation of prostatic lobes. A = anterior fibromuscular stroma; C = central zone; P = peripheral zone;
S = seminal vesicles; T = transition zone;
PU = proximal urethra; DU = distal urethra;
E = ejaculatory duct

grossly to distinguish carcinoma from non-neoplastic prostate, and benign lesions such as granulomatous prostatitis, atrophy, PIN and some nodular hyperplasias may mimic carcinoma. It is not mandatory to submit the entire prostate for microscopy even when a gross lesion is not identified. Stage A carcinomas (incidentally discovered at transurethral resection for urinary outlet obstruction) tend to arise in the central and anterior regions and involve the anterior margin more often than Stage B carcinomas (palpable tumour at rectal examination) which are usually posteriorly located and tend to spread posteriorly, postero-laterally and through the apex. For Stage A tumours with or without gross tumour, block the entire lesion if visible, and sample alternate grossly normal 3 mm slices in their entirety, typically requiring four blocks per slice, identifying one edge with a notch. Sections are shaved from the proximal bladder base and distal urethral margins, and taken off the base of both seminal vesicles and vas deferens margins.

For Stage B tumours with gross tumour, section the entire lesion, the proximal bladder base and distal urethral margins, the most apical slice adjacent to the distal margin and the base of both seminal vesicles and the vas deferens margins. For Stage B tumours with no visible carcinoma, block alternate posterior slices and take samples as described above for Stage B with gross tumour. The urethra may retract within the apical prostate making the assessment of transverse sections difficult. In such a situation it may be necessary to treat the apex of the specimen like a cervical cone biopsy and block it entirely as longitudinal sections.

The prostatic apex is the only consistent site where undetected carcinoma is prognostically significant and is one of the most frequent sites for positive margins. This is due to the growth characteristics of prostatic carcinoma as well as the difficulty in dissecting the apex in the radical prostatectomy procedure. The importance of sampling the apex cannot be over-emphasised. The routine addition of just the most apical slice, regardless of its gross appearance, identifies virtually all cases with positive resection margins and established capsular penetration which are diagnosed by complete histological sectioning.

## Penis and scrotum

### Clinical indications

Skin biopsies are performed for condylomas, inflammatory conditions, benign and malignant neoplasms.

In childhood circumcision, the foreskin is usually normal, whilst in adults the foreskin may be removed for phimosis, balanitis, lichen sclerosis and squamous dysplasia/in situ squamous cell carcinoma.

Penile amputations may be performed for infarction and gangrene, malignant tumours, trauma, as part of a sex change procedure and very rarely for distorting, painful inflammatory conditions such as fibromatosis.

The penile urethra may be removed for multifocal urothelial tumours.

### Examination and dissection technique

The rugose foreskin is sectioned transversely. The specimen often wrinkles and may need to be pinned flat and fixed for a short time on corkboard before cutting if unusual pathology is anticipated.

If infection is suspected, fresh tissue should be submitted for culture. Otherwise, the penis should be well fixed before sectioning. Attached inguinal lymph node dissection, if included, is separated and dissected as described elsewhere. The penis resection margins including the urethra and skin are inked. Photograph the specimen, particularly if removed for a traumatic injury, and draw block key diagrams. Most carcinomas involve the glans and coronal sulcus, and may spread into and along the corpora cavernosa. Take transverse sections of margins, before dissection, to assess involvement by tumour or, in the case of trauma, viability. The urethra is opened with blunt-ended scissors, from the external meatus, along the ventral aspect. Alternatively, it can be bisected longitudinally with a long-bladed knife using, as a guide, a metal probe placed in the urethra. Further cuts as needed can be made perpendicular to this first cut.

# Osteoarticular system and soft tissues

## Bone and cartilage

### Clinical indications

Needle core biopsy of bone is performed to investigate radiological and/or clinically symptomatic, sclerotic or osteolytic bone lesions, particularly when metastasis is suspected, and to diagnose primary bone neoplasms. They are also used to examine haematological diseases (see 'Lympho-reticular system' p. 79), metabolic bone disease (typically iliac crest biopsies) and suspected chronic infection. Curettings may be received from bone tumours and suspected osteomyelitis. Open wedge biopsies are employed to provide sufficient-ly large samples (to reduce sampling error) in metabolic bone disease, and are taken to screen for malignancy and infection in donor bone for bone banks. Fragments of fractured bone may be submitted for the exclusion of pathological fracture, and bone and joint capsule around loose or infected prostheses may be received for examination (see 'Joint and synovium' p. 87). Segmental bone resections are generally performed for osseous or joint neoplasia, or soft tissue neoplasms with focal bone involvement, and amputations may be performed for some bone and soft tissue malignant neoplasms, uncontrolled infection or extensive traumatic injury which is beyond surgical correction. Amputations for vascular disease and trauma are discussed elsewhere (see 'Cardiovascular system' p. 48). Hemimandibulectomy and maxillectomy are employed to remove aggressive mucosal or soft tissue neoplasms with bone involve-ment and some primary bone neoplasms arising in the region.

### Examination and dissection technique

Most needle biopsies and curettings are received in formalin. In cases of suspected osteomyelitis, fresh tissue should be sent for microbiological culture. In larger pieces of bone, specimen radiography may be helpful, e.g. to localise the nidus of osteoid osteoma. Gritty bone curettings and trephine biopsies for diseases other than metabolic bone disease require decalcifica-tion. A number of acids and chelating agents are available for decalcification (see Ch. 4). Nine per cent EDTA or nitric acid are commonly used and in conjunction with specimen radiography to determine the decalcification endpoint. After decalcifi-cation, larger bone fragments are trimmed and cut perpendicular to the cortical surface. Biopsies for metabolic bone disease are received in neutral buffered formalin to preserve mineralisation and are embedded in resin and sectioned undecalcified. Tetracycline labelling to study bone mineralisation can be performed by giving the patient two doses of 1 g of tetracycline 10 days apart. This binds to areas of active mineralisation and the two bands labelled with this antibiotic can be visualised with immunofluorescence, allowing the mineral-isation rate and distribution to be assessed.

X-rays, CT and MRI scans, ultrasono-graphs and their reports should be available for review prior to the dissection and reporting of osseous and cartilaginous tumours.

The correct side of amputation is established, previous biopsy sites outlined with a black marking pen and the main draining regional lymph nodes, e.g. inguinal and popliteal for the lower limb, removed and dissected out. Unless the bone has been disarticulated, the proximal bone resection margin and soft tissue should be sampled in cases of tumour. Blunt and sharp dissection with scalpel, scissors and forceps is used to dissect down to the periosteum overlying the area of bone which contains tumour. However, if radiography suggests soft tissue extension, careful dissection of soft tissue to retain continuity with the underlying bone is required. Unless involved by direct spread, joints can be cut through. The entire track of any previous biopsy site should be preserved and sampled for histology. The bone with tumour is X-rayed and sectioned longitudinally with a bandsaw, typically into anterior and posterior halves, but other planes of transection may be employed to best demonstrate the tumour. The cut surface should be washed and brushed with a nail brush to remove bone dust. Photograph the cut surface and draw a block key diagram. Bone cut surfaces are particularly suitable for photocopying. Wood's light can be used to visualise the autofluoresence of tetracycline if necessary. Thinner slices of bone can be made for decalcification prior to sectioning, although in tumours with little or no calcification/ossification, preliminary sections can be taken. Finally, inspect the peritumour soft tissues, joints, skin and other bones, the latter preferably by transecting with a bandsaw.

The mandibulectomy specimen must be well fixed before dissection and the margins of resection are inked. For bone neoplasms, the bone and soft tissue is sectioned parallel at 1 cm intervals with a bandsaw before decalcification. For mucosal or soft tissue neoplasms, the soft tissue is dissected from the mandible with scissors and scalpel. A radical neck dissection may be attached and this is dissected as previously described (see 'Radical neck dissection' p. 80). If direct spread is apparent, ink the upper neck dissection resection margins. Maxillectomy specimens

also are fixed before examination and resection margins inked and sampled. The specimen is cut at parallel 1 cm intervals in the coronal plane with a bandsaw. Preliminary sections of mucosal and soft tissue neoplasms are taken and the bone is decalcified. Specimen photographs, photocopies and block key diagrams are advisable and X-rays may be helpful.

Undecalcified bone sections to investigate metabolic bone disease can be stained with von Kossa (for phosphate and carbonate) with H & E or van Gieson as a counter-stain, acid phosphatase (for osteoblasts), Goldner Trichrome (for osteoid), Irwin's Aluminon (for aluminium), PAS and Alizarin Red S (for calcium). The mineralisation rate is assessed by tetracycline labelling on 10 $\mu$ unstained sections with immunofluorescence and computer image analysis allows quantitation of multiple bone parameters.

## Joint and synovium

### Clinical indications

Femoral heads are removed mainly for osteoarthritis and may be replaced by a variety of prosthetic joints.

Synovial biopsies are employed to investigate conditions such as acute and chronic synovitis, infection, crystal arthropathy, pigmented villonodular synovitis, trauma, degeneration and synovial chondrometaplasia.

Menisci may be removed following tears with incomplete repair.

Tendons and tendon sheaths are biopsied primarily for inflammatory conditions.

Capsules and synovium around loose prosthetic joints are removed at the time of revision surgery to rule out infection and assess wear particle dissemination from the prosthesis.

*Examination and dissection technique*

The femoral head is measured, the side indicated if known and an X-ray taken. The adherent joint capsule is removed, the articular surface inspected and the bone is cut into parallel 1 cm slices through the articular surface in the longitudinal plane with a bandsaw. The cut surface is examined for eburnation, erosion, pannus, fissuring and subchondral cysts. A handsaw can be used with the bone held in a clamp, but this is a time consuming process. Photographs can be taken of the intact or cut surface. The slices are decalcified prior to sectioning.

Synovial biopsies are usually submitted in formalin but may be sent fresh for bacterial culture, or in alcohol to diagnose gout.

Menisci are cut transversely across any tear and sampled.

Joint capsular biopsies are sent for frozen section assessment of neutrophil presence to diagnose infection. A portion is taken under sterile conditions and submitted for culture. The rest of the tissue is cut at 5 mm intervals perpendicular to the surface. Small 1 mm fragments may be taken for electron dispersive X-ray analysis to study detritic synovitis. The type and composition of the prosthesis should be known.

Intervertebral discs

*Clinical indications*

Portions of disc are removed where they have herniated and are causing back pain.

*Examination and dissection technique*

The specimen is usually fragmented. An endeavour should be made to orientate the nucleosus pulposus and the outer annulus fibrosis and sections taken across these structures. Vertebral bone may be included, necessitating decalcification prior to processing.

Bursas

*Clinical indications*

Bursal sacs may be excised for chronic inflammation due to trauma, infection, crystal deposition or rheumatoid arthritis.

*Examination and dissection technique*

Bursal sacs are transected as cross-sectional slices at 5 mm intervals. In cases of suspected gout, the specimen should be received fresh or in alcohol to preserve the urate crystals which are water soluble and dissolve in formalin.

Soft tissue including skeletal muscle biopsy

*Clinical indications*

There is a myriad of connective tissue tumours (fibrous, nerve sheath, vascular, smooth muscle, fat, skeletal muscle, synovial), both benign and malignant, which may be biopsied.

Skeletal muscle biopsy has a role in the investigation of muscle weakness or pain due to conditions such as myositis, metabolic diseases, myopathies and dystrophies. Occasionally, biopsy is used to assess the asymptomatic carriers of genetic disease such as the malignant hyperthermia syndrome.

*Examination and dissection technique*

Lumpectomy and excision specimens of lesions other than typical lipomas from the superficial subcutis should have their margins inked. The relationship of the tumour mass to surrounding tissues such as muscle and nerves or other anatomical landmarks should be noted. Some larger resections will be submitted with orientating sutures or staples placed by the surgeon. In the difficult specimen, the surgeon should be requested to orientate the specimen. Weigh larger resections before sectioning. The specimen is then sliced at 1 cm parallel intervals with a long-bladed knife and the slices kept in sequence during further formalin fixation. Photograph the tumour cut surface and prepare a block key diagram. If the tumour is received fresh, freeze a small portion away and fix 1 mm cubes for ultrastructural analysis. Imprints of tumour can be performed and in suspected sarcoma, a sterile piece for cytogenetic studies may yield helpful diagnostic or prognostic information. In wide excisions which include overlying skin in sarcomas from the head and neck or extremities, isolate the track of any previous incision biopsy for histological sampling.

The examination of skeletal muscle biopsies is a specialised procedure and the specimen should be submitted fresh. The vastus lateralis is the usual muscle biopsied if clinically involved but not severely wasted. In distal myopathies, the brachioradialis or gastrocnemius may be sampled. Biopsies should not be taken from sites where EMG needles have been inserted and the surgeon should not inject local anaesthetic into the muscle and should avoid using diathermy. The muscle biopsy must be immediately prepared for histology and should be submitted in three parts: an unclamped $5 \times 5$ mm specimen and two portions stretched between metal clamps each measuring $15 \times 5$ mm. Part of the unclamped portion is cut into 1 mm cubes and fixed for ultrastructural examination,

whilst the rest is cut into transverse sections and snap frozen in isopentane/liquid nitrogen and stored for immunofluorescence. One clamped portion is placed into 10% formalin and, following fixation, the clamps are removed and transverse and longitudinal sections taken. The other clamped portion is snap frozen in isopentane/liquid nitrogen, the clamps removed and the muscle cut into three 5 mm thick transverse sections. This frozen tissue is cut in a cryostat and stained for a battery of enzymes and muscle components (see below). In suspected metabolic disease, additional tissue should be kept frozen. At least 100 mg of the specimen is desirable to assess deficiencies such as carnitine palmityl transferase, whilst for complex mitochondrial myopathies, over 1 g is needed.

Besides H & E stains and deeper levels on paraffin embedded tissue, PTAH and trichrome stains are useful. Transverse sections of the frozen muscle are stained with: H & E, Gomori's trichrome pH 3.4 (ragged red fibres, nemaline bodies), myosin ATPase pH 9.4, 4.6 and 4.3 (fibre typing and distribution), PAS, PASD, Oil red O (glycogen and lipid storage disorders, ring and coil fibres), NADH, LDH (fibre type and architecture), alkaline phosphatase (inflammatory response and regenerating fibres), acid phosphatase (phagocytes, necrosis), myophosphorylase, adenylate deaminase and cytochrome oxidase. Histochemically stained frozen sections can be subjected to interactive image analysis.

With limb amputations, review the radiographs to locate the tumour and its extent before commencing dissection. Record the length of the limb and the circumference at different levels, including that of the tumour. Document the location, number and size of previous biopsy sites and scars. Separate the major draining lymph node groups, e.g. inguinal and popliteal nodes for the lower limb, and supratrochlear and axillary nodes for the upper limb, and place in Carnoy's fixative for fat clearance. The sharp and blunt dissection of tissues around a soft tissue neoplasm may be time-consuming and the specimen may be difficult to orientate without the aid of an anatomy atlas. Evaluate the relationship of skin, subcutaneous fat, muscle, major arteries, veins, nerves, periosteum and bone to the tumour and with these landmarks marked if necessary, widely resect this area using a scalpel, forceps and scissors from the rest of the amputation. The removed block must include the track and incision site of any previous biopsy. Depending on the specimen size, either leave the block to fix or make slices into the specimen with a long-bladed knife, keeping any separated slices in sequence. Radiology and photography of the block resection may be indicated and a photocopy or block key diagram is essential. The soft tissues and skin of the rest of the amputation should be inspected for tumour, joints opened and inspected and the long bones divided longitudinally with a bandsaw, examined for tumour foci and other lesions. A small portion of bone adjacent to any soft tissue neoplasm is taken for decalcification and histological examination.

# Respiratory system

## Trachea and lung including bronchi

### Clinical indications

The trachea is rarely biopsied for a variety of inflammatory and neoplastic conditions including lesions around tracheostomy stoma.

Biopsies of lung are frequently small and obtained either via a bronchoscope, mediastinoscope or percutaneously. They are taken for the investigation of pulmonary masses and diffuse lung disease.

Open lung biopsies are generally performed in cases of idiopathic interstitial lung disease which cannot be diagnosed by transbronchial biopsy. They are increasingly performed in immunosuppressed patients for the diagnosis of a variety of infective, iatrogenic and neoplastic conditions.

Lung resections are utilised for the removal of benign and malignant tumours, radiological opacities that remain elusive to diagnosis by other means and some inflammatory conditions such as bronchiectasis.

### Examination and dissection technique

The endoscopic biopsies are small and are embedded whole. In cases of suspected infection, fresh tissue should be submitted for culture. Biopsies for suspected tuberculosis, HIV or hydatid infection require 24 hours fixation prior to handling. The standard biopsy is 2–10 mm long and 2–3 mm across. Submit fresh tissue for frozen section immunohistochemistry or lymphocyte surface markers in suspected lymphoma, and fix for ultrastructural examination in undifferentiated neoplasms and diseases such as Langerhans' cell histiocytosis.

The open lung biopsy has two major advantages: sampling of pathological tissue is performed under direct vision and more tissue is biopsied. Such biopsies are typically taken from surgically accessible areas of peripheral lung such as the right middle lobe and the left lingula. It is important that the specimen is received fresh and tissue can be taken for microbiological culture and other investigations. In some cases of immunosuppression, frozen section examination will be warranted but most diagnoses, e.g. viral inclusions, are more readily seen on permanent sections and rapid processing in intrashort (1½ h) cycles is preferable. Touch imprints of the cut surface are taken and stained with methanamine silver stain for pneumocystis and fungi. Open biopsies for interstitial lung disease in the non-immunosuppressed patient are best evaluated following formalin fixation. This is done by gentle inflation with a syringe and a fine 25 g needle passed through the pleural surface into the parenchyma, until the piece of lung attains the appearance of full distension with the pleural surface smoothed out. Following fixation, the specimen is sliced thinly at 3 mm intervals.

Dissection of the pneumonectomy specimen entails opening the bronchi longitudinally, having taken a transverse section of the bronchial resection margin before commencing. Sample all hilar nodes and submit fresh tissue for bacterial and viral cultures if appropriate. The lung parenchyma and tumour are then cut longitudinally with the lung lying on its hilar surface. Alternatively, the lung or lung segment can be inflamed with formalin via the main or segmental bronchus, sampling a transverse section of the bronchial resection margin before injection. The bronchus is tied or clamped or simply plugged with soaked cotton or gauze following inflation. The lung is inflated until the pleural surface becomes smooth. Following overnight fixation in a large container of formalin, the lung is placed on its hilar surface and sliced in the horizontal plane at 1 cm intervals with a sharp knife.

The method of opening along the bronchi is the preferred technique for assessment of proximal bronchus-based tumours as it allows more accurate assessment of the relationship between neoplasm and bronchus, distance of tumour from the resection margin and changes in the lung parenchyma distal to the neoplasm.

Lungs thought to harbour tuberculosis or other infections such as hydatid are fixed by inflation for a minimum of 24 hours prior to sectioning. In the case of suspected pneumoconiosis where an assessment of particulate load is important, a portion of lung is submitted for electron dispersive X-ray analysis. The same should be done for cases of mesothelioma and a 2 cm cube of tumour and lung tissue can be submitted for digestion and examination for asbestos bodies. Occasionally a rib is received with lung tissue and this should be measured and decalcified.

In pneumoconiosis whole mount thin slices are useful and the number, severity and distribution of dust lesions, emphysema and interstitial fibrosis is documented grossly and the pleura examined for colour, thickness, exudate and plaques. Detailed discussion of the technique is beyond the scope of this book.

## Pleura

### Clinical indications

Pleural biopsies are performed to investigate radiological pleural thickening, peripheral lung opacities and recurrent pleural effusion, particularly unilateral, due to inflammatory conditions such as tuberculosis and rheumatoid arthritis, and neoplasms including mesothelioma, primary lung carcinoma and metastatic tumours. These biopsies are typically performed in conjunction with cytological examination of effusion fluid.

### Examination and dissection technique

In cases of suspected mesothelioma, if adequate tissue is received, a portion of tissue should be submitted for electron microscopic examination which is very helpful in the separation of mesothelioma from carcinoma.

The thoracoscopy decortication specimen comprises strips and flat sheets of pleura which are cut transversely.

# Salivary glands

## Clinical indications

The salivary gland is biopsied or excised for chronic sialadenitis with or without sialolithiasis and salivary gland tumours.

## Examination and dissection technique

The external surface of parotid specimens is examined for the deep fascia, the presence or absence of the facial nerve and attached lymph nodes. In glands involved by tumours, the margins are inked as many tumours can extend beyond what appears to be a delineating capsule. The gland is serially sliced in parallel sections at 4 mm intervals. Intrasalivary gland lymph nodes and nerve bundles should be sampled. Photograph the specimen if appropriate. Accompanying radical neck dissections are dissected as previously described. If calculi are suspected, consider specimen radiography and the calculus can be submitted for biochemical analysis. Blocks with calculi will need decalcification.

In the case of neoplasms, the tissue blocks should include the tumour periphery with capsule and the surrounding gland as well as samples of resection margins. Sample the facial nerve if included in the resection and examine all lymph nodes present.

# Skin and lip

## Skin

### Clinical indications

There is a myriad of inflammatory and degenerative lesions, neoplasms both benign and malignant, cysts, hamartomas, sinuses and dysplasias which involve the skin.

### Examination and dissection technique

Curettings, scrapings and shave biopsies are employed to remove superficial skin lesions which are mainly benign conditions such as seborrhoeic keratosis, verruca and naevi, but are also occasionally used to sample superficial basal cell carcinoma and well differentiated squamous cell carcinoma. These specimens are difficult to orientate and the fragments are embedded whole. Larger shave biopsies are cut into parallel transverse sections. As further treatment such as cautery to the base and edges of the lesion is often performed, clearance of excision margins is not necessary.

Many medical skin diseases are sampled by punch biopsies or by incisional biopsies, often multiple and from different body locations. Punch biopsies of less than 3 mm in diameter are not satisfactory as tissue shrinkage in formalin makes assessment difficult and the risk of sampling error dramatically increases. Both punch and incisional biopsies should be directed at the growing edge of the rash and are best bisected prior to embedding. Punch biopsies can be bisected using the tip of a sharp scalpel blade, cutting from the deep aspect through to the epidermis. The incisional ellipse is bisected longitudinally to follow the transition from normal to lesional skin, as an assessment of the short axial resection margins is not important in medical skin cases. It is important to remind the technician not to trim the blocks excessively in these biopsies as lesional tissue may be lost. For this reason, very small punch or incisional biopsies are best embedded uncut and levels through the block examined. For vesiculobullous diseases, keeping the vesicle intact by embedding the specimen uncut and cutting levels is the preferred technique. Rarely, larger punch biopsies are used to excise small benign lesions such as naevi. If the gross appearance is suspicious of a neoplasm, the margins of resection should be inked.

In many inflammatory skin diseases, additional biopsies (either punch or incision) may be sent separately in saline or a transport media such as Michell's medium for direct immunofluorescence which is important in the investigation of the vesiculobullous diseases, lupus, vasculitis and photosensitivity eruptions. Fresh biopsies are required for bacterial and viral cultures and for flow cytometry and molecular studies.

The margin of clearance in skin biopsies is dependent on the clinical nature of the lesion, the site, patient age and the need for further treatment. Generally speaking, the margins will be greater for suspected malignant tumours such as squamous cell carcinoma, compared to benign lesions such as a melanocytic naevus. Melanocytic lesions felt clinically to represent melanoma are often initially excised with narrow margins so that the need for wider excision can be determined by microscopic examination. The skin should be well fixed before cutting and the margins of potentially malignant lesions should be clearly inked, particularly if they are close to the tumour.

The commonest method for sampling surgical skin lesions is to cut the skin in transverse sections so that the lesion and its relationship to the closest short axial

resection margin and deep margin can all be determined. The sections are embedded on edge. In small lesions of 2–6 mm, the biopsy, cut in transverse sections, is embedded in toto in one block (Fig. 6.8). It is useful to bisect small lesions asymmetrically or to cut on either side of the lesion and have levels cut into the lesional block to ensure the lesion is not lost when the block is trimmed. Lesions smaller than 2 mm are often best embedded whole, sacrificing the ability to assess the short margins of the biopsy. Lesions larger than 6 mm are also best cut transversely. The extent of sampling is dependent on the macroscopic appearance. For a well-defined keratinising squamous cell carcinoma, it is acceptable to take a few representative transverse sections of the tumour; however, it may be necessary to block all lesional tissue in cases of large pigmented lesions. The ends of most

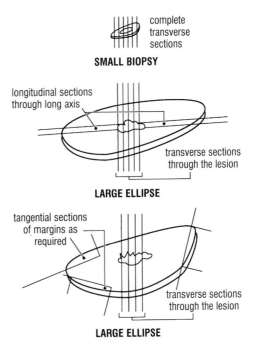

**Fig. 6.8**   Skin biopsy

skin biopsies are readily recognised, as in the transverse sections, these are the smallest pieces.

Another approach to sampling intermediate-sized well-defined lesions is to use the hot cross bun method where transverse sections are taken centrally through the lesion and longitudinal sections are taken from the edge of the lesion to the ends of the ellipse (Fig. 6.8). This method should not be used in melanocytic lesions and when the margins are narrow, as assessment of margins is inadequate.

Many skin excisions will contain two or more apparently discrete lesions which are best assessed using transverse sections, sampling each lesion in separate blocks.

For large lesions on broad skin excisions, it is not practical to block the entire lesion or biopsy. As with biopsies from other body organs, the tumour should be sampled and the closest resection margins need to be examined. In cases where the tumour is close to an edge, a transverse section to include tumour and the margin is recommended. If the margins are well clear of the lesion, they can be sampled as longitudinal or tangential blocks of the margins (Fig. 6.8). If necessary, multiple tangential sections of the entire margin can be taken circumferentially. Specific margins should be identified by the clinician for microscopic examination.

Photographs should be taken of unusual skin lesions and pigmented lesions suspected of being malignant melanoma. Routine PASD stains of 'medical' skin biopsies are useful.

## Lip

### Clinical indications

Wedge excision of the lip is performed to remove tumours, typically squamous cell carcinoma, whilst vermilionectomy is used

to treat more widespread solar cheilitis/squamous cell carcinoma which has failed to respond to other treatments such as cryo- or laser therapy.

### Examination and dissection technique

The specimen should be well fixed and laid out flat before cutting. To achieve this, pin out the specimen on a corkboard and fix for a few hours or overnight. Margins are inked and the specimen cut in parallel transverse sections at 2–3 mm intervals. There are two main ways to handle such wedge biopsies and both entail blocking of all the tissue. One method involves cutting sagittal sections at 3 mm intervals, with the medial and lateral edges in separate blocks. This method is adequate if the medio-lateral excision margins appear macroscopically well clear of the tumour. The other method involves taking coronal sections through the wedge in the medio-lateral direction. Although this is excellent for assessing margins, it does not provide visualisation of the epidermo-mucosal junction.

## Urinary tract

### Kidney

### Clinical indications

Needle biopsies are used in the investigation of renal disease which presents as haematuria, proteinuria, nephrotic syndrome, nephritic syndrome, acute renal failure and unexplained hypertension. It is also used extensively in renal transplants to assess graft failure.

Nephrectomy is typically performed for neoplasia (renal cell carcinoma or transitional cell carcinoma of the renal pelvis in adults, and Wilm's tumour in children), chronic hydronephrosis or reflux with chronic pyelonephritis, calculi and for the treatment of hypertension induced by renal artery stenosis which is unsuitable for corrective surgery. Partial nephrectomies are uncommon and are generally reserved for patients with small tumours and who have pre-existing impaired renal function and require conservation of all functioning renal tissue. Transplant nephrectomies are performed for graft failure due to rejection, hypertension or recurrent renal disease.

*Examination and dissection technique*

The handling and processing of renal needle core biopsies require a number of special techniques. Most needle biopsies are examined by light microscopy, direct immunofluorescence and transmission electron microscopy. The ability to distribute representative tissue for these procedures is enhanced by the use of the dissecting microscope. With the aid of the dissecting microscope or hand lens, the renal cortex and medulla are identified by the respective presence of pinhead-size vascular balls corresponding to glomeruli and red stripes corresponding to the vasa recta. Having determined the tissue to be renal, the technician takes approximately 1–3 mm off the cortical end for ultrastructural examination. If a dissecting microscope is not available, tissue should be taken from both ends of the needle core for electron microscopy and immunofluorescence with the hope that one end would be cortical tissue. Often a separate core is taken for immunofluorescence, and if the sample is assessed as adequate by gross examination, it is snap frozen in isopentane cooled with liquid nitrogen. The core for light microscopic examination is fixed in 10% buffered formalin or formal-saline.

Mercuric chloride fixative has been used but mercury is an environmental pollutant which is difficult to dispose of safely and should no longer be used when alternatives are available. Renal cores may be embedded in resin instead of paraffin wax.

If insufficient tissue is available, a decision has to be made on its allocation. For example, with a biopsy taken a few days after transplant for graft failure, the primary consideration of acute rejection versus cyclosporin toxicity would determine that light microscopy is the preferred examination. However, in the situation of a young man with haematuria and proteinuria, immunofluorescence would be important to rule out an immune complex mediated glomerulonephritis such as IgA nephropathy. Tissue can always be retrieved from the tissue employed for immunofluorescence and reprocessed for light microscopy.

The weight and dimensions of the partial or complete nephrectomy, with or without perinephric fat, should be noted. In active infection, a portion of lesional tissue can be taken for culture. With renal cell carcinoma, an unfixed portion may be taken for cytogenetic studies, and in cases of childhood nephroblastoma (Wilm's tumour), unfixed tumour can be sent for cytogenetics, frozen and fixed in glutaraldehyde, and imprints of the tumour surface should be made. In a radical nephrectomy, lymph nodes in fat around the hilum and attached adrenal gland (separately weighed) should be sampled. The hilar vessels and ureter should be located and a transverse section taken of the renal artery/vein and ureteric resection margins. In renal cell carcinoma, the renal vein is opened longitudinally to examine for tumour spread. If the ureter is not obstructed by tumour, a 1 mm metal probe can be pushed up the ureter to perforate the renal pelvis and renal capsule. The kidney is bisected in the sagittal plane with a sharp long-bladed knife, using the probe as a guide. The probe causes minimal if any trauma to the ureteric lining epithelium and allows the kidney and pelvicalyceal system to be exposed with the first cut. This plane of sectioning exposes the lesion in most cases. It is preferable not to peel off the renal capsule, especially in renal tumours where capsular penetration is of prognostic significance, and keeping the capsule intact allows proper microscopic examination. The hilar vessels should be sampled in tumour cases and transplant rejection.

Transitional cell carcinoma may also show extrarenal spread and the perinephric fat resection margin over the tumour needs to be inked. Photograph the specimen. In cases of hydronephrosis, the specimen can be fixed by injecting with formalin via the ureter and renal artery, both of which are then tied. In transplant nephrectomy, pieces of renal tissue should be snap frozen and fixed in glutaraldehyde for immunofluorescence and electron microscopic examination respectively.

Needle biopsies are embedded intact, with 20 serial levels cut. Special stains are required and, as an example, levels 1, 5, 10, 15 and 20 can be stained with H & E, levels 2, 8 and 19 with silver methenamine, level 11 with Masson's silver, levels 9 and 17 with Masson's trichrome, levels 3, 7, 13 and 18 with AB/PAS and levels 4, 6, 12, 14 and 16 kept as spares. A Congo Red stain is performed if amyloidosis is suspected, e.g. in multiple myeloma.

## Ureter

### Clinical indications

The ureter is removed as part of nephrectomy and cystectomy, and for strictures and rarely for tumours.

### Examination and dissection technique

The ureter is conveniently cut as transverse sections at approximately 3 mm intervals with the resection margin as separate blocks. The ureter may be opened longitudinally in cases of tumour but there is a risk of cutting through the tumour with this method. The Swiss roll method of fixing the rolled-up length of ureter before cutting serial cross-sections of the roll, allows evaluation of the entire ureteric epithelium (see next section).

## Bladder and calculi

### Clinical indications

Cystoscopic biopsies are often taken to investigate chronic cystitis and to diagnose neoplasia. Cystectomy, either partial or total, is reserved for tumours that are poorly differentiated, invade deeply into the bladder wall or have failed to respond to conservative treatment such as cystoscopic resection, intravesical BCG or chemotherapy. Partial cystectomy may be employed for urachal carcinoma where the bladder dome, urachus and umbilicus is excised. Cystectomy is occasionally performed for obstinate chronic interstitial or radiation cystitis and dysfunctional neurogenic bladder. Calculi are sometimes removed from bladders, particularly those with diverticula.

### Examination and dissection technique

The biopsy fragments or curettings are embedded uncut in toto as they are difficult to orientate. Occasionally separate biopsies from the tumour base are submitted to assess muscle invasion. The fresh biopsy can be evaluated for blood group antigens, cytogenetics, flow cytometry or various growth factor receptors which may be of prognostic relevance in bladder tumours. If an unusual neoplasm is suspected, glutaraldehyde fixation for electron microscopy is advisable.

The cystectomy specimen is orientated by using the ureters, attached organs and peritoneal reflections as landmarks (the peritoneum covering of the bladder descends further posteriorly). The ureters, vas deferens and seminal vesicles should be identified prior to opening the bladder. There are two basic methods for opening the bladder. One method involves opening the specimen, soon after receipt, with scissors along the urethra and anterior bladder wall in a T or Y shape, pinning out the specimen on a corkboard, and sampling after complete fixation. The second involves formalin inflation of the intact bladder to enhance fixation. This is done by tying or clamping the urethra and ureters and injecting formalin through the bladder wall at the apex with a 22 gauge needle and a 50 ml syringe, or passing a catheter into the urethra and instilling formalin via this route. Prior to clamping or tying the ends, transverse sections of the urethra/ureter resection margins should be taken. After overnight fixation, the cystectomy is bisected into anterior and posterior halves, opening the lateral walls first. Cut the prostate (if present) with a long-bladed knife guided by a probe placed in the urethra. Sagittal cuts are best avoided as they distort the trigone and ureteric orifices. If the tumour extends close to perivesical resection margins, ink the latter. Similarly, the periprostatic excision margin should be clearly marked. Photographs of tumours are recommended and a diagram or photocopy of the specimen will help map the site of blocks taken. Parallel cuts are made through the bladder wall in the region of tumour to assess the depth of

invasion, and the prostate, if included, is examined by serial antero-posterior directed cuts, leaving the slices attached by a thin rim of prostatic capsule posteriorly. The ureteric orifices can be probed from the trigone unless distorted or involved by tumour. The openings are located at the limits of the interureteric bar. The ureters are opened either longitudinally with a pair of fine scissors or by serial transverse sections. The latter method enables more informative sections to be taken of the ureteric orifice. An alternative method to examine the ureters which are not distorted by fibrosis or tumour is the Swiss roll technique, which enables inspection of the entire ureteric length in one block with accurate localisation of any abnormalities. The ureter is opened longitudinally with a pair of fine scissors and rolled, mucosal aspect innermost, around a pair of fine forceps or a clamp. The rolled specimen is gently pried off the forceps and its shape maintained by pushing a pin along the equator of the roll. The specimen is allowed to fix in this position for several hours or overnight, the pin is removed, and the roll is either placed flat uncut into a cassette or bisected. The seminal vesicles, if included, are cut longitudinally, whilst the vas deferens are cut transversely. Attached vagina, uterus, fallopian tubes and ovaries, if uninvolved by tumour extension, are separated from the bladder and dissected as outlined for the individual organs under 'Female genital tract' (see p. 64). They are maintained with the bladder if involved by tumour spread and invasion.

Diverticula are cut with parallel longitudinal sections. If tumour is visible, ink the margins. Calculi are photographed and may be submitted for biochemical analysis.

Bladder calculi are occasionally sent for examination. Photograph the specimen and describe the calculi in terms of size, shape, colour, consistency, external appearance and number. Urate calculi are smooth, brown to yellow and oval to round, whilst oxalate calculi are hard and may be irregular, spiculated, multilobular or smooth and round. Phosphate calculi are typically white or grey, vary considerably in hardness and may be large. The rare cystine calculi are yellow, hard, smooth and somewhat waxy. Routine sections are not necessary and calculi are rarely sent for chemical analysis.

## Miscellaneous

### Pelvic exenteration

*Clinical indications*

This radical debulking surgical procedure removes the pelvic organs and is used for widely but locally infiltrative tumours of the female genital tract, bladder and rectum. The specimen comprises the bladder, rectum, sigmoid colon and pelvic lymph nodes, and includes the prostate and seminal vesicles in men, and the vulva, vagina, uterus, tubes and ovaries in women. Modifications include anterior exenteration which excludes the rectosigmoid colon, and posterior exenteration which excludes the bladder.

*Examination and dissection technique*

The approach to this specimen will vary depending on the site of the primary tumour. The rectal contents are expressed and, if not opened, the lumen can be packed with gauze or formalin-soaked cotton. The vagina can be similarly packed. If the bladder is not opened, it can be inflated with formalin using a syringe or via a catheter as described previously and the endometrium can be exposed to enhance fixation by cutting into the uterine fundus. Surgical margins are inked. The complete specimen should be well fixed before dissection. Following removal of packing material, the entire specimen can be bisected in the sagittal plane. The large bowel, bladder and vagina are best cut with scissors whilst the uterus is sectioned with a knife. Photograph the cross-section of the specimen and prepare a block key diagram. Lymph nodes are dissected out and orientated into groups: perivesical, right and left parametrial, retrorectal and mesosigmoid.

Indicate the type of exenteration, i.e. total, anterior or posterior, and document the organs removed and their dimensions. The tumour characteristics are described with relation to its primary site, size, colour, configuration, consistency, haemorrhage, necrosis, involvement of adjacent organs, fistulas, perforation, proximity to resection margins and signs of radiation damage. Also note the number, size and cut surface appearance of lymph nodes resected.

The aim of the examination is to diagnose the tumour, assess its primary origin, spread and local clearance. Examine for complications such as fistula, perforation, sinus tracts and effects of previous treatment such as radiation.

### Immotile cilia syndrome

Electron microscopy is necessary in the identification of the primary defects underlying the ciliary dyskinesia syndrome. Patients with this syndrome have varying combinations of sinusitis, respiratory infections, bronchiectasis, infertility in males due to immotile sperm and sometimes have situs inversus. The diagnosis requires ultrastructural examination of either ciliated cells or spermatozoa. Suitable cells can be obtained by brushing the upper nasal passages. In vitro assessment of motility of spermatozoa can be used to select cases requiring ultrastructural examination. Infection and injury can induce a number of secondary abnormalities in cilia which often cannot be separated from primary structural abnormalities, so that confident identification of the latter is fraught with difficulties.

# 7 Special investigative procedures

# Introduction

There are a number of specialised procedures in surgical pathology which are of
diagnostic or prognostic importance and
with which the trainee pathologist should
be acquainted. Some of these have been in
use for many years but others, particularly
with the advent of molecular techniques,
are relatively recent. This chapter outlines
many of these procedures and briefly
discusses their use in routine surgical
pathology. It should be read in conjunction
with Chapter 9 which is devoted to
histochemistry and immunohistochemistry
and Chapter 13 which describes special
techniques in light microscopy.

# X-ray studies

X-ray studies may be performed in conjunction with the radiology department or
within the pathology laboratory if there is
access to a Faxitron X-ray machine.

## Bony specimens

Bone tumours should never be reported
without reference to the X-rays. Whilst
these are usually performed in vivo, X-rays
of the surgical specimen may allow higher
resolution and better orientation, although
with the use of modern computerised
tomography, these are no longer such
important considerations. Lytic lesions and
inflammatory erosions may be best demonstrated by X-rays which serve to guide the
pathologist in the taking of appropriate
samples.

X-rays are essential in assessing skeletal
abnormalities in the investigation of
stillbirths and fetuses. While such cases
may be included in surgical pathology or
autopsy pathology, as a rule, stillbirths and

fetuses of less than 20 weeks' gestation fall
within the sphere of surgical pathology.

Soft tissue calcification and bone formation may be seen in soft tissue tumours and
reactive processes and the X-ray pattern
may be of help in their differentiation.
Most commonly, bony X-rays are performed in the laboratory to determine the
end-point of bone decalcification.

## Breast tissue

Mammographs performed prior to surgical
resection may accompany the specimen and
be used to indicate the site of the lesion.
They may be performed on the resected
specimen, especially in the examination of
impalpable breast lesions as described in
Chapter 6.

## Cardiac valves

The aetiological diagnosis of cardiac
valvular disorders depends mostly on the
macroscopic appearances. Macrophotography, mandatory in all cases, may
be augmented by X-rays to depict the
extent of calcification present. Stenosis in
chronic rheumatic valve disease may be due
to commissural fusion, fibrosis or complicating dystrophic calcification, and X-rays
may be of immense help in assessing which
of these is the dominant feature.

## Foreign bodies

X-rays may be invaluable in detecting and
locating foreign bodies. Bony spicules from
fractures, implants such as prostheses or
radium pellets and metal fragments from
shrapnel or bullets may all be visualised.
Surgical staples may also be detected by X-
ray and avoided in tissue blocks, preventing
damage to the microtome knife.

## Angiography

Angiography is more often used as an autopsy procedure where it is invaluable in assessing the extent and nature of arterial stenoses. However, the investigation of gastrointestinal haemorrhage due to angiodysplasia is one situation in surgical pathology in which angiography is often performed and can be of immense help in diagnosis. Following surgical resection, angiodysplastic lesions may be demonstrated by the injection of a barium sulphate/gelatin suspension into the mesenteric vessels of the fresh intact specimen. A 5% stock suspension is made by dissolving 50 g of gelatine in hot water to give a volume of 200 ml and adding 800 ml of 100% (w/v) barium sulphate suspension. The stock suspension is divided into suitable aliquots, which can be kept frozen or in a cold room until required. Ideally, the mesenteric arterial vessel is identified by a surgical tie at the time of resection. The vascular system is flushed with saline or a fibrinolytic prior to injection of the reheated barium gelatin. Care must be taken not to exert too great a pressure in order to prevent artefactual rupture of small vessels. An in-line sphygmomanometer can be used to monitor the injection pressure although this can be messy and, with practice, is unnecessary. Subsequent X-rays will demonstrate a vascular 'blush' which is often grossly visible through the mucosa.

## Immunofluorescence

The principles of fluorescent microscopy and immunofluorescence are outlined in Chapter 13. Direct immunofluorescence refers to the detection of a specific tissue antigen by a fluorescent-labelled antibody. In this situation, the antigen may be any protein, including immunoglobulins. The antibody is raised against the specific antigen in an animal host, e.g. in the case of mouse anti-human IgG, the antigen is human IgG the antibodies to which have been raised in a mouse and subsequently labelled. Indirect immunofluorescence refers to the detection of circulating antibodies through incubation of an appropriate section of tissue with the patient's serum. The antibody is then detected with a fluorescent-labelled anti-human antibody. This is sometimes referred to as the sandwich technique whereby the circulating antibody requiring detection is sandwiched between the tissue antigen and the fluorescent-labelled anti-human antibody. However, the sandwich technique is more accurately applied to the detection of an antibody producing cell by antigen which is subsequently detected by fluorescent-labelled anti-human antibody. Direct immunofluorescence is still widely employed in the biopsy investigation of the glomerulonephritides and bullous skin disorders where it is generally a more reliable and more rapid technique than immunohistochemistry. Indirect immunofluorescence is still commonly used in immunology laboratories for the identification of circulating autoantibodies, e.g. anti-neutrophilic cytoplasmic antibodies (ANCA) in certain cases of vasculitis, anti-nuclear factor in systemic lupus erythematosus, rheumatoid factor in rheumatoid arthritis, anti-mitochondrial and smooth muscle antibodies in liver disease and anti-microsomal and long-acting thyroid stimulator (LATS) antibodies in thyroid disease.

Immunofluorescence studies are generally performed on fresh frozen tissues. While the procedure can be employed on fixed tissues, it loses much of its sensitivity.

# Electron microscopy

In microscopy, decreasing the wavelength of the energy source leads to greater resolution and the ability to resolve objects at higher magnifications. An electron beam has a far shorter wavelength than that of light, and when used as the energy source has a resolving power over 1000 times that of the light microscope, thus allowing the use of high magnification without loss of resolution.

## Transmission electron microscopy

Transmission electron microscopy may be used in diagnostic surgical pathology whenever knowledge of cell ultrastructure is important. Recognition of specific cellular ultrastructural features may provide a specific diagnosis in an otherwise undifferentiated tumour, e.g. the presence of premelanosomes in a melanoma, the differential length of microvilli in distinguishing between adenocarcinoma and mesothelioma and the presence of Z-bands in a rhabdomyosarcoma. Although the increasing use of immunoperoxidase has obviated the need for electron microscopy in many cases, it remains an extremely useful adjunct in tumour diagnosis. Electron microscopy is of routine use in the examination of renal biopsies and, in some cases, is the sole technique on which a diagnosis is made, e.g. thin membrane or minimal change nephropathies. It is also invaluable for the examination of skeletal and cardiac muscle biopsies where certain myopathies, e.g. due to mitochondrial abnormalities, can be specifically recognised.

It must be appreciated that in the examination of ultrastructure, preservation of cellular organelles is of vital importance. Ideally, specimens should be placed in the appropriate fixative as soon as possible to prevent cellular changes due to autolysis. Gluteraldehyde is the most frequently used fixative for electron microscopy although specimens fixed in formalin may give adequate results, and even material chipped from a paraffin block may provide the necessary information to arrive at a diagnosis. It should be remembered that fixation in glutaraldehyde is slower then formalin and that the penetration of the fixative is minimal, necessitating the provision of diced fragments of tissue of not more than 1 mm in any one dimension. This is best obtained as a shave from the cut surface of the lesion. A variety of reagents and processing protocols have been developed for transmission electron microscopy. The most commonly used fixative is 2.5% glutaraldehyde in 0.05 M cacodylate buffer at 4°C. The fixation time may be varied from 2 to 24 hours, after which the tissue is transferred to sodium phosphate or cacodylate buffer at 4°C until ready for processing.

## Scanning electron microscopy

In transmission electron microscopy, the image is obtained by electrons transmitted through the specimen, whereas in scanning electron microscopy, images are obtained through interaction of the electrons with the surface of the specimen by detecting secondary and backscattered electrons. High-energy primary electrons are emitted from a probe which scans the specimen in a square raster pattern. Low-energy secondary electrons are produced by inelastic scattering through electron–electron interactions originating from the surface of the specimen. Their emission is determined by the surface characteristics of the specimen and differences in emission can be used to build a three-dimensional topographical image of the specimen, allowing localisation of areas of interest for specific X-ray microanalysis.

Scanning electron microscopy is ideally suited to surfaces such as those of the skin and mucosa, and structures which may be exposed on the surface of cleanly sectioned tissues including glomeruli, alveolar spaces and blood vessels. Formalin-fixed tissues can be used and these must be dehydrated through alcohols and dried. Critical point drying with liquid carbon dioxide is employed before coating with carbon or a thin layer of gold or palladium to reflect the electron beam off the surface of the specimen.

Modern microscopes are capable of resolving topographical details from 5 to 10 nm and have a working range of magnification from ×10 to ×100 000. Unlike conventional transmission micro-scopes which utilise ultrathin sections, the scanning microscope can be used on solid, unsectioned specimens.

Currently, the scanning electron micro-scope has only a small role in surgical pathology, but as a research tool it has greatly increased our knowledge and understanding of normal structure and disease processes.

## Energy dispersive X-ray analysis

In a different mode, the scanning electron microscope can be used for elemental analysis of materials within a specimen. When the electron beam interacts with the specimen, X-rays are produced and these may be measured as the total number of specific X-ray energy levels (energy dispersive) or X-rays of a certain wave-length (wavelength dispersive). The specific X-rays produced when an electron from the probe interacts with an electron of a specific element in the specimen can be used to identify that element. Combining energy dispersive X-ray analysis (EDXA) with scanning electron microscopy allows the identification and quantitation of the elemental and chemical composition of selected surface tissue structures. Some scanning microscopes can also be switched to transmission mode and conventional transmission microscopes which are fitted with electron probe microanalysers allow analysis of ultrathin sections used in conventional electron microscopy.

EDXA is occasionally used in diagnostic surgical pathology. It may be employed to analyse particulate matter and material present in foreign body reactions such as calcium, beryllium, lead and silicon in tissues such as skin, lung, liver and kidney.

Backscattered electrons are deflected electrons which emerge without energy loss from the surface through which they entered. These result from electron–nucleus interactions and can escape from depths of several micrometres. The number of backscattered electrons produced is proportional to the atomic number of the surface elements within the specimen and provides information regarding the types of atoms in the specimen.

Tissues for EDXA can be formalin-fixed, although it is preferable to employ glu-taraldehyde for fixation.

## Immunoelectron microscopy

Tissue antigens may be located at a subcellular level by an immunolabelling technique which employs an antibody labelled with a marker which electron dense. This technique has made a signifi-cant contribution to our understanding of the molecular structure of cells and tissues. The iron-containing protein ferritin was one of the first electron-dense markers to be conjugated to antibodies, allowing identification at, or near, the site of interaction with tissue antigens. Since then, the horseradish peroxidase and diaminobenzidine reactions have been modified for use with electron microscopy, utilising the formation of osmiophilic reaction products with either conjugated or non-conjugated antibodies. More recently, colloidal gold has been used to label the primary antibody and the immunogold staining technique is now the most commonly used technique for transmission and scanning electron microscopy. Because immunolabelling is conveniently performed on paraffin sections, immunoelectron microscopy is seldom employed in diagnostic pathology but is widely utilised in research.

Immunostaining for electron microscopy can be performed before or after embedding. In pre-embedding techniques, the tissue is immunostained before it is embedded and sectioned so that the tissue antigens are exposed to antibodies before they are denatured or even eluted by processing and embedding. However, in some situations it may only be possible to stain for antigens by using the post-embedding method because the antigens need to be exposed by cutting open the cell and organelle membranes through ultrathin sectioning. As with paraffin section immunohistochemistry, the fixative of choice varies with the antigen of interest but generally a mixture of 1% glutaraldehyde and 1% paraformaldehyde in 0.1 M sodium cacodylate buffer at pH 7.2 is used, although the proportion of glutaraldehyde to paraformaldehyde may vary with the antigen of interest and the antibody used. Immunocryoultramicrotomy is an alternative method in which ice provides the rigidity for cutting tissues and cells into ultrathin sections for immunolabelling; however, this procedure is largely a research tool.

# Quantitation and image analysis

Quantitative assessment in some form or another is becoming a part of routine in specialised areas of surgical pathology. It is useful in those cases where the structural features of a disease deviate only slightly from the normal state or where an objective assessment of morphological parameters is necessary for diagnostic or therapeutic reasons. Morphometry may be defined as the measurement of the forms of organisms, whereas histometry more specifically refers to the measurement of tissues. Stereology is the quantitative study of the three-dimensional properties of objects from two-dimensional planes using geometrical procedures. Many measurements applicable to histology fall under the heading of stereology, since the aim is to provide information on volumetric parameters from a study of a two-dimensional tissue section without the need to resort to laborious three-dimensional reconstructions. The French geologist, Delesse, in 1847 established the fundamental principle relating to stereology: the volumetric composition of a material composed of two or more randomly distributed components is proportional to the area of a surface that is occupied by those components. Thus, from analysis of a two-dimensional tissue section plane, estimations of the volumetric composition can be made.

## Applications in surgical pathology

Histometric measurements that are in everyday use include assessment of mitotic rates and linear measurements of depth and clearance of tumours, e.g. assessment of microinvasive versus overtly invasive carcinoma of the cervix, Breslow thickness of invasive malignant melanoma and depth of myometrial invasion of endometrial carcinoma, as well as linear measurements of the thickness of the subepithelial collagen plate in suspected cases of collagenous colitis and of the glomerular basement membrane from electron micrographs in suspected cases of benign familial haematuria (thin membrane nephropathy) and diabetes mellitus. Measurement of surface area unrelated to volumetric analysis may also be of use in assessing the aetiology of cardiac valvular disease.

More complex stereological measurements are useful in estimating mineralised bone and osteoid in the study of metabolic bone disease; haemopoietic components of bone marrow; mucosal volume and mononuclear cells of gastrointestinal mucosa; the ratio of parenchyma to air space in lung biopsies; nerve cells and dendrites in cerebral tissue; villi, capillaries and intervillous space in placental tissue; spermatic tubules and Leydig cells in testicular biopsies; steatosis in the liver; fibre type and size in muscle biopsies; and in the study of various fetal tissues.

Currently, quantitation involving computerised image analysis is a research procedure, but with the increased use of immunohistochemical assays of prognostic markers, applications of image analysis in diagnostic histopathology are becoming apparent. If appropriately controlled, staining intensity can be objectively assessed and quantified by image analysis rather than subjectively by inspection. Densitometry allows quantification of immunoperoxidase reactions for hormone receptors and tumour markers, although inter-laboratory standardisation and comparisons cannot be made because of existing differences in fixation and immunostaining protocols.

## Simple histometric measurements

Strictly speaking, assessment of the mitotic activity of a tumour is a stereological measurement and is usually made by counting the number of mitoses per 10 high power fields. It is one of the most important parameters in the diagnosis of some tumours but is not without its pitfalls and is discussed more fully later in this chapter.

Linear measurements such as margins of tumour clearance and depth of invasion can be easily made by using a graticule eyepiece inserted into the eyepiece lens of the microscope. The graticule is calibrated against a microscope slide on which a micrometer scale is engraved. The eyepiece must be calibrated for each objective magnification but once this has been done for the particular microscope in use, linear measurements can be quickly calculated on all future occasions. The calibrations obtained for one microscope cannot be transposed to another and any accessory lens, e.g. polarising or multihead facility, inserted between the objective and the eyepiece may alter the calibrations significantly.

Linear measurements may be made without the use of an eyepiece graticule. The vertical and horizontal Vernier scales on the microscope stage are graduated in millimetres and may be used to provide a fairly accurate measurement to two decimal places. The trainee pathologist should be acquainted with the use of the Vernier scale. An advantage of this method is that measurements are independent of objective magnification; the disadvantage is that the distance to be measured must be aligned with either the vertical or the horizontal scale and this is not always easy. With an eyepiece graticule, the microscope stage or graticule may be rotated so that the distance to be measured aligns with the graticule scale.

Some linear measurements can be estimated by reference to an object of known dimensions, e.g. a red blood cell or lymphocyte. The division of the thickness of the myometrium into thirds or halves in assessing the depth of invasion of endometrial carcinoma can be done visually.

## Stereological measurements

Volume proportions, surface areas, particle numbers and particle dimensions may all be estimated in tissues using various combinations of planimetry and eyepiece graticules.

Delesse's theorem states that the area proportion of a component in a random cut surface is equal to its volume proportion. There are three basic ways of measuring areas in a tissue section:

1  Measurement of traced images which entails tracing an image on a uniform thickness and weight paper, cutting out the shapes and weighing the pieces. Alternatively, a planimeter may be used to trace the area of the profile under consideration. Microscope images are projected onto a screen, or a camera lucida attachment is used to project the image onto the work surface for tracing.

2  Linear integration whereby a system of parallel lines placed over the section is used to express the length of the line contained within the structure being considered, as a proportion of the total length of the line covering the tissue. With the use of an eyepiece graticule, area measurements may be made without the need to construct time consuming tracings.

3  Point counting is the most efficient way of obtaining area measurements of tissue sections. Eyepiece graticules using a randomly disposed arrangement of points or test points placed at the angles of equilateral triangles are used to score the various components of a tissue section.

With all of these methods, calculation of volume proportion is susceptible to error from section thickness. However, in comparing the volume proportions of the same tissue components under different conditions, this effect may be disregarded provided that tissue section thickness, from slide to slide, is constant.

The surface area of well-defined structures, such as the villi of small intestinal mucosa or the placenta, may be measured in tissue sections using a linear intercept method. The surface density or surface area per unit volume may be calculated from a recording of the number of intercepts a test line makes with the contours of the structure under consideration. Various grids are available for these surface area measurements depending on whether or not the component is randomly arranged. The Weibel multipurpose grid or Zeiss type II integrating eyepiece are suitable for randomly arranged objects, but for non-randomly arranged features such as jejunal mucosal villi and placental villi, the Weibel type I grid or Merz curvilinear grid is preferred. The total surface area of a component is obtained by multiplying the surface density by the organ volume and this may provide a more accurate measurement than the surface density alone. Surface to volume ratios and perimeter measurements may also be made using the linear intercept method.

The numerical estimation of different particles in a tissue section is not as straightforward as volume and surface area measurements, owing to variations in size, distribution and fragmentation. Numbers of large particles can generally be estimated accurately, but an accurate count of particles with a size less than 10 times the section thickness can only be made on spherical bodies of uniform size. Estimation of volume proportions is more accurate for non-spherical or variably sized small particles. A squared grid or Weibel's multipurpose grid is suitable for estimating the numbers of large particles. Dimensions of particles may also be difficult to obtain especially if they are of differing sizes and shapes. In this instance, complicated analyses are required.

## How many recordings?

An important consideration in interpreting the significance of quantitative methods is the number of measurements that should be performed. Whilst sample size must be adequate, it is not infrequent for an unnecessarily high number of counts to be made. Variance in measurement numbers relates to numbers of tissue blocks, sections, microscope fields and readings within a field. The sample size required for significance depends on the frequency and distribution of the feature under consideration. If the feature is randomly distributed and occupies a large proportion of the tissue, a small sample size will be sufficient and vice versa. A percentage standard error of 5% is an acceptable target, and for point counting is calculated as a percentage of the standard error divided by the fraction of test points lying over the feature.

## Computer-assisted histometry and image analysis

The methods of quantitation described above are often laborious and time consuming. These measurements may now be performed automatically or semi-automatically with computers, depending on the nature of the quantitation and the level of sophistication of the system. Desktop computers may be linked to a digitising pad for computer-assisted planimetry. Point counting, linear and area measurements may all be easily performed through projection of the microscope image onto a digitising pad which generates XY coordinates from traces made over its surface with a special pen or cursor. From these coordinates, the computer is able to generate measurements. The use of a camera lucida attachment allows tracings to be transferred directly from the microscopic tissue section to the computer via the digitising pad without the need to provide a hard copy. Many such systems provide software packages which enable statistical analyses to be carried out on the stored data.

In contrast, digital image processing systems use images stored within the computer memory and allow automatic analysis of the image by a computer program. These systems may utilise desktop computers and specially written software programs or dedicated image processing computers which are more complex but optimised for rapid image processing and analysis. Image input, digitisation and display usually employ a television camera mounted on the microscope. The output voltage analogue signal produced is proportional to the image brightness and is converted into a digital representation of the image by an analogue-to-digital converter. The resulting pixels can be stored in a computer memory for future use. Each pixel in the digitised image is represented by a numerical intensity value or grey-level which may be manipulated to alter the original image as required. In this way, background or unwanted features can be eliminated from analysis and boundaries can be better defined. Such systems are now capable of quantifying enzymatic and immunohistochemical reactions. It must be appreciated, however, that these techniques introduce their own sources of problems and errors and every attempt must be made to control and calibrate all stages if the recordings are to be reliable.

## Analytical cytology

Techniques for quantitative analysis of cellular parameters have been developed in an effort to provide prognostic information in tumour diagnosis. The discipline that aims at such analysis has been termed analytical cytology. Approaches based on image analysis of cytological preparations on glass slides are known as image cytometry, whilst those based on interaction of a cell suspension as it passes through a beam of light fall under the area of flow cytometry.

### Image cytometry

Morphometric analysis of cytological preparations is subject to the same principles as morphometric analysis of tissue sections. Subjective criteria such as enlarged cells, nuclei and nucleoli, anisokaryosis, pleomorphism, disturbed nucleocytoplasmic ratios, altered chromatin pattern and decreased cellular cohesion may be objectively quantified as an increase in cytoplasmic area, nuclear area and nucleolar area, an increased standard deviation of nuclear area, an alteration of shape factors, an alteration of nucleocytoplasmic ratio area, an alteration of nuclear texture parameters and an expression of a small cluster size respectively.

The development of sophisticated computerised video-image analysis systems has allowed more automated and accurate cell image analysis, including the subtle photometric analysis of variable staining intensities. In turn, this has allowed an estimation of ploidy through analysis of cells stained specifically for DNA. A prerequisite of all quantitative techniques is the need for standardised conditions which include sample preparation, fixation, staining and calibration of digitised imagery. Information so obtained may be of diagnostic importance in the consideration of borderline malignancy, of prognostic importance and of therapeutic importance in monitoring tumour response to radiotherapy or chemotherapy.

Computerised image analysis systems with algorithmic and neural network capabilities have been developed for screening of cytological smears (discussed in Ch. 14).

### Flow cytometry

Flow cytometry is an automated technique which allows the simultaneous measurement of several cellular parameters as a suspension of cells flows past stationary detectors through a beam of light usually produced by a laser. The light is scattered at various angles by the cells, detected and converted to electronic signals which are digitised and analysed by computer. The typical analysis rate is in the order of several thousand objects per second. The cellular features that can be evaluated include cell size, cytoplasmic granularity, cell viability, cell cycle time, DNA content, surface marker phenotype and enzyme content. The main limitation of flow cytometry is the requirement for the sample to be in a single-cell suspension. This is readily achieved for blood and body fluids and has become a routine technique for analysis of leukaemias and lymphomas in many institutions. Although single-cell suspensions are more difficult to obtain with solid tumours, suitable techniques have been developed so that flow cytometry may be adapted for preparations obtained from thick sections of routine formalin-fixed paraffin-embedded tissue.

The principal uses for flow cytometry in the evaluation of solid tumours are to support a diagnosis of malignancy in borderline lesions and when the morphological changes are equivocal, to provide prognostic information independent of stage and grade, to monitor response to therapy and to establish development of tumour relapse.

## Cell kinetic studies

Following completion of mitosis, daughter cells enter the Gap (G1) phase of the cell cycle which varies in length according to the type of tissue. The next phase in the cell cycle is the DNA synthesis (S) phase during which cellular genetic material is doubled. A second Gap (G2) phase occurs before the cell undergoes mitosis again (M phase). The time between two mitoses is often referred to as the cell cycle time and this varies according to the length of the G1 phase. Tritiated thymidine uptake is the gold standard for the determination of S-phase cells but the technique is cumbersome, laborious and requires the use of fresh tissue, culture techniques and radioisotopes. A number of simpler methods have been devised to assess the phases of the cell cycle and to correlate these measurements with the biological behaviour of the tumour cell.

### Mitotic count

One of the most widely used methods to assess cell proliferation, assumed to have prognostic implication in oncological pathology, is the mitotic count. This is usually given as the number of mitoses per ten high-power fields (HPF). Although accepted as being the single most reliable predictor of behaviour in some tumours,

e.g. smooth muscle tumours, there are a number of pitfalls which should be avoided if this parameter is used. It cannot be assumed that all mitotically active tumours are necessarily aggressive. Basal cell carcinomas are amongst some of the most mitotically active tumours and yet they rarely, if ever, metastasise. It is essential, therefore, in using the mitotic count as a prognostic parameter, to know those tumours to which it should be applied and the site of origin of a particular tumour, e.g. a smooth muscle tumour of a given mitotic count may be regarded as malignant in the gastrointestinal tract but benign in the uterus.

In assessing mitotic counts, further factors need to be considered. The area included in a HPF may differ markedly depending on the objective and eyepiece lenses used. To overcome this problem, the mitotic count is best expressed per square millimetre of tissue but this is seldom performed in practice. Failure to distinguish between mitoses and pyknotic nuclei, failure to locate the most active region or 'hot spot' on the slide, variation in the number of fields counted and variation in the thickness of the section are further reasons for inter-observer variation. Furthermore, the mitotic count fails to take into account the cell size: a tumour composed of large cells will contain fewer cells and thereby fewer mitoses per HPF than a tumour composed of small cells having the same mitotic index.

The mitotic index is the fraction of cells undergoing mitoses expressed as a percentage of the total number of cells. Whilst this is a more accurate measurement, the method is more time consuming and its role in routine diagnostic histopathology has not yet been fully evaluated. If the mitotic count is to be used as a prognostic parameter, it must be considered in conjunction with other pathological and clinical findings.

## Nucleolar organiser regions

Nucleolar organiser regions (NORs) are loops of DNA which are present in the nucleoli of cells and which transcribe to ribosomal RNA. They are of relevance in the ultimate synthesis of protein. The numbers and configurations of these NORs may reflect the activity of the cell. NORs are readily identified by argyrophilic staining techniques (AgNORs). When applied to metaphase chromosome spreads, their demonstration has been used by cytogeneticists in the analysis of genetic disorders. Modifications of the stain enable the identification of AgNORs as black intranuclear dots in paraffin sections.

Although it is not known exactly what the AgNOR count measures, the results of many studies show a significant difference between benign and malignant lesions and between low and high grade tumours. More recent studies, however, indicate that the count is not likely to be of help in differentiating borderline lesions and the significance and practical application of the AgNOR count requires further evaluation.

## Ki-67 nuclear antigen

The Ki-67 mouse monoclonal antibody recognises a nuclear antigen present only in proliferating cells at all stages of the cell cycle except G0. The number of cells labelled by the antibody is said to represent the number of cells cycling at any one time. Various workers have reported good correlation between Ki-67 positivity and cell proliferation data obtained through other techniques including tritiated thymidine uptake. The Ki-67 antibody suffers from the handicap of being reactive only in frozen sections, but newer antibodies such as polyclonal Ki-67, MIB-1, Ki-S1 and Ki-55 have been made to identify the formalin-resistant epitope of the Ki-67 antigen. Antibodies to proliferating cell nuclear antigen (PCNA) have also been produced but several studies have suggested that PCNA may be expressed in non-cycling cells. A recently produced antibody, statin, stains non-cycling cells so that both cycling and non-cycling cells can now be assessed by immunostaining. The ability to stain for proliferating cells in paraffin sections promises to be a potentially powerful biological parameter for some tumours.

## Flow cytometry

In addition to providing information on morphometric cellular parameters, flow cytometry may be used to quantify cellular DNA content and to analyse cell cycle distribution. The DNA index or ploidy status of a cell may be analysed by flow cytometry of a cell suspension which has been stained with DNA-specific fluorochrome dyes. The DNA index is the ratio of the G0/G1 test cells compared to a standard diploid cell population. A diploid cell has an index of 1.00 compared to an index of 2.00 for a tetraploid cell and >2.00 for an aneuploid or polyploid cell. The S-phase content and proliferative activity of the sample can also be determined from the histogram produced.

The majority of tumours display homogeneity of ploidy status although some tumours, e.g. colorectal carcinomas, may display heterogeneity. The finding of a diploid population within an otherwise aneuploid tumour is usually due to incorporation of benign diploid stromal or inflammatory cells. Such contamination is a major drawback of homogenised suspensions, but the identification of tumour cells with antibodies makes it possible to overcome this problem.

A number of studies have shown that ploidy correlates well with overall survival rates, risk of recurrence and clinical stage for a variety of tumours including breast carcinomas, ovarian tumours, bladder cancers and non-Hodgkin's lymphomas. However, other studies indicate that at best, ploidy is a weak predictor of tumour behaviour. Ploidy has also been shown to be a useful adjunct in the diagnosis of ovarian borderline lesions. Borderline tumours are diploid whereas aneuploidy implies aggressive behaviour. However, again, care is required with the interpretation in some lesions, e.g. as many as 16% of melanocytic naevi have been shown to be aneuploid and some malignant tumours may be diploid. Flow cytometry is a useful tool in assessing the S-phase fraction of a tumour cell population, a parameter of established prognostic relevance for a variety of tumours.

## Other prognostic parameters

In addition to the cell kinetic markers outlined above and routine immunohistochemical methods in use for tumour diagnosis, the estimation of basement membrane integrity and confirmation of vascular or lymphatic permeation, and a number of other markers, have been shown to be of prognostic and therapeutic significance in tumour pathology.

### Receptors for hormones and growth factors

Hormones and growth factors have trophic effects on tissues and may influence the behaviour of tumours. Biochemical assays for such receptors performed on tumour homogenates are now being replaced by immunohistochemical techniques on formalin-fixed, paraffin-embedded tissue sections, the latter having the important advantage of morphological correlation.

The most characterised receptors of prognostic significance are the steroid receptors for oestrogen (ER) and progesterone (PR) in breast carcinoma and several other tumours. Patients whose tumours express ER survive longer than those whose tumours are ER poor or negative, and ER positive tumours show a higher rate of response to hormonal manipulation and therapy. A variety of other oestrogen-induced proteins such as PR and pS2 have been shown to be of prognostic relevance in breast cancer and the expression of growth factor receptors such as epidermal growth factor receptor (EGFR) and *c-erbB*-2 correlate with poor outcome and tumour aggressiveness in tumours such as breast and bladder cancers.

### Oncogene and tumour-suppressor gene expression

Most data on the prognostic significance of oncogene expression have been obtained from the immunohistochemical demonstration of the oncoprotein (oncogene product) rather than detection of the amplified gene (oncogene) or its message (mRNA).

*c-erbB*-2 (HER2 or neu) encodes for an oncoprotein located on the cell membrane. Invasive breast carcinomas expressing this oncoprotein are associated with a poorer survival and strong expression correlates with high nuclear grade in ductal carcinoma in situ of the breast.

The oncoprotein *c-myc* interacts with nuclear DNA to stimulate DNA synthesis. Increased expression may be associated with tumour development and progression in terms of a more aggressive behaviour, a shorter disease-free interval and reduced survival.

Increased expression of the p21 *ras* oncoprotein has been reported in hepatocellular and colonic carcinomas. As yet, studies have failed to show correlation of expression with clinical outcome. The p53 gene located on chromosome 17p is an example of a tumour suppressor gene. It is a DNA binding protein that inactivates gene transcription and the loss of this function correlates with loss of the ability to suppress transformation. Loss of p53 function occurs by loss of both p53 alleles, by loss of one allele with a mutation which inactivates the other, or by a dominantly acting mutation in one allele which suppresses the wild-type protein encoded by the normal allele. Germline p53 mutations are associated with familial cancer syndromes such as the Li–Fraumeni syndrome.

Other cancer-associated genes such as the anti-apoptosis genes represented by the *bcl*-2 gene and p53 gene, the anti-metastasis gene represented by the nm 23 genes and multidrug resistance genes may have important prognostic and therapeutic relevance and can now be assessed by immunohistochemical staining.

## Biochemical assays and enzyme techniques

With the development of antigen (epitope) retrieval methods for immunoperoxidase detection of receptors and tumour markers and the development of sophisticated computerised quantitative analysis techniques, biochemical assays for quantitative assessment of prognostic and therapeutic parameters such as hormone receptors in breast carcinoma are gradually becoming redundant, obviating the need for the rapid submission of fresh frozen material for biochemical analyses. Enzyme histochemistry, however, is still used in surgical pathology laboratories, particularly for the assessment of skeletal muscle biopsies, the rapid detection of ganglia and nerves in suspected cases of Hirschprung's disease, the demonstration of specific lactase or sucrase deficiency in jejunal biopsies and the demonstration of various white blood cells and mast cells. Although some enzyme techniques may be carried out on formalin-fixed, paraffin-embedded tissue sections, the majority require cryostat sections of fresh frozen tissue.

## Cytogenetic studies

Cytogenetics is the study of chromosome morphology and function and requires the examination of dividing cell populations. Human cytogenetics was developed in the mid 1950s using colchicine to arrest cells in metaphase, and a hypotonic solution to spread the chromosomes on glass slides. More recent developments in molecular biology and recombinant DNA technology have allowed correlation of chromosomal morphology at the light microscope level with molecular events at the gene level. Although most specimens submitted for cytogenetics are usually sent directly by the clinician, there are a number of situations where specimens submitted for diagnostic histopathology may require submission of tissue for cytogenetic studies.

Cytogenetic studies may be performed on tissue from patients or fetuses with congenital anomalies or abnormalities of sex differentiation. Peripheral blood provides a ready source of lymphocytes that can be stimulated to divide. Skin biopsy specimens or other tissues obtained at surgery may be processed for tissue culture on which cytogenetics can be performed. Prenatal diagnosis of fetal disorders, e.g., Down's syndrome, can be made from cytogenetic studies of amniotic fluid or chorionic villus sampling. Amniotic fluid has the additional advantage of being able to be analysed for alpha-fetoprotein content, an indicator of neural tube defects. Cytogenetics may also be used to identify chromosomal abnormalities in certain neoplastic states, e.g. Philadelphia chromosome in chronic myeloid leukaemia, various translocations in acute myeloid leukaemia, acute lymphoblastic leukaemia, certain lymphomas and solid tumours, and chromosomal deletions in solid tumours such as retinoblastoma and Wilm's tumour. Cytogenetics is particularly useful in some soft tissue tumours and aids in diagnosis. A list of common cytogenetic abnormalities in such tumours is provided in Table 7.1.

**Table 7.1** Specific translocations of diagnostic relevance in soft tissue tumours

| Tumour | Characteristic cytogenetic abnormality |
|---|---|
| Alveolar rhabdomyosarcoma | t(2;13)(q35–37;q14) |
| Ewing's sarcoma/ Askin's tumour/peripheral neuroepithelial tumour | t(11;22)(q21–24;q11–13) |
| Intra-abdominal desmoplastic small round cell tumour | t(11;22)(p13;q11.2–12) |
| Synovial sarcoma | t(x;18)(p11.2;q11.2) |
| Clear cell sarcoma | t(12;22)(q13–14;q12–13) |
| Myxoid liposarcoma | t(12;16)(q13;p11) |
| Extraskeletal myxoid chondrosarcoma | t(9;22)(q22;q11–12) |

The specimen for cytogenetic studies should be an aseptic sample of viable cells that can be later stimulated to grow.

Mitosis is subsequently arrested and the chromosomes examined in prometaphase or metaphase spreads. Although specimens for consideration of cytogenetics must be received unfixed and generally should be placed in appropriate tissue culture transport media such as RPMI 1640 as soon as possible upon receipt, some delay in transfer and transport of the specimens is often not crucial. Many viable specimens will survive transport for up to a week whilst specimens collected at post-mortem often yield satisfactory results, although this depends on the nature of the tissues.

Numerical abnormalities, when the number of chromosomes differs from the normal 46,XY or 46,XX, is referred to as aneuploidy. Care must be taken to ensure that aneuploidy is not a consequence of an artefact in preparation or part of mosaicism. Mosaicism refers to the presence of two or more cell lines in the one individual, e.g. 45,X/46,XX. Examples of numerical chromosomal aberrations include 45,X or monosomy for X; 47,XY + 13 or trisomy for chromosome 13; 69,XXY or triploidy and 92,XXXX or tetraploidy. The analysis of structural abnormalities is often more difficult.

Chromosomes may be recognised by their length, arm ratios, presence of secondary constrictions and the presence of satellites. The chromosomes are photographed and the karyotype constructed by fitting the cut-outs of the photographed chromosomes to a karyotype form which lists them according to size and number. Banding techniques allow the distinction of different regions as recognised by lighter and darker staining intensities. Bands are identified according to the chromosome number, arm symbol, region number and band number, e.g. 2p23 refers to chromosome 2, short arm (p), region 2 and band 3. Structural abnormalities include isochromosomes, deletions, inversions, duplications, translocations, insertions, rings and dicentrics.

# Molecular studies

Central to the rapidly advancing field of molecular pathology are the nucleic acids DNA and RNA. Each is composed of four building blocks known as nucleotides which in turn consist of a base and a triphosphate group attached to a 5-carbon sugar. The nucleotides are connected to form a chain that comprises the nucleic acid sequence. DNA is composed of two paired chains which are complementary to each other while RNA is composed of a single strand. For DNA, the bases are adenine (A), cytosine (C), guanine (G) and thymine (T) and the sugar is deoxyribose. For RNA, the bases are A, C, G and uracil substitutes for thymine and the sugar is ribose. Complementary strands of DNA are held together by hydrogen bonds between the matched pair bases A and T, and C and G.

## Nucleic acid hybridisation

When two DNA strands meet, they orient each other in an antiparallel direction to allow base pair matching. If there is sufficient base pair matching, they will join together or hybridise. The degree of base pair matching or homology determines whether the strands stay together. The term stringency refers to conditions which favour hydrogen bond formation and thus hybridisation. High stringency refers to conditions that do not favour the formation of hydrogen bonds and require greater homology for the strands to remain hybridised. Under low stringency conditions, strands remain hybridised unless homology is very low. Denaturation is the separation of DNA strands. The ratio of hybridised/denatured DNA depends on the degree of homology and any condition that influences hydrogen bonding, e.g. temperature. The melting temperature (Tm) refers to the temperature at which one half of the strands remain hybridised and one half is denatured for any given reaction conditions. In hybridisation assays, the probe is a labelled complementary sequence of DNA which is capable of hybridising to the target sequence of DNA under investigation. The target sequence of heat-denatured DNA will hybridise to the labelled probe when the temperature is lowered. This forms the basis of hybridisation-based analyses.

## Hybridisation assays

Several hybridisation techniques are available for detection of nucleic acid sequences. DNA extracted from a tissue may be bound to a filter (filter hybridisation) or placed on a filter with the aid of a vacuum manifold that has slot-like spaces for each sample (slot or dot blot hybridisation) and hybridised with the labelled probe. Alternatively, the DNA may first be separated according to size and configuration by gel electrophoresis and then transferred to a filter for hybridisation (Southern blot hybridisation). Northern blot hybridisation refers to hybridisation of RNA with complementary DNA. In these techniques, the tissue is destroyed, precluding direct histological correlation.

In in situ hybridisation, the target DNA is not extracted from the tissue but kept in the intact cell where it binds to the probe. This can be carried out on tissue sections where direct morphological correlation may be made. Furthermore, in situ hybridisation is more rapid and requires less tissue but is less sensitive than Southern blotting.

## Polymerase chain reaction

The polymerase chain reaction (PCR) amplifies specific DNA targets exponentially and is a more sensitive system than Southern blot hybridisation but requires that at least part of the DNA sequence to be targeted is known. However, the partial or complete sequences of various oncogenes and many viruses are now available so that the technique has extensive diagnostic potentials. Extracted DNA or, in some cases, whole cell lysates may be added to the PCR mixture. Specific DNA oligonucleotide primers which are homologous to regions at each end of the DNA target sequence to be amplified, are allowed to anneal with the target sequence following initial DNA denaturation. The original targets are then duplicated by addition of bases to the primer through the action of a thermostable DNA polymerase (Taq DNA polymerase). The reaction products are again denatured and the whole procedure repeated for many cycles. By using primers that hybridise to both strands of the target DNA, repeated cycles of denaturation, annealing and DNA synthesis result in a geometric amplification of the target sequence. The procedure is conducted in a thermal cycler which heats up to 95°C, causing DNA to denature into two strands. When cooled to 55°C, the primers bind to the complementary sites on the single-stranded DNA. When the temperature is raised to 72°C, new DNA strands are synthesised starting from regions where the primers have bound to the DNA template. Repeated heating and cooling cycles result in this denaturation–synthesis–annealing process. Theoretically, after 30 cycles there will be 109 copies of a single original target and the whole process can be fully automated.

The PCR product can be subsequently separated on agarose or polyacrylamide gels and visualised by staining with ethidium chloride or bromide. PCR is an extremely sensitive, simple and rapid technique requiring only a small amount of DNA which does not need to be fully intact. The main disadvantage is that, because of its sensitivity, contamination of the PCR reaction by very small quantities of extraneous DNA, as little as one part in a million, may give rise to false positive results. Strict precautions to prevent contamination must be taken.

It is now possible to perform PCR in tissue sections and to combine this with in situ hybridisation. In this way, it is possible to identify probe-specific DNA at its sites of production in tissue sections and cell preparations following initial amplification.

## Diagnostic applications

The greatest impact of in situ hybridisation and PCR has been in the identification of organisms which cannot be easily cultured in vitro. PCR has been used for the detection of human pathogens such as human papilloma virus, cytomegalovirus, Epstein–Barr virus, herpes viruses, hepatitis viruses, human immunodeficiency viruses, mycobacteria, toxoplasma, *Trypanosoma cruzi* and malaria.

In the area of oncology, the ability to perform in situ hybridisation and PCR on formalin-fixed, paraffin-embedded tissues has enabled identification of oncogenes, anti-oncogenes and growth factors in a variety of neoplasms. Both nucleic acid hybridisation and PCR can be used to identify rearrangements between single genetic loci. For example, the translocation t(14;18) is a common feature of follicular lymphomas and can be readily detected using these techniques. The extreme sensitivity of PCR has provided the opportunity for detection of residual or recurrent tumour cells (minimal residual disease). Such studies are in their infancy and, as yet, it cannot be assumed that such residual tumour cells have prognostic significance. The identification of oncogenes in morphologically normal tissues may form the basis of identifying persons susceptible to specific tumours. Some amplified genes have been shown to be of relevance in predicting the behaviour of tumours such as the *c-erbB*-2 gene in breast cancer and the p53 mutation in a variety of tumours, including breast cancer, colonic cancer, thyroid cancer and lymphomas.

PCR can detect all of the common genetically inherited diseases in which the defective locus has been identified. It can also trace the inheritance of disease in which the defective locus has only been defined in terms of linkage to other cellular genes and allows more detailed linkage studies than have previously been possible using restriction fragment length polymorphism (RFLP) analysis.

Applications for molecular techniques in forensic pathology are extensive. Identification of minute amounts of DNA from hair, blood, body fluids and exfoliated cells offers enormous advances in forensic medicine. In situ PCR may be applied retrospectively to formalin-fixed, paraffin-embedded tissues obtained from deceased persons who have undergone autopsy many years previously.

The sensitivity and simplicity of these techniques should enable the pathologist to actively participate in the diagnostic, therapeutic and research applications of molecular technology.

## Tissue banks

Various tissue banks serve different functions. Some tissue banks, e.g. bone,

skin and eye banks, serve as reservoirs for transplant purposes; others serve as a source of material for research, retrospective analysis and control tissue samples.

### Bone bank

Bone for transplantation purposes is normally obtained from femoral heads removed during prosthetic replacement for arthritis or fracture. Occasionally, knee joints undergoing prosthetic replacement and long bones removed under sterile conditions from autopsy material may also be used. The collected bone is screened for infection and occult disease, particularly tumours, prior to being irradiated and stored at −70°C for future use. The non-viable transplanted bone acts as a scaffold around which new bone is laid down by the recipient. Femoral heads are used as bone chips packed into the appropriate defect, e.g. a curetted benign osseous lesion. Removal of entire long bones for some osseous neoplasms and replacement with autopsy harvested long bones may obviate the need for amputation. In time, the non-viable transplanted bone is replaced by new bone from the recipient. Submitted bone in which occult malignancy or infection is identified is discarded despite the knowledge that the subsequent irradiation would eradicate any viable disease. It should be emphasised that management of a bone bank for transplantation purposes demands scrupulous attention to detail and close liaison between clinicians, pathologists and bone bank personnel.

### Skin and eye banks

As yet, skin banks are less common than bone banks but skin harvested under sterile conditions at autopsy may be stored and used to provide covering and protection in burns victims. Corneal grafting is now common-place and eye banks have been set up to harvest and store corneas removed at autopsy under sterile conditions. Many of the safety precautions pertaining to bone banking will apply also to skin and eye banking although there is seldom the necessity for routine histological examination. Other organs for transplant such as kidney, liver and lung may require microscopic examination for pathology, particularly infections.

Organ and tumour banks

The storage of other organs and tumours serves to provide a reservoir of tissue for research and retrospective analyses. New techniques having an impact on prognosis and therapy may be applied retrospectively to such tissues. Extraction of hormones for human use from endocrine organs collected at autopsy, e.g. growth hormone from pooled pituitaries, is no longer performed. Many of these hormones can now be synthetically produced in pure form, thus overcoming the danger of transmissible diseases such as Creutzfeldt–Jakob disease.

## Further reading

Heim S, Mitelman F 1992 Cytogenetics of solid tumours. In: Anthony PP, MacSween RNM (eds) Recent advances in histopathology, No 15. Churchill Livingstone, Edinburgh

Leong AS-Y, Lee AKC 1995 Biological indices in the assessment of breast cancer. Journal of Clinical Pathology: Clinical Molecular Pathology 48: M221–M238

Nuovo GJ 1994 PCR in situ hybridisation: protocols and applications. 2nd ed., Raven Press, New York

Polak JM, Varndell IM 1984 Immunolabelling for electron microscopy. Elsevier, Netherlands

# 8  Fixatives, tissue processing and stains

# Tissue fixation

The production of permanent tissue sections comprises several steps. Firstly, the fresh tissue is fixed; next, water and lipids are removed from the tissue during the processes of dehydration and clearing respectively, and the tissue is finally penetrated with paraffin wax. The latter provides a rigid support to enable the cutting of thin sections of high quality.

Cell death with destruction and autolysis is inevitable following the removal of tissue from the body. Autolysis is independent of any bacterial action and is retarded by cold temperature. It is greatly accelerated at temperatures above 30°C and is inhibited by heating to 50°C. Tissue autolysis is more severe in organs rich in enzymes such as the liver, brain and kidney and is less rapid in tissues such as elastic fibre and collagen. There is no accompanying inflammatory or cellular response.

The purpose of fixation is to prevent autolysis and bacterial decomposition and to preserve cells and tissue constituents in as close a life-like state as possible. Fixation is also necessary to allow tissues to undergo, without change, further processing procedures. To achieve this, the process of fixation denatures proteins and preserves other tissue substances, allowing them to undergo the subsequent stages of dehydration, clearing and impregnation for the preparation of thin sections which can be stained with dyes and other reagents. The primary goal is to produce good quality tissue sections, but increasing interest in cell constituents and the extensive use of immunohistochemistry to augment histological diagnosis have imposed additional requirements on the process of fixation, including the preservation of cellular substances and proteins.

A wide variety of fixatives is available but no single substance or combination has the ability to preserve and allow the demonstration of every tissue component; some fixatives have only limited and special applications. The selection of a fixative is based on considerations such as the structures and substances to be demonstrated and the effects of short- and long-term storage.

Various classifications of fixatives have been proposed with major divisions according to function as coagulants and non-coagulants, or according to their chemical nature. Fixatives may also be classified as follows:

1  *Aldehydes:* e.g. formaldehyde, glutaraldehyde.
2  *Oxidising agents:* metallic ions and complexes, e.g. osmium tetroxide, chromic acid.
3  *Protein-denaturing agents:* e.g. acetic acid, methyl alcohol, ethyl alcohol.
4  *Unknown mechanism:* e.g. mercuric chloride, picric acid.
5  *Combined reagents.*
6  *Microwaves.*
7  *Miscellaneous:* excluded volume fixation, vapour fixation.

## Aldehydes and other cross-linking fixatives

### Formaldehyde

Formaldehyde, as 4% buffered formaldehyde (10% buffered formalin), is the most widely employed universal fixative for routine paraffin-embedded sections. It is a colourless liquid or gas with a very pungent odour. It is soluble in water to a maximum extent of 40% by weight, a state known as formalin. Formaldehyde can also be obtained in a stable solid form composed of high molecular weight polymers, and is known as paraformaldehyde. Heated paraformaldehyde generates gaseous formaldehyde which, when dissolved in water, reverts mainly to a monomeric form. Aqueous formaldehyde exists primarily in the form of its monohydrate, methylene glycol, which has been suggested to be the reactive component.

Ten per cent buffered formalin is commonly made up of 100 ml of 40% formaldehyde in 900 ml distilled water with 4 g sodium phosphate, monobasic, and 6.5 g sodium phosphate, dibasic (anhydrous). For effective fixation, specimens need to be submerged completely in five to ten times their volume of fixative for variable periods depending on the size of the specimen. Generally, 2 mm thick tissue blocks are fixed for 4–8 hours in buffered formalin, possibly followed by a further period in formol sublimate.

Ten per cent buffered formalin requires a relatively short fixation time but can also be used for long-term storage. Tissues left in formalin for long periods show no deleterious effects on cell morphology, and nuclear and cytoplasmic details remain adequately preserved.

It is thought that the fixing action of aldehydes is due to the formation of cross-links between proteins, forming a gel which retains cellular constituents in their in vivo relationships to each other. The reaction between protein molecules is mostly with the basic amino acid lysine residues which are situated on the exterior of the protein molecule. Although the degree of protein denaturation is not of importance in routine surgical pathology, denaturation is of particular relevance in the detection of antigens both by immunofluorescence and immunoenzyme techniques, as well as in high resolution electron microscopy. Similarly, the shapes of large molecules must not be changed if they are to be

recognised by biochemical analysis. Unlike formaldehyde, glutaraldehyde can cause a loss of up to 30% of the alpha helix structure of protein.

Formalin does not precipitate proteins and only slightly precipitates other components of the cell. It neither preserves nor destroys adipose tissue and is a good fixative for complex lipids but has no effect on neutral fats. It is not the fixative of choice for carbohydrates but preserves proteins so that they hold glycogen.

Formalin becomes acid on storage by oxidisation to formic acid. This reduces its effectiveness as a preservative and solution neutralisation is essential. In addition, formalin produces acid formalin haematin pigment which deposits in sites containing blood. Neutralisation is usually achieved with phosphate buffers, producing a pH-stable solution for many months. Formalin should not be used with chromates because it readily oxidises to formic acid. Concentrated formalin may revert to paraformaldehyde on storage but can still be utilised following filtration.

Formaldehyde is an immediate irritant to the eyes, upper respiratory tract and skin. If spilt on skin or mucosa, the tissues should be thoroughly washed with water and work with this fixative should be undertaken in areas with proper ventilation and exhaust.

*Glutaraldehyde*

Aqueous solutions of glutaraldehyde (glutaric dialdehyde) are complex and consist of approximately 4% free aldehyde, 16% monohydrate, 9% dihydrate and 70% hemiacetal. Free glutaraldehyde may form polymers which are favoured by some as representing the reactive species, whilst others believe pure monomeric glutaraldehyde is the best fixative. The large range of molecules available in the solution has also been suggested to be responsible for the success at protein cross-linking. Glutaraldehyde is best refrigerated to reduce precipitate formation and a fall in aldehyde levels.

Glutaraldehyde penetrates tissues more slowly than formaldehyde and is mainly used in electron microscopy, enzyme histochemistry and in the biomedical area (e.g. for the chemical sterilisation and preparation of tissue xenografts such as cardiac valves). Due to slow penetration of the fixative, it works best on small blocks of 1–2 mm at cold temperatures of 1–4°C. Fixed tissue specimens can be stored in buffer solutions for many months. The slow penetration, requirement for cold temperature, and need for a storage medium have greatly limited the use of glutaraldehyde as a fixative for routine diagnostic histology, apart from electron microscopy.

## Other aldehyde fixatives

Another aldehyde fixative is acrolein which is a compound acrylic aldehyde sometimes employed as a fixative for enzyme cyto-chemistry. Labile enzymes such as glucose-6-phosphatase are retained in tissues fixed in 4% acrolein. Other cross-linking aldehydes include glyoxal (ethanedial, diformyl), malonaldehyde (malonic dialdehyde), diacetyl (2,3-butanedione) and the polyaldehydes. These have been rarely employed to retain specific enzymes or proteins for histochemistry.

## Oxidising agents – metallic ions and complexes

Even less is known of the action of this group of fixatives with cellular proteins.

## Osmium tetroxide

Osmium tetroxide was once employed as a fixative for cytology but poor penetration limited its use. Currently, its main role is as a secondary fixative for electron microscopy. The rise in viscosity of a protein solution when osmium tetroxide is added suggests that cross-linking has occurred, but its prime reactivity is with lipids. Osmium tetroxide is reduced by unsaturated lipids with the formation of black compounds containing hexavalent osmium. For electron microscopy, osmium tetroxide is used for the preservation of fine structure. If used as a fixative for light microscopy, the tissues often crumble when embedded in paraffin and there is interference with many staining procedures.

## Chromic acid

Chromic acid (chromium trioxide) is a strong oxidising agent and is used with other ingredients. It has no effect on fats and penetrates slowly so that tissues are susceptible to shrinkage during subsequent processing steps. Chromium salts form complexes with water which combine with reactive protein groups to form a cross-linking effect similar to that of formaldehyde.

## Potassium dichromate

Potassium dichromate reacts with adrenal medulla catecholamines to produce black or brown water-insoluble precipitates. The dichromate-oxidation product is visible grossly and is also seen in tissue sections. It is employed as a rapid means of identifying tissues containing aromatic amines such as adrenal medulla tumours. If used other than for amine demonstration, thorough washing is required to remove the oxide that forms otherwise it cannot be removed during subsequent processing.

## Protein-denaturing agents

### Methyl and ethyl alcohols

Methyl and ethyl alcohols function as fixatives by bringing about alteration of the structure of the protein molecule primarily due to disruption of the hydrophobic bonds which are important in the maintenance of the tertiary structure of proteins. Hydrogen bonds appear to be more stable in methanol and ethanol than in water, so that while affecting the tertiary structure of proteins, these alcohols may preserve their secondary structure. Both methanol and ethanol are closely related in structure to water and replace bound and unbound water molecules in the tissues during the process of fixation. Absolute alcohol (ethanol) preserves glycogen but can cause distortion of nuclear detail and shrinkage of cytoplasm. If fixation in alcohol is prolonged, histones will be removed from the nuclei, followed later by RNA and DNA.

### Methacarn

Methacarn, a 6 : 3 : 1 mixture of absolute methanol, chloroform and glacial acetic acid, has been used to preserve helical proteins in myofibrils and collagen. More recently, it has been employed as the fixative of choice for the demonstration of intermediate filaments by immunostaining.

Acetic acid is never used alone as a fixative, but is often combined with other fixatives that cause shrinkage such as ethanol and methanol. Acetic acid penetrates thoroughly and rapidly but produces lysis of red blood cells.

## Fixation by unknown mechanisms

### Picric acid

Picric acid is often used in combination with other reagents and produces precipitation of all proteins. It penetrates well and leaves the tissues soft. The acid continues to react with tissue structures and causes a loss of basophilia, so that thorough washing following fixation is essential.

### Mercuric chloride and other mercuric salts

Mercuric chloride and other salts of mercury were frequently used as fixatives due to their rapid penetration and precipitation of all proteins, reacting with a number of amino acid residues including thiol, amino, imidazole, phosphate and hydroxyl groups. Production of hydrogen ions makes the fixative solution more acidic and deposition of mercuric crystals in the tissues requires removal by iodine and then sodium thiosulphate, prior to staining. Mercuric chloride is contained in Zenker's, Helly's, Ridley's and B5 solutions. These fixatives penetrate poorly so tissue blocks must be thin. Over-fixation causes tissue brittleness, so that as soon as fixation is complete blocks should be placed in 70% alcohol. Mercury-based fixatives amplify stains but interfere with certain reactions such as the detection of esterase. Mercuric salts have lost their popularity as fixatives as they are highly poisonous and require special disposal. One method of disposal involves precipitating the salts with thioacetamide. Because mercury is a toxic environmental pollutant, its use in the laboratory should be strictly restricted.

## Other heavy metal salts

Recently, heavy metal salts such as zinc have been employed as protein precipitants in an attempt to enhance immunostaining of cellular antigens. Zinc sulphate in formalin tends to deposit formalin pigment by lowering the pH. This can be avoided by using zinc chloride.

## Acetone

Acetone has been exploited as a dehydrating agent in tissue processing and is more volatile than the alcohols and other dehydrants. It is a clear, colourless and inflammable liquid which is miscible with water, ethanol and most organic solvents. Although rapid, it causes tissue brittleness on prolonged exposure and its volatility prevents its use in automated processing schedules. Acetone has a greater solvent action on lipids and is rapidly removed by most clearing agents, making it very useful in manual tissue processing.

Of late, acetone has been employed as a fixative in the acetone-methylbenzoate-xylene (AMEX) technique designed for the preservation of labile lymphocyte membrane antigens. The method requires overnight fixation of tissues in acetone at −20°C, clearing in methylbenzoate and xylene before paraffin embedding. The result is claimed to show improved histological preservation over that of cryostat sections which are normally required for the demonstration of many labile lymphocyte antigens.

## Microwave irradiation

Microwave irradiation (MW) can be used as a primary fixative or employed to accelerate the action of conventional cross-linking fixatives such as formaldehyde and glutaraldehyde. Although it has been known for a long time that heat can denature protein, it was not until the arrival of microwave technology that the primary problem of non-uniform tissue heating was overcome. There is a variation in optimal temperatures for the fixation of different tissues but satisfactory fixation of most tissues is obtained by heating to a temperature range of 52–72°C. This is achieved by immersing tissue blocks contained in cassettes in a container of normal saline and irradiating in a domestic microwave oven to a saline temperature of about 68°C. The time required will vary with the volume of tissue being fixed and the voltage of the microwave oven. Domestic MW ovens operating at 2.45 GHz and at 600 W output will accomplish fixation of a small volume of tissue in about 120 seconds. The use of a rotating plate or carousel allows a more even distribution of the electromagnetic waves and a digital timer improves accuracy. The temperature attained for a fixed volume of tissue and saline is proportional to the duration of electromagnetic flux and ovens may thus be readily calibrated; however, models with temperature probes make operation even easier.

Specimens should continue to be transported in 10% buffered formalin to prevent autolysis and the problems which are inevitably encountered in the transportation of fresh unfixed tissue. Two millimetre thick tissue samples are placed in cassettes, completely immersed in normal saline and irradiated to a temperature of 68°C. For convenience, 20 cassettes are placed in each of three glass containers of normal saline, equidistantly located at the periphery of the rotating dish of a 2.45 GHz and 600 W output domestic microwave oven. The best compromise temperature for optimal morphological preservation and retention of tissue antigens is 68°C. On attaining this temperature, tissues are held in the hot saline for a further 30 seconds and then processed through cycles of absolute alcohol, chloroform or xylene, and wax in a vacuum-assisted automated processor. The elimination of formalin from routine processing aids in the preservation of tissue antigens. Cycles of 1.5 and 3.5 hours are used, the former for endoscopic and other small biopsies, and the latter for virtually all other tissue blocks. For convenience, an overnight cycle of 16.5 hours can still be used. In the interim between microwave irradiation and commencement of tissue processing, the tissue blocks can be contained in 70% alcohol, Carnoy's solution, 10% buffered formalin, or even normal saline. The first two solutions are particularly useful for tissues that contain large quantities of adipose tissue, whereas 10% formalin is useful for larger pieces of skin and dense tissue such as myometrium whose morphological preservation appears to be enhanced by a brief period of immersion of about 30 minutes in formalin. This exposure to formalin can also be done prior to MW irradiation.

MWs can also be employed to harden large specimens such as stomach, solid organs and segments of bowel by irradiating in normal saline to 68°C. MWs have limited penetration in solid tissues and temperature gradients make it impossible to accomplish uniform fixation in large specimens so that MWs are employed primarily to harden the specimens to allow easy handling and dissection avoiding the necessity of overnight formalin fixation. Optimal fixation is achieved by further irradiating the sampled tissue blocks to 68°C in the manner described above.

MW fixation does not result in any deleterious effect on special stains and cellular antigen preservation is better than that obtained with 10% formalin. Skin and myometrium is best placed in 10% buffered formalin for 30 minutes prior to MW fixation in saline. Lipid-rich tissues should be briefly cleared in 70% alcohol before exposure to microwaves.

MWs can also be used to accelerate fixation by 10% formalin or by alcohols. This accelerated fixation, however, results in the generation of formalin fumes within the oven. Fixation by glutaraldehyde can similarly be accelerated by MW irradiation. Following irradiation to 50°C, requiring about 5–10 seconds, the tissue is either stored in 0.1 M sodium cacodylate buffer with 0.02% sodium azide or immediately processed.

The mechanism of fixation by MWs, a form of non-ionising radiation, is controversial. Heat is considered to be the primary factor responsible but the rapid movement of molecules within the electromagnetic flux may itself have a direct role in accelerating chemical reactions. The diffusion of monomers or dimers in aldehyde solutions is enhanced by exposure to MWs and low intensity MW fields may affect the integrity of non-covalent secondary bonding.

## Other methods of fixation

These are all not commonly used. When polymers are added to a reaction mixture, small diffusible molecules are fixed, their capability to diffuse dependent on molecule size and polymer concentration. This process is called excluded volume fixation and 20% polyvinyl alcohol or 20% polyethylene glycol (Carbowax 6000) have been used.

Another method is vapour fixation. It is possible to retain soluble materials in situ by converting them into insoluble products before contacting water or non-aqueous solvents. Formaldehyde has been mainly used in this method and its primary application, at raised temperature, is to convert catecholamines and 5-hydroxy-tryptamine in freeze-dried tissue to produce fluorescent condensation products.

Freeze-drying can preserve labile lymphocyte antigens but the method is cumbersome, the resultant tissues brittle and morphology suboptimal. A recently developed alternative with improved morphology utilises freeze substitution with low temperature plastic embedding.

## Post-fixation

Wet tissue may be subjected to post-fixation or secondary fixation when the primary fixation process is not optimal. For example, mercuric chloride fixation may follow buffered formalin fixation with improvement to subsequent staining. Osmium tetroxide is often used after glutaraldehyde as a post-fixative to improve cell membrane staining for ultrastructural examination. Post-fixation in heavy metal salt solutions such as zinc formalin precipitates proteins and may enhance immunostaining.

## Fixation mixtures and additives

A mixture of osmium tetroxide and glutaraldehyde is a useful fixative for neutral fat and the fine structural localisation of acid phosphatase. Osmium tetroxide-zinc iodide post-fixation has been used to delineate synaptic vesicles and Langerhans' cells. Tannic acid is sometimes added to fixative solutions to enhance precipitation of proteins and act as a mordant for heavy metal staining. Two per cent phenol accelerates the action of formaldehyde as a fixative, improves morphological detail, reduces shrinkage

and removes formalin pigment. The salts of transitional metals such as zinc sulphate can be added to formalin to enhance antigen preservation and immunostaining. Detergents such as saponin may be added to primary fixatives but their deleterious effect on cytological detail restricts their application to special situations.

## Factors influencing fixation

### Temperature

Temperature affects fixation. Whilst most surgical specimens are fixed at room temperature, the optimal fixation temperature for specimens for electron microscopy and some histochemical procedures is 0–4°C. Lower temperatures may retard autolysis and diffusion of cell components but a contrary argument is that the fixation reactions are accelerated at high temperature, albeit with increased tissue distortion.

### Specimen size

The specimen size influences the fixation rate as the penetration of fixatives into tissue is a relatively slow process. Tissue blocks should therefore be cut small or thin and large specimens such as bowel need to be opened and pinned on corkboard or sliced before immersion in a container of formalin to achieve optimal fixation. Alternatively, they may be hardened by microwaves to allow immediate dissection so that the sampled tissue blocks can then be properly fixed by further exposure to microwaves or by formalin. For electron microscopy, tissues must be diced before fixation in glutaraldehyde.

### Fixative concentration

Some fixatives are effective within a range of different concentrations.

Glutaraldehyde, normally used at a 4% solution, is effective as low as 0.25%, provided pH is maintained in the physiological range.

The process of fixation alters tissue volume due to factors such as inhibition of cell respiration and changes in membrane permeability and ion transport. It has been estimated that tissue fixed in formaldehyde and embedded in paraffin wax shrinks by around 33%. The buffering of fixative solutions alters the osmotic pressure exerted by the solution. Hypertonic solutions cause cell shrinkage whilst hypotonic solutions result in cell swelling and poor fixation. For electron microscopy, slightly hypertonic solutions are best and sucrose is commonly added to osmium tetroxide.

### pH of fixative

Fixation is altered by changes in pH and for most fixatives the hydrogen ion concentration is kept in the pH range 6–8 by buffer systems such as phosphate, s-collidine, bicarbonate, Tris, veronal acetate and cacodylate.The buffer should not react with the fixative or inhibit enzymes, otherwise histochemistry stains would be affected.

## Fixation of specific tissue substances

### Glycogen

Identification of glycogen is helpful in the investigation of glycogen storage disorders and some tumours, e.g. renal cell carcinoma. Many glycogens show varying degrees of polymerisation in their natural state and the smaller molecules are readily lost in routine fixatives. Glycogen retention is

thought to result from trapping in a matrix of fixed protein or covalent binding to protein which renders it insoluble in water. Dehydration of cells decreases the solubility of glycogen and alcohol remains the main method of fixing glycogen. Bouin's fixative is also useful.

### Lipids

Lipids are largely lost with routine tissue processing. Osmium tetroxide and chromic acid are the only true lipid-fixing reagents, rendering them insoluble. Several other fixatives preserve lipids, e.g. Baker's fixative for phospholipids, but they do not alter their solubility in lipid solvents used later in tissue processing. The demonstration of lipids is best performed in cryostat sections which are fixed with reagents containing mercuric chloride and potassium dichromate such as Elftman's fluid, with fixation of unsaturated lipids completed over 3 days at room temperature. For electron microscopy, lipids are demonstrated by mixing additives with glutaraldehyde. These include digitonin for cholesterol and Malachite Green or Karnovsky's fixative for phospholipids and glycolipids. Imidazole has been used as an additive for the demonstration of unsaturated fatty acids and phospholipids following glutaraldehyde fixation.

### Proteins

Tissue proteins are preserved adequately by most fixatives if the process is allowed to proceed for 1–2 days. Glutaraldehyde is a more rapid fixative of proteins whereas formaldehyde reacts reversibly over the first 24 hours. Prolonged exposure to osmium tetroxide causes the breakdown of proteins.

## Nucleic acids

The nucleic acids exist in many different states of polymerisation and any method of fixation induces changes in their physical state. Formalin is not a good fixative for nucleic acids as it blocks a number of reactive groups, resulting in reduced stainability by both basic and acid dyes. This can be improved when mercury or chromium salts are added. The precipitant fixatives such as alcohol, acetic acid and Carnoy's give excellent nuclear morphology by breaking the bonds between nucleic acids and proteins, increasing the available acid groups and increasing basophilic staining. Long fixation in acid fixatives damages nuclear proteins.

## Mucosubstances

Mucosubstances tend to be lost during fixation. They include the homoglycans (glucose, starch and cellulose), heteroglycans (keratosulphate, sialoglycans, hyaluronic acid, chondroitin sulphate and heparin) and the protein-polysaccharide complexes known as proteoglycans. Four per cent basic lead citrate or 1% lead citrate are used as fixatives for acid heteroglycans whilst alcoholic 8% lead nitrate with or without 10% formalin has been employed for connective tissue glycosoaminoglucoronoglycans. For acid mucins, formalin-alcohol mixtures with calcium acetate have been used whilst formalin has always been a fixative component for the demonstration of proteoglycans. Seventy to eighty per cent ethanol for 3–6 days before clearing reduces the diffusion of the soluble hetero- and proteoglycans. Freeze-drying followed by hot formalin vapour is more successful in preserving all types of mucin compared to other fixation methods. Cationic dyes such as toluidine blue have been introduced for electron microscopic demonstration of mucosubstances without prior fixation with glutaraldehyde.

## Biogenic amines

These comprise two main groups: the catecholamines, noradrenaline and adrenaline, and the indolalkylamines, dopamine, DOPA and 5-hydroxytryptamine. The chromaffin reaction may be demonstrated by fixing the tissue in a solution of formalin with sodium acetate and potassium dichromate. The biogenic amines can also be visualised by formaldehyde-induced fluorescence. The most effective method to retain biogenic amines for ultrastructural examination is a three-stage fixation procedure, with primary fixation in 1% glutaraldehyde, 0.4% formaldehyde, sodium chromate and potassium dichromate, followed by 18 hours storage in sodium chromate and potassium dichromate, and post-fixation in 2% osmium tetroxide, sodium chromate and potassium dichromate.

# Decalcification

Undecalcified bone biopsy samples are important in the investigation of metabolic bone disease but in most non-specialised histopathology laboratories, bone and other heavily calcified tissues require decalcification prior to processing. The calcified specimens need to be thoroughly fixed before decalcification otherwise poor nuclear staining results.

There are two main types of decalcifying agents: acids and chelating agents. The choice is influenced by the case urgency, the extent of specimen mineralisation and the possible additional techniques that may need to be employed. Any acid has some effect on the stain uptake of tissues, increasing with acidity and duration of exposure. Thus, the more rapid the decalcifier, the more injurious are its effects on staining.

## Acid decalcifiers

These are categorised into strong and weak acid groups, the former represented by hydrochloric acid and nitric acid, and the latter by formic, acetic and picric acid. An aqueous solution of 9.5% nitric acid decalcifies rapidly. The acid should be changed two to three times during the first 24 hours. Fresh or urea-stabilised solution should be used to prevent tissue yellowing. Three millimetre bone trephine specimens decalcify in 3.5–5 hours whist solid bones may take up to 3 days. Formic acid is much slower and gentler to the tissue, and is used as a 5–10% aqueous solution or with additives such as formalin or a buffer. It is used mainly for non-urgent cases, decalcification taking 1–10 days depending on the size and type of calcified specimen. Carnoy's fixative contains acetic acid and has been used in urgent cases where the tissues are only lightly calcified.

## Chelating agents

EDTA (ethylenediaminetetra-acetic acid) is the most commonly used chemical. It does not act as a mineral or organic acid but removes metallic ions, mainly calcium, by chelation, progressively from the surface. The process is slow but has no effect on cell morphology and some enzymes remain active. EDTA takes 7 days to decalcify 2 mm bone trephines.

The rate of decalcification is accelerated by changing the solution daily, increasing the concentration of the solution and raising the temperature. The effect of agitation, suspension, microwaves and ultrasonics is more controversial. Ion exchange resins have also been employed to speed up decalcification by removing liberated calcium from the solution.

## Decalcification endpoint

It is desirable to minimise the time tissues spend in decalcifying solutions and a number of methods have been devised to assess the decalcification endpoint to achieve this objective. The two most reliable are radiological and chemical. Physical tests such as cutting, trimming, needling and bending will damage the tissue and, at best, are only a guide. Taking daily radiographs of specimens in a Faxitron is a convenient and accurate method.

The chemical methods detect residual calcium by the precipitation of visible calcium salts and the endpoint is a negative test. For example, the addition of ammonium hydroxide and ammonium oxalate to a solution with calcium salts produces white calcium oxalate. Chemical endpoints cannot be assessed following decalcification by EDTA.

Following decalcification, specimens should be neutralised with 6% aqueous sodium sulphoxide or washed in tap water to remove acids before dehydration, and secondary fixation in mercuric chloride-formalin will do much to counteract the deleterious effect of acids used in decalcification.

# Dehydration

After fixation, complete dehydration of the tissues can be effected with any of several dehydrants. Most laboratories use graded alcohols. Dehydration is part of all processing methods except those employing a water miscible embedding medium.

### Alcohols

Alcohols used for dehydration include ethanol (ethyl alcohol), industrial methylated spirit (denatured alcohol), methanol (methyl alcohol) and isopropyl alcohol. The most commonly used is denatured alcohol. This is ethanol to which has been added some methanol to make it unpalatable for consumption and to avoid excise duties. It is a clear, colourless, flammable, hydrophilic liquid which can effectively be regarded as absolute alcohol for dilution purposes. Tissues are typically first immersed in 50–70% alcohol, progressing through 95% alcohol to several cycles of absolute alcohol. Contamination of absolute alcohol by lower grade alcohols results in incomplete clearing and paraffin infiltration, with section disintegration. Isopropyl alcohol is not commonly used but it does not harden tissues like ethanol.

### Acetone

Acetone is a liquid which is colourless, clear, inflammable and has a pungent odour. It is miscible with water, ethanol and the majority of organic solvents. Although fast in action and cheap, it is not generally used due to its volatility and tendency to cause tissue shrinkage, distortion, hardness and brittleness. Its main role is in some manual processing schedules.

### Dioxane and tetrahydrofuran

Both these liquids can be used as simultaneous dehydrating and clearing agents. Dioxane is fast but its fumes are highly toxic. Tetrahydrofuran is less toxic but expensive.

### Solid dehydrants

Anhydrous copper sulphate can be added to dehydration containers, and following water absorption from the tissue the fluid turns blue.

### Chemical dehydration

These techniques dehydrate tissue by a chemical reaction between water and materials such as 2,2-dimethoxypropane. Acidified dimethoxypropane is hydrolysed by water with the production of methanol and acetone. Prolonged use induces tissue shrinkage. Dimethoxypropane has been used as a fixative and dehydrant due to its chemical by-product activity and is miscible with most resins and paraffins.

## Clearing

This step in tissue processing refers to the phase during which the tissue is treated by a fluid that removes the dehydrating agent and is miscible with the material used in the subsequent embedding step which is usually paraffin wax. Removal of the dehydrating agent renders the tissues translucent. It is essential, therefore, that the clearing agent is miscible with both the dehydrating and embedding agent. Most clearing agents are inflammable liquids and are removed from hot paraffin wax at a speed which is greatest for those with a low boiling point. Vacuum-assisted processing accelerates clearing.

*Xylene (Xylol)* is most widely used and is the agent of choice on 3–5 mm blocks although it may harden tissue if clearing time is prolonged. *Toluene* is similar to xylene and is more forgiving to tissues on prolonged clearing. *Chloroform* has a slower action than xylene and is satisfactory on tissue up to 1 cm. Lymphoid tissues are often rendered brittle by chloroform which, when heated, releases the toxic gas phosgene. *Benzene* and *carbon tetrachloride* give good technical results, but, like *dioxane*, are too toxic for use. Offensive odour has restricted the use of agents such as *amyl acetate*, *methyl benzoate* and *carbon disulphide*. Other liquids used for clearing have included *cedarwood oil*, *clove oil* and *citrus fruit oils*. Low volatility leads to less complete removal by vacuum processors. Derivatives of citrus fruit oils such as Histoclear have an advantage of being essentially non-toxic but their odour is unpleasant and causes headaches in some people. They also tend to partially leach dyes if used prior to section mounting.

## Tissue embedding

This process involves surrounding and impregnating tissue with a firm substance such as wax to facilitate the cutting of thin sections for microscopy. Paraffin wax is the most popular method but others such as celloidin, ester wax and other water-soluble embedding media are available. Different types of resins have been described as alternatives to wax.

### Paraffin wax

Paraffin is colourless or white, mostly translucent and odourless. It is a mixture of solid hydrocarbons derived from petroleum and is available with varying melting points between 45 and 60°C. The soft paraffins are best suited for soft tissues whereas those with higher melting points are best employed for hard tissues such as bone. Most pathology laboratories use paraffin with a melting point around 56°C for routine use. The choice is also influenced

by local climate. Rises in temperature more than 5°C above the melting point of the paraffin result in excessive shrinkage and hardening of tissue whilst slow cooling induces crystallisation and difficulties in sectioning with loss of differential staining.

Plastic polymers have been added to paraffin to increase consistency and provide greater elasticity. This allows tissue ribbons to be cut more easily and aids in preventing section compression. Commercial products such as Paraplast, Bioloid and Tissuemat are available. Rubber additives have also been used. Bees wax mixed with paraffin smooths consistency and adds elasticity. Diemethyl sulphoxide (DMSO) is hygroscopic and promotes paraffin infiltration. It should be used when vacuum-assisted processing is not available.

### Celloidin

Celloidin provides better support for hard specimens like uterus and bone, or fragile tissue such as eye, compared to traditional paraffin waxes. Celloidin is a purified form of nitrocellulose obtained by treating cellulose with sulphuric and nitric acids. It does not require heat at any stage of processing and can be used for specimens that would be heat sensitive. Low viscosity nitrocellulose is a substitute for celloidin.

Both celloidin and low viscosity nitrocellulose unfortunately need 7–10 days to infiltrate a specimen and tissue blocks have to be stored in 70–80% alcohol. Moisture prevents celloidin from solidifying. It is difficult to obtain sections thinner than 10 μm and flammable ether is required.

### Water-soluble embedding media

These include carbowax, gelatin, agar and Optimum Compound Temperature (OCT).

Using these media, specimens can be transferred directly from the fixative into the infiltrating solution, avoiding the need to dehydrate and clear the tissue. OCT is the most commonly employed medium for cryostat rapid frozen sectioning. These media are also valuable when it is necessary to demonstrate fat which is dissolved during tissue processing or other substances denatured by heat.

### Resins

A variety of resins are available as alternatives to paraffin for embedding tissues. The epoxy group are generally used to embed tissue primarily for electron microscopy and include those based on glycerol (Epons), cyclohexane dioxide (Spurrs) and bisphenol A (Araldites). Acrylic resins such as glycol methacrylate have been increasingly employed to embed tissue for light microscopy. Advantages over wax include the ability to cut thinner sections, greatly enhanced morphological detail and less tissue shrinkage. Furthermore, calcified tissue can be processed without prior decalcification and tissue blocks do not need to be completely dehydrated as the resin is water miscible. Wax embedding media are unable to withstand the energy beam of the electron microscope. In addition, the activity of most enzymes can be preserved in resin if temperature rises during polymerisation are minimised, paraformaldehyde is used as the fixative and acetone is employed for dehydration. Freeze drying with low temperature resin embedding is advantageous for retention of fixation-fragile enzymes such as the dehydrogenases. Many antigens are retained in resins and tissue blocks which can be stored for prolonged periods at room temperature with preservation of enzymes and antigens. The thin 1–2 μm

sections obtained from resin-embedded tissue has facilitated the morphological diagnosis of diseases of the renal glomerulus and lymphoreticular system.

## Automated tissue processing

Most histopathology departments now utilise machines to process tissues; however, there remain rare circumstances such as the very urgent specimen, unusually large tissue blocks such as whole brain slices, and in cases of electrical power failure or machine breakdown where manual processing is needed.

The automated tissue processing machines fall into two major groups:

1  Carousel type.
2  Enclosed vacuum pumped fluid type e.g. Shandon, VIP 3L.

The enclosed machines use vacuum and heating at all stages which can dramatically speed up processing. Temperatures of over 37°C can result in the hardening of tissues such as skin and muscle. Such machines cost about A$54 000 and process up to 300 blocks.

All tissues to be processed need to be fixed first, commonly with cross-linking fixatives, 10% formalin being the most popular, or with microwaves. Ultrashort, short, standard and long automated processing cycles can be employed, enabling same day sections to be prepared from most specimens.

Gastrointestinal and bronchial endoscopic biopsies no greater than 1 mm in total thickness are processed on an ultrashort cycle lasting 1 hour and 41 minutes. All other tissues can be processed through 3.5 hour cycle. For convenience, to accommodate late specimens and weekends, two long cycles can be employed, taking 12 hours 36 minutes and 18 hours and 36 minutes. The automated cycle schedules are provided in Tables 8.1–8.4.

**Table 8.1** Ultrashort 1.5 hour cycle schedule

| Step | Reagent | Vacuum | Temperature | Time | Drain |
|---|---|---|---|---|---|
| 1 | 100% ethanol | Yes | 45°C | 5 min | 15 |
| 2 | 100% ethanol | Yes | 45°C | 10 min | 15 |
| 3 | 100% ethanol | Yes | 45°C | 10 min | 15 |
| 4 | Chloroform | No | 45°C | 10 min | 15 |
| 5 | Chloroform | No | 45°C | 10 min | 15 |
| 6 | Wax | Yes | 65°C | 10 min | 30 |
| 7 | Wax | Yes | 65°C | 10 min | 30 |

**Table 8.2** Short 3.5 hour cycle schedule

| Step | Reagent | Vacuum | Temperature | Time | Drain |
|---|---|---|---|---|---|
| 1 | 100% ethanol | Yes | 45°C | 20 min | 15 |
| 2 | 100% ethanol | Yes | 45°C | 10 min | 15 |
| 3 | 100% ethanol | Yes | 45°C | 15 min | 15 |
| 4 | 100% ethanol | Yes | 45°C | 30 min | 15 |
| 5 | Chloroform | No | 45°C | 20 min | 15 |
| 6 | Chloroform | No | 45°C | 10 min | 15 |
| 7 | Chloroform | No | 45°C | 20 min | 15 |
| 8 | Wax | Yes | 65°C | 30 min | 30 |
| 9 | Wax | Yes | 65°C | 20 min | 30 |

**Table 8.3** Long cycle of 12 hours 36 minutes

| Step | Reagent | Vacuum | Temperature | Time | Drain |
|---|---|---|---|---|---|
| 1 | 70% ethanol | Yes | 37°C | 1 h | 15 |
| 2 | 100% ethanol | Yes | 37°C | 1 h | 15 |
| 3 | 100% ethanol | Yes | 37°C | 20 min | 15 |
| 4 | 100% ethanol | Yes | 37°C | 20 min | 15 |
| 5 | 100% ethanol | Yes | 37°C | 20 min | 15 |
| 6 | 100% ethanol | Yes | 37°C | 30 min | 15 |
| 7 | 100% ethanol | Yes | 37°C | 1 h | 15 |
| 8 | Chloroform | No | 37°C | 1 h | 15 |
| 9 | Chloroform | No | 37°C | 1 h | 15 |
| 10 | Chloroform | No | 37°C | 1.5 h | 15 |
| 11 | Wax | Yes | 60°C | 2.5 h | 60 |
| 12 | Wax | Yes | 60°C | 2 h | 60 |

**Table 8.4**   Ultra long cycle of 18 hours 36 minutes

| Step | Reagent | Vacuum | Temperature | Time | Drain |
| --- | --- | --- | --- | --- | --- |
| 1 | 70% ethanol | Yes | 37°C | 1 h | 15 |
| 2 | 100% ethanol | Yes | 37°C | 2 h | 15 |
| 3 | 100% ethanol | Yes | 37°C | 1.5 h | 15 |
| 4 | 100% ethanol | Yes | 37°C | 30 min | 15 |
| 5 | 100% ethanol | Yes | 37°C | 30 min | 15 |
| 6 | 100% ethanol | Yes | 37°C | 30 min | 15 |
| 7 | 100% ethanol | Yes | 37°C | 1.5 h | 15 |
| 8 | Chloroform | No | 37°C | 2 h | 15 |
| 9 | Chloroform | No | 37°C | 1.5 h | 15 |
| 10 | Chloroform | No | 37°C | 2 h | 15 |
| 11 | Wax | Yes | 60°C | 3 h | 120 |
| 12 | Wax | Yes | 60°C | 2.5 h | 120 |

## Tissue block orientation

The process of positioning tissue in molten paraffin blocks to obtain an optimal section is a highly skilled process undertaken by the technician. If difficulty with orientation is anticipated, the problem should be clearly explained to the technician and it may help to mark with ink the surface opposite that to be cut. Blocks need to be embedded promptly as prolonged exposure to air allows a thin layer of paraffin to solidify around the specimen producing trapping of air spaces.

Most tissue sections are embedded flat. Large rectangular or dense tissue specimens such as prostate and uterus should be embedded at a slight angle to the knife edge to allow the knife to start cutting with less resistance. This decreases vibration and reduces the risk of gouging tissue from the block. In the case of multiple small biopsy specimens with epithelial surfaces, the tissue pieces are best placed side by side with the epithelium all facing the top of the block. Multiple soft tissue fragments and lymph nodes should be placed side by side with space between and not one above the other.

Cystic structures, when bisected, are dome-shaped and should be embedded with the cut surface down so the knife cuts through all layers of the cyst wall. Small rectangular tissue should be orientated parallel to the knife edge to minimise pressure distortion and wrinkling. When ink has been used to identify a surgical margin, the block should be placed on edge so the ink will be visible on the section.

## Section cutting (microtomy)

Practical details of microtomy are beyond the scope of this book and only the basics will be discussed. All microtomes, apart from those used to cut ultrathin sections for electron microscopy, work on the principle of a moving screw thread advancing the knife or tissue block through a preset number of microns. The screw thread motion is directly applied in some freezing microtomes whilst the others use an arrangement of gears or levers to magnify the movement. The types of microtomes include the Hand, Rocking, Rotary, Freezing, Base sledge and Vibrating knife. Some microtomes have built-in motor drives. For routine sections, rotary microtomes are used with freezing microtomes employed for the production of frozen sections. Sledge microtomes are particularly useful in cutting large hard specimens, such as undecalcified bone embedded in resin. The vibrating knife microtome enables sections to be obtained without fixation, impregnation or freezing, and has been used for enzyme histochemistry.

Microtome knives are available in stainless steel, carbide, diamond, glass or as disposable blades. The choice is dependent on the structure of the specimen to be sectioned and the medium used for embedding. Stainless steel and tungsten carbide knives are used for sectioning paraffin and resin-embedded specimens respectively, whereas, disposable blades provide an excellent cutting edge for paraffin sectioning and are available in different sizes and thicknesses. Specimens embedded in resins such as epoxy and glycolmethacrylate require the use of diamond, sapphire or glass knives that have harder edges. The former two are very expensive whilst glass knives used for electron microscopy are time consuming to make and require skill.

The knife for microtomy must be sharp and free of nicks. Knife lines account for many of the laboratory-generated artefacts seen in tissue sections.

Most paraffin blocks are cut at about 3–4 $\mu$m for routine sections whilst resin-embedded thin sections are often cut at 1 $\mu$m.

# Tissue section staining

Staining is essential for visualisation of the otherwise transparent sections and the routine stain for most sections is the haematoxylin and eosin (H & E) stain.

## Haematoxylin and eosin stain

Haematoxylin is a natural dye whose active blue colouring agent, formed by the oxidation of haematoxylin, is haematin. Oxidation is accelerated by the use of oxidising agents such as sodium iodate or mercuric oxide. Light exposure induces oxidation and haematoxylin should be stored in dark bottles until ready for use. Haematoxylin is an excellent nuclear stain, particularly when combined with aluminium, iron, chromium, copper or tungsten salts which increase the dye's affinity. There are two methods of haematoxylin staining known as the progressive and regressive procedures.

The progressive method, e.g. Mayer's haematoxylin, stains nuclei only and enhancement of the blue colour is accomplished by washing the slides in running tap water. The regressive method, e.g. Harris' method, stains all tissue structures including nuclei, cytoplasm and connective tissue and is followed by controlling decolourisation (differentiation) and blueing to produce the optimal nuclear staining. Eosin is applied after haematoxylin as a counterstain. Eosin-phloxine gives a wide range of contrasts from pink to bright red. Alcohol used as a dehydrating agent after H & E staining, also serves to remove excess eosin.

H & E staining can be carried out on automated linear staining machines.

## Special stains

Stains applied to tissue sections other than the routine H & E are conventionally known as 'special stains', although in many instances there is nothing particularly special or complex about their methodology or applications. Their main uses are to confirm and/or assess tissue components that are either invisible or poorly visible with routine H & E staining. A listing of tissues, substances and organisms and useful stains for their demonstration is provided below and Chapter 9 lists special stains and their uses.

## Connective tissue stains

Connective tissue is a collective term applied to cells and extracellular fibres and proteins which make up the ground substance. The cellular components include fibroblasts, adipocytes, mast cells, chondrocytes and osteocytes whilst the fibres are collagen, reticulum and elastin. The ground substance includes hyaluronic acid, chondroitin sulphate and dermatin sulphate as well as aqueous material through which nutrients and waste products are transported.

### Collagen
This is readily seen on H & E stain as eosinophilic fibres. Trichrome stains such as the Masson's and Gomori's enable distinction of collagen (green) from muscle (red).

### Reticulum
These branched fine fibres are argyrophilic and stain black with ammoniacal silver solutions such as the Gordon and Sweets, and Snook's.

### Elastic fibres
These are best demonstrated with iron haematoxylin in the Verhoeff's stain, resorcin fuchsin in Hart's or Miller's elastic stain, or aldehyde fuchsin in Gomori's aldehyde fuchsin stain. The elastic fibres stain black and other connective tissue elements can be visualised by counterstain-

ing with van Gieson (collagen—red; muscle—yellow; fibrin—yellow; mast cell granules—black).

Glomerular basement membrane basal lamina can be highlighted with the Jones' hexamine-silver stain.

### Mast cells
Mast cells contain granules which are not easily seen on H & E stained slides. The granules are readily visualised with dyes such as methylene blue in the Giemsa stain or toluidine blue. The reaction is metachromatic, i.e. the colour product is different to the colour of the stain, the granules staining purplish red with the blue dye.

## Carbohydrate complexes

Glycogen is normally found in liver, cardiac and skeletal muscle; sialomucins are found in the salivary glands, intestinal goblet cells and gastric lining cells; sulphated acid mucosubstances are found in goblet cells of the intestine; neutral mucosubstances are present in gastric lining cells and in duodenal Brunner's glands; heparin sulphate is seen in mast cells, aorta and cardiac connective tissue; chondroitin sulphate is contained in cartilage, aorta, heart valves, umbilical cord and the dermis; and hyaluronic acid is found in the connective tissue of the dermis and umbilical cord.

Glycogen is detected by periodic acid Schiff (PAS); sialomucins and sulphated mucosubstances by Gomori's aldehyde fuchsin at pH 1.7 and pH 1.0; neutral mucosubstances by PAS with diastase (PASD); acid mucosubstances by Alcian blue at pH 2.5 and 0.4 which can provide differential staining of non-sulphated and sulphated mucosubstances respectively; acid mucosaccharides by colloidal iron and chondromucins by safranine O. The mucicarmine stain has been employed to demonstrate acid mucosubstances but the results are not specific although it is more consistent in the staining of epithelial rather than connective tissue mucosubstances. Combined PAS and Alcian blue simultaneously demonstrate neutral and acidic mucins, whilst Ravetto's Alcian blue/yellow delineates acidic from neutral mucins. Pretreatment of sections with enzymes such as diastase, sialidase, hyaluronidase and chondroitinase allows the specific identification of some carbohydrate complexes.

## Lipids

Lipid stains need to be performed on unfixed fresh frozen tissue or on cryostat sections of formalin-fixed tissue. Such stains include the oil red O, Sudan red and Sudan black in which the dyes are more soluble in the lipid to be demonstrated than the vehicular solvent. Osmium tetroxide can be used on frozen sections, as can Baker's acid haematin for phospholipids and Schultz's method for cholesterol.

## Pigments and minerals

Human tissues contain several pigments, the most important of which are lipofuschin (ceroid), melanin and the breakdown products of haemoglobin (bilirubin and haematoidin). Lipofuschin and melanin are brown to black non-birefringent pigments. Melanin does not stain with the PAS, oil red O or acid fast stains and is reduced by ammoniacal silver, whereas lipofuschin generally does not stain with these procedures. The most common stain for melanin is the Masson–Fontana which stains melanin black and works on the principle that melanin can reduce solutions of ammoniacal silver nitrate to metallic silver without the use of an external reducing agent. It is not specific, as argentaffin granules and some lipofuschins stain. Both melanin and lipofuschin pigments can be removed by bleaching using 0.25% potassium permanganate and 5% oxalic acid.

Although many minerals may be encountered in human tissues, most cannot be suitably stained as they are highly water soluble. Inorganic compounds such as silica are water insoluble but are unreactive to reagents used for tissue preservation and fixation. The mineral apatites found in bone, teeth and pathological calcifications are fairly insoluble and some inorganic elements bound to proteins can be stained in formalin-fixed tissues. The commonest stain is the Perls' Prussian blue for ferric ions. The ferric salts, invariably haemosiderin, stain deep blue whilst ferrous ions are not stained. Copper deposits can be stained by the DMAB-rhodamine method. The latter is a chelating agent with a strong affinity for proteinaceous copper deposits. Bile pigments can be demonstrated as green deposits with Fouchet's method and Hall's method. Calcium deposits are highlighted as black with a von Kossa stain although the calcium is picked up indirectly as the method, in reality, stains the calcium-associated carbonate and phosphate ions. A specific method for calcium is the Alizarin red S stain where most calcium salts stain as birefringent red precipitates. However, calcium oxalate has no reaction. Formalin and malarial pigments are sometimes seen in sections, the former commonly in areas of erythrocyte aggregation. Both pigments are gold brown and birefringent, and can be removed from sections by a saturated solution of alcoholic picric acid, the malarial parasites remaining unchanged.

Electron-dispersive-X-ray analysis offers a more sensitive and specific technique for identification of elemental and mineral deposits in human tissues.

## Neurosecretory granules

A wide variety of tumours of neuroepithelial and neuroendocrine origin are characterized by cytoplasmic membrane bound granules which are not visualised on routine staining but whose positive identification is essential for correct diagnosis. These granules are subdivided into argentaffin and argyrophil types. The former have the ability to reduce silver salts and trap the precipitated silver whilst the latter are dependent on the addition of an external reducing agent to enable trapping of the silver. Both the Masson–Fontana and Diazo stains are employed to detect argentaffin granules whilst the Churukian and Schenk method is used for demonstration of argyrophil granules. Known positive control tissues are essential in interpreting these special staining reactions.

## Bacteria, fungi and other organisms

The use of stains to render invisible microorganisms visible or to highlight sparse numbers of difficult to identify organisms is an important aspect of the diagnosis of a number of infectious diseases.

### Bacteria

Some bacteria are visible in H & E stained sections but the Gram stain readily divides bacteria into blue/black Gram positive and red Gram negative groups. Bacteria such as spirochaetes and Proteobacteria species including *Afipia* and *Rochalimaea* and Donovan bodies (*Calymmatobacteria donovani*) can also be demonstrated by silver impregnation methods such as the Warthin–Starry stain. The organisms are coated when the silver is reduced to its metallic state, enlarging their appearance. Such silver stains can be greatly accelerated by exposure to microwaves. Mycobacteria are acid fast bacteria, so called because their waxy coat is resistant to dilute mineral acid differentiation. *Mycobacterium tuberculosis* are visualised as red bacilli with the Ziehl–Neelsen technique whilst *Mycobacterium leprae* is less acid resistant and is best demonstrated with the Fite's method in which dilute HCl is employed instead of $H_2SO_4$. Giemsa staining can reveal Gram positive and negative coccobacilli, acid fast bacilli, helicobacter, Donovan bodies and actinomyces.

### Fungi

Fungi exist as hyphae and/or yeasts or yeast-like spores. Their cell walls may contain chitin so they may be stained with silver stains or may be PAS positive. Silver stains are more uniformly reliable if the background is kept clean. The more common stains employed for fungi are Grocott's methenamine silver nitrate, PAS, Gram, colloidal iron and Giemsa.

### Viruses

Viruses cannot be seen by light microscopy although aggregates of viral particles may be seen in paraffin sections. Some, such as herpes simplex and cytomegalovirus, are observed in H & E preparations, but generally, specific identification of viral proteins is performed with immunohistochemical techniques. The hepatitis B surface antigen can be demonstrated by orcein or aldehyde fuchsin and others are seen with the Giemsa stain.

### Rickettsia

These are obligate intracellular arthropod-borne parasites carried by ticks, mites or lice and appear in paraffin sections as small cocco-bacilli forms. The elementary bodies of rickettsia stain pale blue to violet in H & E preparations, reddish/purple with Giemsa and are Gram negative.

### Parasites

This group of organisms ranges from one-celled protozoans to grossly visible worms. The identification of microscopic parasites can be aided with stains such as Giemsa, silver impregnation and PAS. Amoebae can also be demonstrated with Hale's colloidal iron stain.

### Miscellaneous stains

A large number of stains are available for specialised areas of pathology such as for neural tissues, bone and cartilage. A highly selected list includes: methyl green-pyronin for DNA and RNA, Luna's method for mast cells, Cresyl violet (Vogt's) method for Nissl substance, Bielschowsky method for neurofibrils, Bodian's method for nerve fibres and nerve endings, Holmes' method for nerve cells and fibres, Luxol fast blue stain for myelin and nerve cells, phospho-tungstic acid haematoxylin (PTAH) for muscle, myelin sheaths and glial cell processes, and Holzer's method for glial fibres.

With all special staining procedures, it is essential that control sections of known positive cases are included. It is preferable to have the control and test section on the same slide to indicate that both sections were stained simultaneously.

## Mounting media and coverslipping

The final step in the preparation of a slide is the application of a coverslip to cover the portion containing the tissue on the glass slide. This protects the tissue, makes the slide permanent and allows microscopic examination. The three main types of mounting media are synthetic resins, natural resins and aqueous media. All are chosen with refractive indices close to glass to improve optical resolution.

Synthetic resins are the most common mounting media used for routine H & E preparations as well as for most special stains. DePeX (Gurr, BDH Laboratory Supplies, Poole, UK) is a common mounting medium.

Canada balsam was a widely used natural resin but it is impractical due to long drying time. Eosin staining intensity is reduced after several years and Prussian blue reactions fade.

Aqueous media are used when dyes such as crystal violet or structures such as lipid are altered or destroyed by dehydration or by xylene-based media. Examples of these media are glycerine jelly, polyvinyl alcohol mounting medium and Apathy's mounting medium.

## Further reading

Bancroft JD, Stevens A 1995 Theory and practice of histological techniques, 4th edn. Churchill Livingstone, Edinburgh

Leong AS-Y 1994 Fixation and fixatives. In: Wood A, Ellis R (eds) Laboratory histopathology: a complete reference. Churchill Livingstone, London, pp 4.1–4.26

Leong AS-Y 1994 Microwave technology in morphological diagnosis and research. Cell Vision 1: 278–288

Pearse AGE 1985 Histochemistry, theoretical and applied, vols 1, 2, 4th edn. Churchill Livingstone, Edinburgh

Prophet EB, Mills B, Arrington JB, Sobin LH 1992 Laboratory methods in histotechnology. American Registry of Pathology, Washington

# 9 Immunohistochemistry and special stains

143

## Introduction

The development of the immunoperoxidase and hybridoma techniques are two major milestones of technological advancements in diagnostic histopathology. Coons and associates applied the fluorescent antibody method to tissue sections in 1941, signalling the commencement of a technique that would permit specific identification of cells according to their antigenic constituents or cellular products. Immunofluorescence methods were very successful in some areas of pathology such as the study of renal diseases, but the technique did not achieve widespread application because of two principal disadvantages: it was unsuitable for use in conventional formalin-fixed, paraffin-embedded tissues and morphological details in cryostat sections were poor, the inability to study fine cytomorphological features being a major handicap.

By substituting horseradish peroxidase for fluorescein-isothiocyanate as the label for the specific antibody, it became possible to stain for the horseradish peroxidase by adding a suitable chromogenic substrate to produce a coloured reaction product visible by ordinary light microscopy. This was the basis of Sternberger's peroxidase-antiperoxidase technique (1970). The development of the hybridoma monoclonal antibody technique by Kohler and Milstein (1975) propelled immunohistochemistry into an era of exponential growth which has been called the 'brown revolution'. This modality of examination has produced an enormous impact on the diagnosis, classification and understanding of many diseases and neoplasms.

Refinements in cancer treatment have made it necessary to have a precise morphological diagnosis prior to the selection of the optimal therapeutic regimen, making it necessary to employ all ancillary investigations which aid in arriving at this diagnosis. Immunohistochemistry has rapidly established such a role, making major contributions in the area of tumour diagnosis.

While immunoperoxidase histochemistry can act as 'magic markers', the technique is beset by many technological and interpretative pitfalls, and knowledge of problems encountered, particularly in initial specimen handling, is important regardless of whether immunostaining is done in-house or by a reference laboratory.

## Immunofluorescence techniques

These techniques are discussed in detail in Chapter 12. Because of the need for fresh frozen tissue and poor morphological preservation, immunohistochemistry has replaced immunofluorescence as the method of choice in many areas of pathological diagnosis. Traditionally, immunofluorescence procedures are still employed in the diagnosis of glomerular diseases and bullous skin lesions because of the simplicity and rapidity of the technique. Immunofluorescence methods are still extensively employed for the detection of serum antibodies and in flow cytometry.

## Immunoenzyme techniques

Immunohistochemical techniques are based on the attachment of an enzyme to a specific antibody. The enzymatic activity induces a visible colour change in the substrate and chromogen at the sites of localisation of the antibody–enzyme complex within the tissue. Horseradish peroxidase is the prototype of the immunoenzyme method but other enzymes such as glucose oxidase and alkaline phosphatase have been employed.

## Direct immunoenzyme staining

The direct immunoenzyme technique utilises an enzyme-conjugated antibody to bind an enzyme to antigens in the section. The section is then incubated with an appropriate substrate such as hydrogen peroxide and a chromogen such as diaminobenzidine (DAB) to produce a brown reaction product which is identifiable by light microscopy. Although simple, it is less sensitive than the indirect or bridge techniques.

## Bridge techniques

These have the main advantage of increasing the sensitivity of the immunoenzyme stain by augmenting the amount of reaction product deposited at the antigen sites. In the *enzyme–anti-enzyme technique* the primary antibody is not labelled. Instead, anti-enzyme antibodies are used to form a bridge between the primary antibody and the enzyme, avoiding the necessity of conjugating enzyme to antibodies, a procedure which can reduce antigen-binding avidity and is often technically difficult.

The *peroxidase antiperoxidase system* (PAP) is reported to have a sensitivity of 100- to 1000-fold greater than comparable conjugate techniques. The PAP complex, which is the tertiary reagent, consists of a soluble and stable pre-formed complex of antibody against horseradish peroxidase and horseradish peroxidase antigen. This immune complex typically consists of two antibody molecules and three peroxidase molecules in a cyclic arrangement. The primary antibody, specific to the human antigen, binds through its Fab portion. The secondary or bridge reagent, in turn, forms a molecular bridge between the primary antibody and the immunoglobulin incorporated into the PAP complex. Both the primary antibody and the PAP reagent have to be of the same species, so that the bridge reagent, derived from a second species, can have specificity for the constant components of both primary and tertiary reagents.

Endogenous peroxidase in the sections has first to be blocked with hydrogen peroxide or a mixture of hydrogen peroxide and methanol. Non-specific binding is also blocked with diluted non-immune serum from the same species from which the bridging antibody was obtained. The bridging antibody is then added in excess so that free antigen binding sites will remain for linkage to PAP complexes. Unbound bridging antibody is rinsed away before soluble PAP complexes are incubated with the specimen. The final step is the reaction of the PAP complex with substrate and chromogen to form a product visible by light microscopy at the site of antigen in the tissue section.

Both the *alkaline phosphatase–anti-alkaline phosphatase* (APAAP) and the *glucose oxidase–anti-glucose oxidase* (GAG) systems are claimed to produce less background staining because of the restricted tissue distribution of these enzymes. These systems are similar to the PAP, except the tertiary reagents (antibody–chromogenic enzyme complexes) comprise two IgG molecules bound to alkaline phosphatase or glucose oxidase in place of horseradish peroxidase.

The *avidin–biotin technique* exploits the high affinity binding between biotin and avidin. Biotin, a low molecular weight vitamin, can be covalently linked to the primary antibody to produce a biotinylated conjugate which localises to the sites of antigen in the section. Avidin, an egg-white glycoprotein, has four binding sites for biotin and can be used as a bridge between the components of multilayered immunoenzyme systems. Avidin, chemically conjugated to horseradish peroxidase, allows tight binding to the biotinylated antibody, locating the peroxidase moiety at the site of antibody–antigen reaction in the tissue section. The method is rapid and can be employed as an indirect procedure but is not as sensitive as the PAP method.

A refinement to the avidin–biotin system is the *avidin–biotin–peroxidase complex* (ABC) which employs a pre-formed complex of avidin bound to biotinylated peroxidase molecules. The method is used as an indirect technique, whereby the primary antibody is linked to the avidin–biotin–peroxidase conjugate by a biotinylated secondary antibody. The complex is a lattice-like, three-dimensional structure which serves to localise several molecules of peroxidase at the antigen site, endowing the technique with more sensitivity than the PAP procedure.

Streptavidin has been introduced as a substitute for avidin. The former has no charge at neutral pH and does not produce the non-specific binding associated with egg-white avidin. Many of the commercially available streptavidin–biotin peroxidase kits can be applied at dilutions many times more than the manufacturer's recommendations. Kits such as the Elite ABC (Vector PK6100) and the Super Sensitive (Biogenix ZP000-UM) are claimed to be more sensitive and have modifications to the procedure such as sequential overlaying of the ABC-stained section with an avidin-rich and biotin-rich complex or the use of a streptavidin- or avidin–horseradish peroxidase conjugate and sequential application of the PAP and ABC techniques (ABPAP).

A potential problem with biotin–avidin procedures is the presence of endogenous biotin that may produce non-specific or false-positive staining. This can be blocked by incubating the specimen with free avidin followed by free biotin.

## Protein-A-peroxidase conjugate method

Staphylococcal protein A has an ability to bind with the constant portion (Fc) of immunoglobulin molecules from several different species. This binding capability enables a rapid immunoperoxidase procedure in which protein A is substituted for the secondary antibody in the PAP method. Protein A is able to bridge between primary antibodies and antiperoxidase antibodies derived from different species. Whilst the technique works well in paraffin sections, in cryostat sections, the protein A–peroxidase conjugate can bind both to the Fc component of the primary antibody and the Fc fragments of intrinsic immunoglobulins within the section.

## Immunogold-silver staining

Metal irons and metal–protein complexes such as ferritin, gold and mercury have been used as markers of immunohistochemical reactions because they are visible by light microscopy when deposited in tissue. Other metals can be superadded on such complexes to enhance their visibility. The immunogold-silver technique is a highly sensitive indirect method in which the secondary antibody is adsorbed to colloidal gold particles. The latter are in the range 5–10 nm, generally not visible by ordinary light microscopy. A silver solution enhances the gold particles which turn black with the silver precipitation and are visible by light microscopy. Immunogold-silver techniques can also be employed in double labelling procedures in combination with chromogens where the immunogold-silver precipitate clearly contrasts with the brown reaction product of DAB.

# In situ hybridisation and in situ polymerase chain reaction

The ability to detect specific nucleic acid sequences is a considerable technological advancement as cellular antigens and other protein components are dependent on both DNA and RNA for their synthesis and protein expression may be a relatively late event and may represent only incidental changes in the histogenesis of the disease or neoplasm. DNA is much more stable than the protein antigen, surviving both fixation and paraffin embedding. Recombinant DNA technology has enabled the development of DNA probes which bind to complementary DNA gene sequences in tissue through hydrogen bonds. Until recently, these hybridisation reactions were performed using radioactive DNA probes with subsequent autoradiography of the probe-target DNA immobilised on cellulose membranes. DNA probes can now be labelled with non-radioactive methods and in situ hybridisation (ISH) can be performed directly on tissue sections and cytological smears. Non-radioactive probes have the advantages of being easier to use, costing less, show higher resolution and do not require radioactive waste disposal facilities.

The methodology is analogous to that of immunohistochemistry in that the DNA probe is rendered immunologically detectable by the attachment of a hapten molecule which can be recognised by specific antibodies. For example, N-acetoxy-2-acetyl-aminofluorene (AAF) which reacts with guanine residues in

nucleic acid can be incorporated directly into a pre-existing DNA or RNA probe, or immunogenic proteins can be bound covalently to DNA and detected by antibodies following hybridisation. Nucleotide analogues can be linked to fluorescent dyes such as fluorescein and rhodamine and it is possible to produce one-step detection systems. Horseradish peroxidase and alkaline phosphatase can also be conjugated covalently to single-stranded DNA probes. The reduced sensitivity of fluorescinated probes compared to other methods and the carcinogenicity of AAF have not made these techniques popular. The peroxidase and phosphatase enzymes lose their activity under the higher temperatures used in hybridisation procedures.

Biotin may be conjugated directly to uridine triphosphate and deoxyuridine triphosphate to enable detection of nucleic acids as in immunohistochemical reactions. Detection of the hybridised biotinylated DNA probe can be accomplished by either antibiotin antibodies or avidin complexed with fluorescent molecules, chromogenic enzymes or electron-opaque plastic spheres. Commercial sources of biotin-labelled probes are available to various organisms, including adenovirus 2, cytomegalovirus, Epstein–Barr virus, hepatitis B virus, herpes simplex viruses I and II, *Chlamydia trachomatis*, human papilloma virus and some oncogenes (Bethesda Research Laboratories, Maryland, USA; Enzo Biochem, New York, USA; Vector, California, USA; Tako Inc., California, USA). ISH with biotinylated probes is performed on deparaffinised tissue sections following proteolytic digestion of the formalin-fixed tissue to expose intracellular nucleic acid targets. mRNA is preserved optimally with cross-linking aldehyde fixatives such as formalin and precipitating fixatives such as Carnoy's, Bouin's and Zenker's retain less. The targets are immobilised in the tissue and breakdown of RNA by endogenous ribonucleases restricted by brief post-fixation in buffered 4% paraformaldehyde. Pre-treatment of tissue sections with proteolytic enzymes or detergents such as Triton X-100 just prior to hybridisation optimises the probe/target nucleic acid interaction. In general terms, the longer the primary fixation time, the greater is the need for digestion. This step is followed by denaturation of the probe and target DNA at high temperature, hybridisation at physiological temperature, and detection of the hybridised probe using either a two-step avidin–peroxidase complex, or a four-step goat antibiotin antibody followed by biotinylated anti-goat antibody and avidin–peroxidase complex procedure.

Other non-radioactive reporter molecules such as digoxigenin, bromodeoxyuridine and acetylaminofluorene can be used with diaminobenzidine or alkaline phosphatase to produce results of at least equivalent sensitivity to radioactive methods. Sites of hybridised biotin can also be visualised by avidin or streptavidin conjugated to fluorochromes or colloidal gold particles or, alternatively, antibiotin antibodies may be used. Probes are available to a wide variety of viruses, chromosomes, mRNA and DNA. ISH of mRNA is valuable in the study of tumour heterogeneity and for the mRNA which encodes hormones, oncogenes, cytokines, secretory proteins and other cell products. The ability of ISH to localise mRNA to cells in a heterogenous background is a clear advantage over Northern blotting and multiple studies can be performed on small tissue samples. The morphological resolution of ISH allows single copy genes to be localised to individual chromosomes, can

identify translocations or other chromosomal abnormalities and enable study of gene expression at the cellular/subcellular level.

The *in situ polymerase chain reaction* (IS-PCR) enables the detection of low levels of gene expression at the cellular level, such as viral DNA, single gene copies and immunoglobulin gene rearrangements in tissue sections and cytospin specimens. Selected segments of DNA are amplified many times in situ and hybridisation with non-isotopic probes can be performed to label the amplified protein. Such methods of DNA analysis of paraffin-embedded tissues are powerful tools for genetic analysis and are likely to be a routine component of the surgical pathologist's diagnostic armamentarium.

## Fluorescence in situ hybridisation

This powerful new technique uses fluorescent labelled DNA probes to identify and localise chromosome aberrations in both metaphase spreads and interphase (non-dividing) nuclei. Pericentromeric probes can be used to determine chromosome copy number within interphase nuclei, allowing an assessment of ploidy in the tissue section. Other abnormalities are investigated with smaller unique DNA sequence probes. The technique can be applied to cytological preparations and archival paraffin sections although the lack of complete nuclei in the latter is a potential trap in identifying chromosome loss. Fluorescence in situ hybridisation (FISH) is more reliable in detecting chromosome gains. Accurate signal detection is difficult in thick sections without the use of confocal microscopy, but disaggregated whole cells can be extracted from solid tissues or paraffin sections. Fluorescent tagging also permits double labelling studies so that probe cocktails can be employed, providing for internal controls. For example, when a deletion is suspected, the use of a control probe on the same chromosome arm or from the centromeric region of the chromosome of interest can confirm that the deletion is the result of a loss of a small part of the chromosome, rather than loss of the entire chromosome. FISH probes can detect prenatal chromosome disorders, viral sequences, tumour specific chromosome translocations, gene amplification and apoptosis, and can be used to monitor cross-sex transplant recipients. For example, using fluorescent probes for the *bcr* region of chromosome 22 and the *c-abl* region of chromosome 9, close proximity of signals is supportive of a Philadelphia chromosome translocation and the diagnosis of chronic myeloid leukaemia. This method can be employed to detect *minimal residual disease*. Oncogenic probes to the *N-myc* loci can analyse the prognostically relevant gene amplification in neuroblastoma. Morphological preservation with FISH is valuable in enabling correlation of genetic variation with morphology.

## Fixation in immunohistochemistry

Fixation is a paramount factor in antigen preservation, and routine processing and paraffin-embedding both reduce the amounts of immunohistochemically detectable antigen. Frozen section remains the gold standard for antigen preservation and cell surface antigens, detectable in small amounts in fresh frozen tissue, may be completely lost during routine processing and embedding. Many lymphocyte surface antigens are particularly labile and cryostat sections are required for their

demonstration. Freezing a portion of fresh biopsy, especially in anticipated problem cases, ensures the availability of the most suitable tissue for antigen demonstration.

Snap freezing techniques are described in Chapter 10. Be careful to cover the sample completely with OCT compound to prevent ice crystal formation and freeze on a metal chuck to obtain an orientable surface. After freezing, the tissue block is pried from the chuck, wrapped in aluminium foil and stored at −20° or −70°C until required.

Material that is not frozen must be promptly fixed or drying will cause denaturation of antigens. Tissue samples should be cut thinly to preserve cells in the centre and since some antigens are destroyed by excessive time in fixative, tissues for immunohistology should be embedded promptly after fixation is complete.

Formaldehyde has remained a widely used fixative in diagnostic pathology but our experience indicates that antigen loss is largely proportional to the duration of exposure to formaldehyde and some antigens are completely lost after fixation of more than 7 days.

Metal salts such as zinc precipitate protein to form insoluble complexes and can enhance immunostaining and antigen preservation. They can be combined with formalin as 1% zinc sulphate in 3.7% unbuffered formalin or the tissues can be post-fixed in zinc sulphate. Heavy metal fixatives are useful for the immunohistochemical detection of nuclear antigens but often produce a high level of background immunostaining.

In the past 10 years, microwave irradiation has become the primary method of tissue fixation in some laboratories. It is not only a rapid and clean method of fixation, but has also been shown to be superior to formalin for the preservation of cellular antigens.

Specimens still arrive in the laboratory in buffered formalin to avoid autolysis due to transport mishaps. The tissues are examined and sampled as 2 mm thick blocks and irradiated in batches of 40 to a temperature of 62°C in normal saline. They are then processed through several cycles of absolute alcohol (75 minutes), chloroform or xylene (50 minutes), and wax (50 minutes) in a vacuum-assisted autoprocessor as described in Chapter 8.

With the exception of S100 protein, the staining for a wide variety of common tissue antigens is superior in microwave-fixed tissues compared to routine formalin fixation. Besides intense immunostaining, morphological preservation in irradiated sections is excellent. Microwave fixation also allows the demonstration of many labile lymphocyte antigens which do not survive formalin fixation and paraffin embedding. Furthermore, with the exception of the cytokeratins and desmin, microwave-fixed tissues do not require enzyme pre-treatment.

No fixative is ideal for all antigens. Ethanol, Carnoy's solution and methacarn appear to optimise the detection of intermediate filament proteins, whereas Bouin's solution provides the best preservation for neuropeptides and biogenic amines.

Periodate-lysine-paraformaldehyde solution oxidises carbohydrate moieties and produces cross-linkage, at the same time stabilising lipids and proteins, allowing the maintenance of morphological integrity. This fixative is used to preserve leukocyte-related membrane receptors and oestrogen receptor proteins.

Antigenic denaturation is greatest in fixatives containing acid substances.

## Decalcifying solutions

Neutral EDTA, 10% formic acid and 10% acetic acid produce little modulation of immunoreactivity, even after several weeks. Five per cent nitric acid, on the other hand, decreases immunoreactivity and necessitates protease treatment. Trichloroacetic acid can be employed as a one-step fixation and decalcifying agent.

## Tissue processing

Detailed studies on the effects of tissue processing on antigen preservation are lacking but temperatures over 60°C may denature antigens and higher temperatures result in a loss of cellular morphology, particularly nuclear detail. Paraffin impregnation is best carried out at temperatures lower than 60°C and the process of tissue fixation and dehydration, rather than the subsequent steps of paraffin embedding, are more likely to cause antigen loss. Fixatives with aldehyde groups, alcohol groups and/or carboxyl groups (e.g. acetic acid) destroy membrane antigens which are preserved with acetone and chloroform. There is a suggestion that dewaxing with Histoclear leads to almost complete loss of antigenic reactivity unlike xylene, although this has not been confirmed.

## Staining

The streptavidin–biotin peroxidase method is a sensitive and convenient method employed by many laboratories. Any step in the immunoperoxidase procedure may conceal a pitfall. For example, failure to block endogenous peroxidase activity may lead to a false-positive result, particularly in fresh frozen tissue. Similarly, undesirable background staining, particularly of connective tissue and collagen, is a nuisance. Pre-incubation of sections with a high concentration of protein solution such as bovine albumin may reduce background staining but it cannot always be avoided. The use of the highest possible dilution of primary antibody will also help to reduce unwanted background reactions.

The incubation time at room temperature for most primary antibodies is 20–30 minutes. Increasing the temperature to 37°C may reduce the incubation time but can lead to false-negative or false-positive results with increased background staining. The optimal method is overnight fixation of the primary antibody at 4°C but room temperature incubation in a humidified chamber is the most convenient. To avoid false-negative results, sections must not be allowed to dry between incubations and washes.

Microwave stimulation reduces the incubation time required for the primary antibody down to a matter of seconds, yielding good morphology and a clean background. All steps of processing can be accelerated by microwaves leading to a stained slide in 16 minutes. The labour intensiveness of this method restricts its use for more urgent cases.

Immunostaining can be performed on previously stained sections and cytological preparations with a wide variety of antigens following removal of the cover glass and brief destaining of the H & E sections in acid alcohol (this step is not necessary for cytological preparations). No significant loss of sensitivity ensues.

To identify weak immunoreactions, the counterstain, typically haematoxylin or methyl green, must be light.

Automation is inevitable in the evolution of immunohistochemistry. Several commercial systems are now available. One popular system utilises a capillary action principle and can perform complete immunoassays from the dewaxing to the nuclear staining stage, analysing 60 slides for 30 different antigens within 2 hours and 35 minutes. Claims of 50% savings on immunochemicals are made and the machine can perform in situ hybridisation procedures. In another system, up to 20 slides can be processed in a 'run', each slide held in a disposable coverplate which regulates the reaction of antibody with the sections.

The ability of automated staining to provide cost savings will depend on the laboratory workload as many of the machines unfortunately do not handle large numbers of slides. Automation has the major advantage of consistency and enables intralaboratory standardisation but the wide variation in tissue fixation makes interlaboratory comparisons impossible at this stage.

## Controls

Controls must form a part of every immunoperoxidase 'run'. Positive controls of normal tissues with large amounts of the antigen in question can be used, but it is also appropriate to have controls of tissues with only small amounts of antigen, corresponding more closely to the levels present in the test section. Many sections have inbuilt positive controls. A negative control is a section from a tissue known to lack the antigen under study. Alternatively, a negative control can take the form of replacing the primary antibody with either non-immune serum or an antibody with irrelevant specificity. Abolition of positive staining by an antibody pre-absorbed by the antigen under study is the best control but is not often practical.

## Reagents

The results obtained in any immunoperoxidase procedure are only as reliable as the antibodies employed. Monoclonal antibodies are very specific and do not show much 'batch to batch' variation. Their reactivity is usually against an epitope rather than the whole antigen and they may be less sensitive than polyclonal antibodies. Some monoclonal antibodies may only react on cryostat sections. All new antibodies should be subjected to in-house testing for sensitivity and specificity on optimally processed tissues. Multitissue blocks are a convenient and expedient way of assessing new antibodies.

Serial dilution studies determine the optimal concentration of the primary antibody. Three- to four-fold dilutions are often required before differences are appreciable. Pathologists must become thoroughly familiar with the staining patterns and intensity of reactions obtained with various antibodies if immunohisto-chemistry is to yield its maximum benefits.

## Chromogens

Different chromogens are available for the different enzyme systems. 3,3-Diamino-benzidine (DAB) is the most widely used chromogen producing an alcohol fast visible brown reaction product, enabling its use with a wide range of counterstains and mounting media. The suspected carcino-genicity of DAB has prompted the trial of other reagents such as 3-amino-9-ethylcarbazole (AEC), tetramethylbenzidine, *p*-phenylenediamine-pyrochatechol, 4-chloro-1-naphthol, alpha-naphthol pyronine and homovanillic acid. AEC has a cherry red colour, is soluble in organic solvents and requires special aqueous media

for mounting. It also tends to fade with storage and recently has also been implicated as a potential carcinogen.

All chromogens are dependent on the ability of peroxidase to mediate an oxidation-reduction reaction in the presence of hydrogen peroxide. The insoluble oxidised visible chromogen precipitates at the sites of tissue-bound antibody–enzyme complexes.

## Enhancement methods

Metallic ions or organic compounds may be used to enhance the visibility of the insoluble, oxidised chromogen products. Immersion of immunostained sections in solutions of 0.5% copper sulphate, 0.125% osmium tetroxide, 1% cobalt chloride or 1% nickel ammonium sulphate will enhance chromogen staining, altering the colour of the reaction product according to the solution used, but do not necessarily increase sensitivity. 0.1 M Imidazole increases the rate of oxidation of DAB by peroxidase several fold at neutral pH and has the advantage of inhibiting the pseudoperoxidase activity of haemoglobin, producing true enhancement of sensitivity.

Where the amount of tissue antigen is low, immunostaining can be enhanced by repeated application of the primary antibody. The initial incubation can be short, followed by washing in PBS, a re-application of the antibody at the same concentration and overnight incubation at 4°C.

### Proteolytic enzyme digestion

Neutral buffered formalin commonly results in cross-linking of antigenic molecules with 'masking' of their immunoreactivity. The treatment of tissue sections with proteolytic enzymes is thought to break the methylene cross-links in the antigenic molecules, reconstituting their immunore-activity. Bovine trypsin and pepsin are commonly employed. The enzymes must be prepared fresh and in a suitable solvent such as 0.01 M NaOH–0.1% calcium chloride at pH 7.8 and applied to rehydrat-ed deparaffinised tissue sections either at room temperature or at 37°C. Tissues fixed for longer periods require longer exposure to proteolytic enzymes and are more resistant to digestion. Tissues fixed in alcohol-based fixatives result in better antigen preservation but the morphology of alcohol-fixed tissue is suboptimal and hand-processing is required.

Enzyme digestion may reduce the background and enhance the immunoreac-tion for certain antibodies but false-negative staining or no enhancement may be observed with other antibodies. Alternatively, enzyme pre-treatment may give increased background staining and false-positive reactivity. Loss of adherence of tissue sections to slides is another disadvantage. Chrome-alum gel, Elmer's glue, polylysine and aminoalkylsilane have been used as binding agents to overcome this problem.

## Heat-induced epitope retrieval (antigen unmasking)

Enzymatic digestion used to be the stan-dard method for antigen unmasking, but over the past 3–4 years the heating of deparaffinised tissues to high temperatures (>100°C) in a liquid medium has lead to the dramatic recovery of many cell anti-gens. With some antibodies such as MIB1 (anti-Ki-67) and the oestrogen receptor antibody 1D5, such a procedure is a pre-requisite for immunostaining.

This method of heat-induced epitope retrieval has greatly improved the sensitivi-ty of immunostaining of fixed tissue and is

effective for a wide range of antigens. Heating to 100°C in saturated lead thio-cyanate or 1% zinc sulphate was first introduced by Shi et al. in 1991 but besides heavy metal solutions, citrate buffer, urea, phosphate-buffered saline and urate have been shown to be effective. Microwave irradiation is a convenient source but alternative methods of heat generation employing pressure cookers and wet autoclaves have also been used. A variety of unmasking solutions are commercially available.

## Interpretation of staining

The interpretation of immunoperoxidase staining requires skill and experience so that the examiner should not only be familiar with the characteristics of a true positive reaction, but should also be aware of possible variability depending on the nature of the tissue and the type of anti-body used. The causes of errors in immunohistochemistry can be either technical or interpretive. A true positive reaction is not only based on the brown staining of cells but also on heterogeneity in distribution within single cells, among groups of cells and throughout the tissue section. In individual cells, the brown granules may occupy all the cytoplasm, the perinuclear area alone, the cell membrane, one pole of the cell, or the nucleus. Diffuse, pale brown or a single tone yellow staining of neoplastic cells is probably non-specific. Most immunohistochemical cell markers are localised either in the cyto-plasm or on the cell membrane with the exception of some viral antigens, Ki-67 antigen, p53, cyclin and hormone receptor proteins which are entirely intranuclear. S100 protein, neuron specific enolase and

LN2 (CD75) are present both in the nuclei and cytoplasm of positive cells.

Some antigens display a specific pattern of distribution which aids in identification. For example, the cells of Merkel cell carcinoma display juxtanuclear whorls of cytokeratin filaments and sometimes neurofilaments. The Reed–Sternberg cell shows a characteristic cell membrane and paranuclear staining pattern with CD15 and the cells of mesothelioma have aberrant, circumferential long microvilli labelled by monoclonal antibodies to epithelial membrane antigen.

It must be appreciated that most importantly, immunostains are used as an adjunct to morphological diagnosis and it is essential to interpret staining in the context of the morphology. This will allow the selection of the appropriate antibodies to make up the panel for sorting out the entities considered in differential diagnosis, the latter derived from morphological examination. This will also reduce the risk of erroneous interpretation such as diagnosing thymoma on the basis of entrapped cytokeratin-positive epithelial cells in a thymic lymphoma.

## Intrinsic and other extrinsic pigments

Pigments such as formalin, melanin and haemosiderin should be differentiated from the brown granules of diaminobenzidine as they are different both in texture and colour. Examination of the antibody control slide will review their true character. Formalin pigment is birefringent and can be removed by treating the pre-stained sections with saturated alcoholic picric acid or sodium hydroxide (1%) in 70% ethanol which does not affect immunostaining. Azure B, instead of haematoxylin, as a counterstain results in green-blue staining of melanin in heavily pigmented lesions,

allowing differentiation from the brown reaction product of diaminobenzidine.

## False positive and false negative staining

Cells in mitosis and necrotic tissue show non-specific staining. There may be passive absorption or active phagocytosis of antigens by histiocytes and other cells which may show false immunoreactivity. For example, macrophages may pick up myoglobin from damaged skeletal muscle or thyroglobulin from thyroid follicles. The stratum granulosum of the epidermis shows non-specific reactivity with many antibodies. The free edges of tissue sections may display non-specific staining and similar artefactual staining may be seen on the membranes of isolated or degenerate cells in cytological effusions. Some antibodies cross-react with antigens different to the target antigen and can lead to false-positive results, a risk which is reduced by the use of monoclonal antibodies. False-positive reactions may also result from the presence of endogenous peroxidase or biotin.

Antigens in tissues held in a condensed or consolidated form, such as Russell bodies or thyroid colloid, may fail to stain with antibodies due to inadequate penetration. Other causes of false-negative staining include inappropriate titre or dilution of reagents, denatured antibody, low antigen levels, masking or loss of antigens and inappropriate incubation time and temperature.

## Quantitation of immunostains

Subjective grading provides semi-quantitative assessment of immunostains. The proportion of specific cells expressing an antigen can be counted and semi-quantitative analysis of immunolabelling can be represented by the product of an assigned grade of staining intensity and percentage of positively stained cells. Image analysis allows a standardised measurement of the concentration, however interlaboratory standardisation is currently not possible because of variations in methods of fixation and immunostaining.

The extensive applications of immuno-histochemistry in diagnostic histopathology are beyond the scope of this book.

## Special stains

The use of enzyme histochemistry in surgical pathology has declined markedly since the 1960s due to the need for fresh frozen tissue, relative non-specificity and the laborious techniques required to demonstrate the enzymes. Histochemistry mainly detects hydrolytic and oxidative enzymes. Many of the hydrolytic enzymes are contained in lysosomes and the process of freezing and thawing leads to some enzyme diffusion. A period of controlled fixation in cold (4°C) formal calcium will decrease enzymatic activity but produces enhanced localisation of the remaining enzymes. Most mitochondrial-based oxidative enzymes are destroyed by any form of fixation.

Currently, the main diagnostic applications for enzyme histochemistry include staining for skeletal muscle related enzymes (ATPase, NADH, LDH, myophosphorylase) to enable fibre typing in the investigation of myopathy/dystrophy, disaccharidase measurements in small bowel biopsies taken for malabsorption, acetylcholinesterase (as an adjunct in the diagnosis of Hirschsprung's disease), chloroacetate esterase (Leder stain) for the identification of myeloid and mast cells, and acid phosphatase to detect prostatic carcinoma and osteoclasts in unfixed trabecular bone. Both the latter two enzymes can be demonstrated following routine formalin

fixation and processing but very few other enzymes resist routine tissue processing. Enzymes are immunogenic proteins and it is more convenient to demonstrate their presence with immunohistochemical methods in formalin-fixed tissue. For example, the Leder stain fails to stain 30% of extramedullary myeloid cell tumours in paraffin-embedded tissue samples, whilst immunohistochemistry with antibodies to myeloperoxidase, neutrophil esterase and other myelomonocytic antigens such as CD68, CD15 and CD30 is clearly more sensitive and detects up to 96% of these tumours.

Plastic-embedding methods following paraformaldehyde fixation have been shown to preserve a number of enzymes such as alkaline phosphatase in germ cell neoplasms, besides retaining excellent cell morphology. Freeze-drying with low temperature resin embedding can also retain certain labile enzymes.

Melanocytes can be identified with the DOPA enzyme histochemical technique which detects tyrosinase in fresh and fixed tissue.

An extensive range of other special stains can be employed to demonstrate various intracellular and extracellular substances. Many of these stains are empirical and are used uncommonly and in special circumstances. In Chapter 8, a list of common tissues, cellular constituents and organisms and useful stains for their demonstration is provided. A list of special stains employed commonly in the diagnostic setting and their reaction products is given below:

### Common special stains

| Stain | Reaction |
| --- | --- |
| Masson's trichrome | Muscle, cytoplasm and keratin stain red, collagen stains blue or |

green and nuclei stain
black

| | |
|---|---|
| Gordon and Sweets' reticulum stain | Reticulum stains black, collagen stains yellow-brown in the untoned section and grey or black after toning, and the background is clear |
| Snook's stain for reticulum | Reticulum fibres stain grey to black and the background remains pink to rose colour |
| van Gieson's stain for collagen and muscle | Collagen stains red, muscle, cytoplasm, fibrin and erythrocytes stain yellow and nuclei stain brownish black |
| Jones' hexamine-silver stains for glomerular basement membrane | Basement membranes stain black and the background is green |

*Stains for carbohydrate complexes:*

| | |
|---|---|
| Periodic-acid Schiff (PAS) stain | Glycogen, neutral mucosubstances or mucin and some basement membranes stain magenta, nuclei stain blue and erythrocytes stain pale pink |
| Alcian blue, pH 2.5, for acid sulphated mucins, hyaluronic acid and sialomucins | Acid mucins stain blue, nuclei stain red and erythrocytes stain yellow |
| Alcian blue, pH 0.4, for strongly acidic sulphated mucins | Strongly acidic sulphated mucins stain blue, nuclei stain pink to red and cytoplasm stains pale pink |
| Combined PAS and Alcian blue | Acid mucins stain blue, neutral mucins stain |

| | |
|---|---|
| for acid and neutral mucins | magenta, while mixtures of acidic and neutral mucins stain blue-purple and nuclei stain deep blue |

*Stains for lipids:*

| | |
|---|---|
| Oil red O for frozen sections | Lipids stain red and nuclei stain blue |
| Osmium tetroxide for frozen sections | Phospholipids stain blue-black and the background stains brown |

*Stains for pigments and minerals:*

| | |
|---|---|
| Masson–Fontana technique for melanin and argentaffin substances | Melanin, argentaffin cell granules, some lipofuschins and chromaffin granules stain black and nuclei stain red. Melanin and lipofuschin pigments are removed by bleaching in the melanin bleach method |
| Diazotised fast red B salt for argentaffin cell granules | Argentaffin granules stain orange red, nuclei stain blue and the background stains pale yellow |
| Churukian and Schenk's stain for argyrophil granules | Argyrophil granules stain black or dark brown, nuclei stain red and the background stains golden |
| Perls' Prussian blue for ferric ions | Ferric salts stain deep blue, nuclei stain red and erythrocytes stain yellow |
| DMAB-Rhodanine stain for copper deposits | Copper deposits stain red and nuclei stain pale blue |

| | |
|---|---|
| Fouchet's stain for bile pigments | Bile pigments stain green, collagen stains red and the background stains yellow |
| Hall's method for bilirubin | Bilirubin oxidised to biliverdin stains olive and emerald green, collagen stains red and muscle stains yellow |
| von Kossa's method for calcium deposition sites | Calcium sites stain black, collagen and osteoid stain red, muscle, cytoplasm, fibrin and erythrocytes stain yellow |
| Alzarin red S procedure for calcium | Most calcium salts stain as birefringent red precipitates. Calcium oxalate has no reaction |

*Special stains for bacteria, fungi and other organisms:*

| | |
|---|---|
| Gram's stain for microorganisms | Blue/black staining microorganisms are Gram-positive, whereas those that are stained red by the counterstain are Gram-negative |
| Ziehl–Neelsen stain for acid-fast micro-organisms | Acid-fast microorganisms stain red, nuclei stain blue and erythrocytes stain pale pink |
| Fite's method for acid-fast bacteria | Lepra and other acid-fast bacilli stain red, nocardia filaments also stain red and the background stains pale blue |
| Giemsa's stain | Bacteria, fungi, parasites stain purplish blue, starch granules and cellulose stain sky-blue, collagen, muscle and bone stain pink, nuclei stain blue and erythrocytes stain salmon pink |
| Giemsa's method for helicobacter | Helicobacter stain dark blue while the background stains light blue |
| Warthin–Starry silver stain for spirochaetes and other micro-organisms | Spirochaetes, bacteria and Donovan bodies stain black and the background stains golden yellow |
| Shikata's modified Orcein for hepatitis B surface antigen | Hepatitis B antigen stains reddish brown and the background stains a much lighter brown |
| Grocott's hexamine-silver stain for fungi | Fungi and histoplasma stain black, mucin stains greyish rose pink and the background stains with the counterstain employed |

*Miscellaneous stains:*

| | |
|---|---|
| Naphthol AS-D chloroacetate esterase (Leder) stain | More mature myeloid cells, tissue mast cells and Chediak–Higashi inclusions stain scarlet red and nuclei stain blue |
| Myeloperoxidase stain | Neutrophils and their precursors stain black to brown |
| Methyl green-pyronin stain for DNA and RNA | Ribonucleic acid (RNA) stains red and deoxyribonucleic acid (DNA) stains blue to blue-green |
| Vogt's cresyl violet stain for Nissl substance | Nissl's substance stains intense purple, nuclei stain purple and the background is clear |

| | |
|---|---|
| Bielschowsky's method for neurofibrils | Neurofibrils and senile plaques stain black and the background stains yellow to brown |
| Bodian's stain for nerve fibres and endings | Nerve fibres, myelinated and non-myelinated, and neurofibrils stain black, background stains blue and nuclei stain black |
| Holmes' stain for nerve cells and fibres | Axons stain black, nerves and nerve endings stain black and the background stains grey to pink |
| Klüver–Barrerra luxol fast blue stain for myelin and nerve cells | Myelin, including phospholipids, stains blue to green and other cells and cell products stain pink to violet |
| Holzer's stain | Glial cells and fibres |
| for glial fibres | stain deep violet and the background stains pale violet |

## Further reading

Elias JM 1990 Immunohistopathology. A practical approach to diagnosis. ASCP Press, Chicago

Leong AS-Y 1993 Applied immunohisto-chemistry for the surgical pathologist. Edward Arnold, London

Prophet EB, Mills B, Arrington JB, Sobin LH 1992 Laboratory methods in histotechnology. Armed Forces Institute of Pathology, Washington

Taylor CR 1986 Immunomicroscopy: a diagnostic tool for the surgical patholo-gist. WB Saunders, Philadelphia

# 10 Frozen section consultation

Sections of frozen human tissue were first cut in the early 19th century, but it was not until much later that the technique was used as a rapid diagnostic method. Welch purportedly was the first to employ intra-operative diagnostic frozen section in 1891 on a patient with a breast lump which was diagnosed as benign. By 1905, the technique was well established at the Mayo Clinic. It soon spread to other hospitals in New York, and later in England where it was employed by workers like E.H. Shaw who described his technique in *The Lancet* in 1910 and 1923. Shaw's first case was that of a breast tumour in 1899. The tumour had clinical growth characteristics of carcinoma or chronic mastitis and frozen section examination confirmed it to be a carcinoma. 'Fortified by this knowledge, the surgeon was then able to proceed with the formidable operation of amputation of the breast with removal of the pectoral muscles and axillary glands, satisfied in his own mind that he was doing the correct operation for his patient' (Shaw 1910). In those days the examination had to be performed under difficult conditions and Dr Shaw described having to use all kinds of odd places for his procedure. He cut his sections on the landing at the top of a flight of stairs, on a board placed across an ordinary bathtub, in the corner of an operating room, on a rickety table in a cottage, on a bed, etc. Sunlight from a window provided the light for his microscope and sometimes a beam from an overhead lamp served as the source of light.

The early methods employed sections cut by hand from frozen tissue and these were stained with polychrome dyes, and it was only in the 1950s that the refrigerated microtome or cryostat became commercially available. By the 1960s, reports of the use of cryostats in diagnostic histopatholo-gy first appeared and it became so popular that in some centres, such as the University of Texas M.D. Anderson Hospital and the Mayo Clinic, frozen sections replaced paraffin sections even for routine surgical pathology.

## Frozen section consultation

The frozen section examination is a consultation between surgeon and pathologist, often carried out during surgery and at short notice. Both the pathologist and surgeon have needs that must be met in this kind of consultation. The need for frozen section can usually be anticipated, and with advanced planning, an optimal consultation can be given. However, frozen section diagnosis has limitations, and, consequently, it is often not possible to provide all the information until permanently fixed and paraffin-embedded sections are available. Requests for frozen sections are occasionally unreasonable because of the lack of knowledge regarding the technical and professional interpretive methodology and limitations of the technique. Most surgeons have never gained any familiarity with the technical aspects of the pathologist's work, much less any insight into the mental processes that result in the formulation of a diagnosis. However, unreasonable requests can be decreased by gradually educating practising surgeons on the intricacies of our speciality. This may require considerable restraint and patience, but we believe that it is a high-priority educational obligation. As surgical pathologists, we must thoughtfully, carefully and repeatedly explain our role as the individuals who are most knowledgeable in the proper handling of tissue for the maximum benefit of the patient. For example, requesting a frozen section on a small breast biopsy for a mammographically detected abnormality in which no gross evidence of invasive carcinoma is present is compromising the care of the patient. In the absence of macroscopic abnormality it is not possible to identify, with any accuracy, where the appropriate section should be taken to include representative histology. Frozen section diagnosis of melanocytic lesions of less than 5 mm diameter is another situation which is fraught with difficulties. Such small lesions are best examined by paraffin sections and frozen section diagnosis should be avoided. Situations such as these provide an opportunity for educating the surgeon regarding problems that are inherent in frozen sections. The pathologist must explain that the random 5 $\mu$m section may not be representative and may not include lesional tissue. Furthermore, the interpretation of non-invasive breast lesions on frozen section is diagnostically hazardous because of the possible suboptimal nature of the section, and the frozen section artefact in subsequent paraffin-embedded tissue sections from the frozen block may also render it inconclusive. Similarly, the diagnosis of soft tissue and bone tumours by frozen section is fraught with difficulties and inaccuracies and should not be encouraged.

Adequate clinical data must always be available when frozen sections are reported and it is just as essential as it is for the more leisurely reporting of paraffin sections. It cannot be over-emphasised that the frozen section is a consultation and for this reason some advocate the use of the term 'intra-operative consultation' instead of 'frozen section'. Surgeon and pathologist should confer before embarking on a diagnostic frozen section in an unusual case. Any previous biopsy material, particularly if neoplastic, should be reviewed beforehand and kept available for reference at the time of doing the frozen section.

It should be remembered that some intra-operative consultations do not culminate in frozen section. The intra-operative decision *not to perform* a frozen section is fully as critical as rendering a diagnosis on a frozen section. The pathologist is in the best position to determine if the frozen section is the best way of obtaining an accurate diagnosis, and other diagnostic techniques such as gross examination, touch imprints, and intra-operative fine needle aspiration may be more appropriately suggested. For these reasons, it has been emphasised that frozen section should never be delegated to trainees, but should always be reported by senior surgical pathologists 'rich in experience, conservative in attitude and, most importantly, he must have judgement' (Ackerman & Ramirez 1959). Trainees, therefore, should always be supervised closely in their performance of frozen sections and should not be allowed to gain their experience by trial and error on their own.

## Indications

There are a variety of reasons for requesting frozen sections. Some relate to the immediate surgical procedure, while others are needed for planning future procedures or treatment. For example, a preliminary frozen section to identify the presence of lesional tissue before processing for electron microscopy, cell surface markers, receptor assays or even paraffin sections can be cost-effective.

One of the most common reasons for frozen section is to determine the nature of the disease. The most frequent application used to be the intra-operative diagnosis of breast lesions, although with the advent of fine needle aspiration biopsies, this use is diminishing. The frozen section diagnosis of breast carcinoma allows the surgeon to proceed with a mastectomy but this has the disadvantage in that the patient may suffer the psychological trauma of not knowing if she would awake from anaesthesia with or without a breast. There is increasing preference for fine needle aspiration biopsy diagnosis which allows the patient time to be mentally prepared prior to the mastectomy if necessary.

Frozen section diagnosis may be requested when the surgeon encounters an unexpected situation during surgery, such as an apparent tumour which was not anticipated. The differentiation of malignancy from inflammatory pseudo-tumours can be very difficult or impossible on macroscopic examination alone. The differentiation of intraperitoneal granulomas due to tuberculosis from disseminated peritoneal deposits of carcinoma is essential as the treatment for these conditions is vastly different, as is the prognosis.

In other situations, intra-operative confirmation of the nature of excised tissue is a common indication for frozen section. For example, frozen section examination is virtually indispensable in parathyroid surgery to distinguish parathyroids from brown fat, peripheral thyroid nodules, lymph nodes and ectopic thymic tissue, all of which can macroscopically resemble parathyroid.

Frozen section is used to determine the extent of a disease. Identification of ganglia in the colon during resections for Hirschsprung's disease determines the limits of the pathological segment of bowel. In cancer surgery, assessment of resection margins is an important method of guiding the surgeon in his extirpative operation.

Lastly, frozen section is used to confirm that lesional tissue has been removed. If the sole purpose of a procedure is to remove tissue for diagnosis, the effort is wasted if the specimen ultimately proves to be inadequate. For example, frozen section examination of lymph nodes is employed to identify abnormal tissue without the need to identify the particular disease process. Another situation arises with biopsies of intrathoracic tissues which frequently occur in a highly vascular setting. As such, the biopsies are small and often may be inadequate or artefactually squashed. A neurosurgeon may request a frozen section to confirm adequacy of diagnostic tissue as there is a high likelihood of sampling error when dealing with brain tumours which are largely necrotic and yield non-diagnostic tissues. Confirmation of adequacy by frozen section is a useful procedure.

## Common applications

### Breast masses

The more common areas in which rapid frozen section diagnosis is employed include the examination of breast lesions which probably still constitute the largest single group in most diagnostic laboratories, despite the fact that pre-operative needle biopsies and aspirates have tended to reduce the need for intra-operative breast frozen sections. It is important to emphasise that frozen section examination should not be performed on impalpable, radiographic-detected breast lesions as very often there is no macroscopic abnormality to direct or guide the sampling for microscopic examination. Errors in frozen section diagnosis of breast lesions tend to result in the over-diagnosis of cancer.

Sclerosing adenosis is the perennial histological mimic of invasive carcinoma. It should be borne in mind that the vast majority of papillary lesions in the breast are benign so that a diagnosis of carcinoma in a papillary tumour should be made with a great deal of circumspect.

## Thyroid nodules

In the case of thyroid nodules, follicular carcinoma can rarely be distinguished from an adenoma or a dominant adenomatous nodule, unless vascular invasion is fortuitously identified. As the vast majority of thyroid lesions tend to be follicular in nature, frozen section diagnosis for the separation of such follicular lesions is usually an unhelpful exercise. In contrast, frozen section consultation is useful for the distinction between Hashimoto's thyroiditis and other inflammatory conditions of the thyroid, although the identification of malignant lymphoma can be a difficult task.

## Parathyroid glands

In the identification of parathyroid tissue, the surgical pathologist is required to decide whether the gland is normal, hyperplastic or an adenoma. This can, on occasion, be a difficult problem. Parathyroid glands should be measured and weighed and the dimensions of normal glands often do not exceed 6 × 4 × 2 mm, with each gland normally weighing about 30 mg. The amount of adipose tissue in each gland increases with age. Density of the gland has been suggested to be a useful guide to the presence of hyperplasia or adenoma. Normal glands float in a mannitol solution of specific gravity 1.049–1.069, whereas, abnormal glands will sink because of the relative paucity of stromal fat.

Adenomas can be distinguished from chief cell hyperplasia with certainty only by the finding of a second gland that is either normal or suppressed. A second enlarged gland strongly favours hyperplasia rather than adenoma and the presence of a compressed rim of suppressed normal parathyroid tissue suggests adenoma. Clear cell hyperplasia invariably produces a diffuse enlargement of the gland and poses relatively few problems. However, a nodular adenomatous configuration, virtually indistinguishable from an adenoma, is seen in chief cell hyperplasia and the other criteria listed above need to be employed. Intracytoplasmic lipid droplets have been suggested to be useful in identifying normal and suppressed parathyroid cells as opposed to their absence in adenomas and hyperplastic glands. However, variable quantities of intracytoplasmic fat can be demonstrated in adenomas and hyperplastic glands and fat droplets tend to smear in frozen sections so that accurate localisation can be difficult.

Lymph nodes, adipose tissue and thyroid nodules macroscopically mimic parathyroid glands and it should also be noted that, microscopically, some parathyroid adenomas can show an acinar arrangement which closely mimics thyroid tissue, even to the extent of containing colloid material.

## Other organs

A variety of other situations may benefit from intra-operative frozen section diagnosis. These include: the distinction between chronic peptic ulcer and ulcerated carcinoma; biopsies from the pancreas and ampullary region for the identification of well-differentiated adenocarcinomas which can show a marked desmoplastic response, tending to simulate chronic pancreatitis; the identification of prostatic carcinoma prior to surgical orchidectomy; the recognition of acute inflammation during the revision of hip and other joint prostheses; the typing of pulmonary tumours, in particular the distinction between oat cell carcinomas and other types of carcinomas which are less responsive to chemotherapy and require extirpation; and the identification of cystic ovarian neoplasms from benign ovarian cysts.

Although surgeons should be advised to avoid frozen section consultation for soft tissue tumours which can be difficult to subtype even with paraffin sections, frozen sections can still be employed in this situation to determine adequacy of resection. It can also be used to confirm the presence of a tumour in order to justify total extirpation of a lesion in which tissue diagnosis was previously unobtainable such as when the lesion is in a relatively inaccessible location like the retroperitoneal space. Soft tissue tumours, like primary malignant bone tumours, are best diagnosed and typed in paraffin sections before definitive surgery is planned.

## Sampling and methods

Sampling of the specimen is governed by the same principles as sampling from fixed tissue for routine paraffin sections. Always wear gloves when handling fresh tissues. Palpate the specimen gently; rough handling of unfixed samples will provide crushing artefacts. Always incise the tissue with a clean sharp blade and endeavour to save at least a small portion for paraffin sections to avoid freezing artefacts.

While the cryostat allows a wide variety of tissues to be cut, some remain difficult to section. Bone poses problems and skin can be difficult. In particular fatty or necrotic tissue tends to fragment and such

specimens should be avoided or trimmed of fat and necrotic areas before sectioning.

A suitable representative tissue block of about 2–3 mm thickness is orientated on a metal chuck so that the best cross-sectional surface for cutting is available. If necessary, the surgical margin can be marked with India ink or some other indelible ink, taking care that the marking fluid does not smear. The tissue block is covered with a water-soluble embedding medium such as Tissue Teck II OCT to prevent ice crystal artefact and it is plunged into liquid nitrogen or isopentane, the process of snap-freezing taking no more than 1 minute. Several suitable sections are cut in a cryostat and stained with a rapid H & E stain. A variety of other quick stains are available, a popular one being Diff-Quick (Lab Aids, Sydney, Australia), which allows the wet section to be examined without a coverslip.

After a diagnosis is rendered, the tissue block is pried from the chuck and fixed in 10% buffered formalin for routine paraffin embedding. The frozen sections and the corresponding blocks should be separately labelled for identification, such as with the letters 'FS'.

Other important practical aspects of performing frozen sections need to be reiterated. Speed and accuracy are of essence in the examination. The total time taken between removal of the specimen and reporting of the findings should not exceed 15 minutes. As soon as the specimen arrives, it should be examined by the attending pathologist and a representative tissue block removed for frozen sectioning. Detailed description and measurements can be recorded after the specimen has been sampled. The surgeon should be notified promptly when technical difficulties are encountered, particularly if they are likely to delay reporting or impede accurate assessment. For example, certain types of specimens such as fatty tissue or bone may interfere with making good sections. There may be problems of adequacy of the specimen such as size or orientation and, at times, delays may occur due to simultaneous requests arriving from multiple operating rooms.

Although speed is of the essence in this procedure, it should not prejudice calm interpretation and accurate diagnosis. Equivocation and fence-sitting are to be avoided. In the case of tumours, either a *definite diagnosis* or a *deferred diagnosis* are the only two acceptable diagnoses which can be given. 'Possibly malignant' is not acceptable as an aggressive surgeon may act on it and proceed with radical extirpation which may prove to be unnecessary. Do not be apologetic if you cannot make a definite diagnosis even when the frozen section is technically optimal. Inform the surgeon of the situation, stating the 'diagnosis is deferred, to await paraffin sections'. However, you should appraise if the tissue removed is representative of the lesion. The surgeon may choose to send more tissue for frozen section or to await permanent sections before proceeding.

## Surgeon–pathologist interaction

It is evident from the above restricted list of clinical situations that rapid frozen section diagnosis provides optimal benefits only when it is employed as a consultative process. Several well-defined steps can be identified. The question must be clearly stated by the clinician requesting the consultation and understood by the pathologist. The pathologist should respond to the question and should have an opportunity to check whether the reply was received and understood. Finally, the

pathologist should also check to see if the reply has generated further questions. Thus, the consultation process clearly involves exchanges of information with the surgeon characterising the clinical problem and indicating the need for the frozen section consultation. The pathologist should know the pertinent history and any previous tissue diagnosis, and should appraise the surgeon of how long the examination will require and, in particular, if technical difficulties are anticipated. In addition, the degree of probability of the diagnosis needs to be clearly stated. It is the *prerogative of the pathologist to recommend against* performing a frozen section when he/she considers that freezing the tissue may render it unsuitable for subsequent permanent sections, or when it is unlikely to produce relevant information and alterative diagnostic procedures such as fine needle aspiration, needle core biopsy or paraffin sections may be more appropriate alternatives. In such circumstances, the pathologist needs to explain to the surgeon why the frozen section should not be done. The frozen section diagnosis is costly, time-consuming and sometimes stressful but despite its established usefulness, it is sometimes misused. Unfortunately, some surgeons use it as a mechanism to communicate the results immediately to the patient's relatives, to satisfy their curiosity or to compensate for their own deficiencies in recognising normal anatomical structures. If the findings of the frozen section examination will not influence the surgical procedure in any way, it should not be performed (Ackerman & Ramirez, 1959).

## Reporting

While the pathologist can often prepare him/herself the day before by examining the operating room schedule and reviewing the charts and laboratory records of patients who may require a frozen section diagnosis, he/she should not hesitate to obtain more information from the clinician when he/she receives an unusual specimen or makes an unexpected observation. This can be done over the telephone, or more conveniently over the intercom, as the surgeon may be scrubbed-up.

In reporting his/her findings, the pathologist must report directly to the operating surgeon or, in the event that he/she is unable to come to the intercom, to another member of the surgical team, such as the anaesthetist, who should be clearly identified. Reports should not be transmitted via theatre orderlies, nurses or other staff.

Clearly identify yourself and give the name of the patient and the nature of the specimen. If you require information from the surgeon, ask your questions before reporting your findings. Use the opportunity to exchange information as the additional clinical information you receive from the surgeon may well influence your interpretation of the specimen. Be clear and concise when speaking on the intercom. Before concluding, ask the surgeon if his/her queries are answered and if he/she plans to send more material for frozen section examination. Record your findings, the time and the name of the recipient of your oral report.

Optimal communication between surgeon and pathologist occurs when the frozen section suite is located within the operating room complex or when the pathologist enters the operating room to receive the specimen or to report his/her findings. This arrangement encourages the pathologist to speak to the surgeon face-to-face and to see the specimen in situ. It provides the best opportunity to resolve questions of orientation and allows the pathologist and surgeon to discuss the plan and limitations of the frozen section consultation. However, this arrangement is not practised in many medical centres as it is a costly and labour intensive exercise to take the pathologist away from the laboratory where he/she is most efficient and productive. It also deprives the pathologist of the experience of other pathologists, who may be consulted, and reference textbooks and other sources of information available in the laboratory.

## Precautions

The cryostat sectioning of a variety of infected tissues should be avoided. For example, tuberculous lesions should not be sectioned and if the diagnosis is made unexpectedly, the contaminated cryostat should be appropriately disinfected before being used again. Other infections such as hepatitis virus B and C, and HIV are definite contraindications to frozen section. However, if clearly unavoidable, full precautions should be employed. These include safety measures directed towards prevention of cuts, and protection of the eyes, nose, mouth and other mucosal surfaces. Protective clothing includes double gloves, eye glasses or goggles, masks, gowns and even a helmet with air supply. Contamination should be confined to a small area of the bench-top and aerosols should not be created, particularly in confined spaces such as the cryostat. The frozen section slide should be briefly immersed in 10% formalin before staining. In the case of hepatitis virus B and C, it may be necessary to immerse the tissue in boiling formalin before frozen sections are performed. All unused tissue should be thoroughly fixed in 10% formalin before it is handled again.

The cryostat should be decontaminated with an appropriate inactivating reagent such as 0.5% sodium hypochlorite or 10% formalin. Details of safety measures are described elsewhere (see Ch. 3).

## Accuracy

The accuracy of frozen section diagnosis has been tested and proven on numerous occasions. Accuracy rates range from 93 to 98% depending on the types of tissue examined. Diagnostic accuracy depends, in part, on active and continuous familiarity with the appearances and artefacts which occur as a result of freezing, proficient technical staff, and close consultation and communication with the surgeons. Diagnostic errors can be minimised both by experience and by seeking a consensus with accessible pathologist colleagues. While errors can occur in all histopathological diagnostic procedures as a result of sampling, technique, communication and interpretation, these can be kept to a minimum with experience, expertise and a good working relationship with the surgeons. If a definitive diagnosis of primary malignancy cannot be made on the available material, diagnosis must be deferred, eliminating unnecessary delay and equivocation. The surgeon must be told to await the interpretation of paraffin sections. Deferring a diagnosis during the examination of margins of resection has different implications than deferring diagnosis of the frozen section from the lesion. A deferred diagnosis of a margin of resection must be followed by the resection of a new margin from the same area. Although speed is important, it must not be allowed to prejudice the accuracy of the given diagnosis. Only calm interpretation of the material will allow a thoroughly

considered diagnosis and judgement should not be adversely influenced by a sense of urgency. Frozen sections should not be performed out of idle curiosity, to fill in a coffee break, to increase a surgeon's, pathologist's or hospital's income, or merely to prove that the pathologist is actually in the hospital (Saltzstein & Nahum 1973).

## Special techniques

### Special stains

A number of special stains have been modified for use in rapid frozen section diagnosis, encompassing only those that have the most contributions in rapid diagnosis. They include Alcian blue, mucicarmine, Papanicolaou and Snook reticulin (Kraemer & Silver 1988). These stains take between 3 and 12 minutes to perform although they can be greatly accelerated with the use of microwaves (reviewed by Kok & Boon 1992).

### Microwave-assisted frozen sections

Exposure of cryostat sections to a brief burst of microwaves produces vastly improved cell form and structure. Freshly cut frozen sections immersed in Wolman's solution (95% ethanol and 5% glacial acetic acid), or in a commercial reagent known as Kryofix, contained in a Coplin jar and irradiated for 15 seconds, with the power setting on 'high', produce noticeable improvement in the quality of the microscopic image without any significant delay in the frozen section procedure. The cytomorphology is greatly improved when compared with sections conventionally fixed in 95% ethanol, in 10% buffered formalin or in formalin vapour (Leong 1992).

## Imprints and scrape cytology

Cytological examination of fresh specimens, particularly of tumours, is a useful ancillary to frozen section diagnosis. It provides additional information to the cryostat section in that cytological morphology is generally better preserved. This is often useful in distinguishing malignant lymphoid cells from small cell carcinomas and can be performed without delaying the frozen section procedure. Indeed, the routine use of imprint cytology as an ancillary to frozen section diagnosis is highly recommended. Clean glass slides should be gently dabbed on fresh cut surfaces of the tumour. If the slide is dabbed on the tissue, it picks up less red cells than if the reverse was done, i.e. the tissue dabbed on the slide. If possible, do not prepare more than two slides per cut surface of tumour as the delicate tumour cells tend to show squash artefact and dry-up if too many imprints are prepared. Use fresh cut surfaces to prepare additional slides. These can be left to air dry for staining with Giemsa and Romanovsky stains, or can be fixed immediately in 95% ethanol for staining with the same rapid H & E procedure performed on the cryostat section, so that there is no delay to the examination process. A mixture of 95% ethanol and 10% buffered formalin in a 1 : 1 volume ratio and staining with the rapid H & E procedure produces a cytomorphological image closest to that seen in the frozen section. Fixation in 95% ethanol results in more shrinkage than observed in the cryostat sections.

In some situations, it is difficult to obtain sufficient cells in imprints and dab preparations so that scrape cytology from the cut surface is a preferred method. A scalpel blade is scraped over a freshly cut surface and air-dried direct smears are made from this material. Diff-Quick (Lab-Aids, Sydney, Australia) is useful for the rapid staining of air-dried smears.

## Resection margins and Mohs' technique

Considering that an ellipse of tissue 2 cm long will provide seven blocks of tissue, each 3 mm thick, and that up to 100 sections can be obtained from each block, it becomes obvious that it is impossible to examine all surgical margins in any specimen. In the excision of skin cancers, especially in the face, there is a great need for conservation and at the same time there is a realisation that the frequent local extension of basal cell carcinoma results in areas of tumour being missed by conventional excision, producing persistence and recurrence of the tumour. In an effort to overcome this problem, a method of total microscopic control of margins of excision has been described by Mohs and modified at the Cleveland Clinic, Ohio, USA (Levine et al 1979). In this technique, the surgeon excises the tumour with the scalpel at a 45° angle towards the centre of the specimen. The excised specimen is divided into marked quadrants with exact orientation, the margins being coded with different coloured dyes. As it will not be possible to examine the entire surgical margin with standard vertical sections, each segment of tissue is flattened with firm pressure applied between glass slides, causing all lateral margins to be forced downward and outward, and ultimately into the same plane as the deep margin (Fig. 10.1) before freezing. Between eight and ten sections are then cut horizontally through the tissue, beginning at the deep surface. Each section so obtained represents a complete view of all margins, both lateral and deep, at which tumour extension might occur. When this is performed on each quadrant of tissue that is excised, total microscopic control of the margins is obtained. It should be remembered that with this technique, it will not be possible to provide a diagnosis of the tumour if it is not present in the margins of excision as only the margins will be sectioned. Diagnosis of the tumour will have to be performed on an incisional biopsy prior to the commencement of this procedure, which is aimed only at the complete examination of all surgical margins. Mohs' method, widely employed in the USA, has several technical drawbacks and should not be routinely employed except in the context of Mohs' surgery.

In the examination of resection margins in other samples, the pathologist must use his/her judgement and experience in determining the appropriateness and extent of sampling. He/she must determine if more pertinent information is to be gained by taking parallel or perpendicular sections, if quadrants should be sampled, if only one area needs to be studied, or if the entire margin should be evaluated. Theoretically, blocks including the margin of excision, whether on a parallel or perpendicular axis, could be entirely sectioned, thereby providing complete information regarding the tumour at the margin and the distance of tumour to the margin. As a general guide, if the lesion is some distance from the resection margin then a parallel section would be more useful as it would sample a larger margin. In contrast, if the margin lies close to the lesion then several perpendicular sections will provide more information and will also indicate the actual distance of the tumour from the margin if the latter is uninvolved. Margins which are hollow cylinders or rings, such as bronchial, urethral or oesophageal margins, can easily be studied circumferentially en face, usually with a single frozen section block. By convention, the majority of excisional

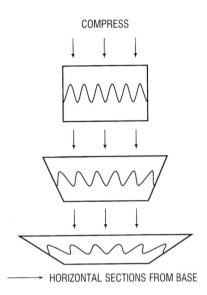

**Fig. 10.1** Moh's technique of examining surgical margins

biopsy specimens examined at frozen section are sectioned perpendicularly to the margin. For larger specimens, one section perpendicular to the closest margin is submitted and, when feasible, the remainder of the margins are examined by parallel sections to the margin (discussed further in Ch. 5).

## Further reading

Ackerman LV, Ramirez GA 1959 Indications and limitations of frozen section diagnosis. A review of 1269 consecutive frozen section diagnoses. British Journal of Surgery 46: 336–350

Kok LP, Boon ME 1992 Microwave cookbook for microscopists. Art and science of visualisation, 3rd edn. Coulomb Press, Leyden, pp 181–183

Kramer BB, Silva EG 1988 The examination of margins of resection by frozen section, Part II. Surgical Pathology 1: 437–446

Leong AS-Y 1992 Microwave techniques for diagnostic laboratories. Scanning 15: 88–95

Levine H, Bailin P, Wood B, Tucker H 1979 Tissue conservation in treatment of cutaneous neoplasms of the head and neck. Combined use of Mohs' chemosurgery and conventional surgical techniques. Archives of Otolaryngology 105: 140–144

Saltzstein SL, Nahum AM 1973 Frozen section diagnosis: accuracy and errors, uses and abuses. Laryngoscope 83: 1128–1143

Silva EG, Kraemer BB 1988 The examination of margins of resection by frozen section, Part I. Surgical Pathology 1: 303–306

# 11 Photography of gross specimens

Macrophotography is performed for a variety of reasons but, if considered necessary, should be regarded as an integral part of specimen examination and may require as much thought and composition as the macroscopic or microscopic description. Thus, although photography of gross specimens is often performed by technical staff or specialist photographers, it is desirable for the pathologist to have a major input into the orientation and composition of the picture since an understanding of the disease process is essential to ensure illustration of the pathology. All surgical pathologists enjoy good photographs of gross specimens and often take great pride in their collection. The photographs may be black-and-white prints for inclusion in the surgical pathology reports or for publication, Kodachrome slides for projection and, less commonly, colour prints.

## Uses

Macrophotography may be used to help in the description and orientation of the surgical specimen. This is especially true for complex specimens such as a block dissection, a total mastectomy with axillary clearance or various other radical resections. The position of positive lymph nodes and clearance margins can be easily described with reference to a black-and-white photograph included in the report. Often, block keys can be more easily understood with the aid of a photograph or line diagram.

There are some specimens for which macrophotography is a prerequisite, e.g. the histological examination of cardiac valves is often unrewarding per se, the definitive diagnosis usually being dependent on the macroscopic description or its substitute, the photograph, particularly if a second opinion is sought. The photograph, if appropriately taken, also acts as a permanent record of the gross specimen and can be reviewed for reassessment of diagnosis or for medico-legal purposes in the same way as a histological section retrieved from archival files.

A common use for the photograph is in publications. Unlike the histological slide which can be photographed months or years later, macroscopic specimens are often not available in a suitable state for photography following dissection and fixation, even if they have not been discarded. Thus, the trainee pathologist must always be vigilant for unusual or interesting specimens which may later be the subject of a case presentation or publication and act appropriately with regard to photography before dissection of the specimen.

Another major role for macrophotography is in teaching and at clinicopathological conferences, where they are excellent aids in the demonstration of pathology. Naturally, it is essential that the point being made is actually demonstrated in the photograph and this is not always as easy as it sounds.

## Equipment

Macrophotography can be organised in different ways with some laboratories providing the service themselves, but with specialist advice, and others relying solely on the services of a specialist photographic unit. We have found that close co-operation with a specialist photographic unit, whereby the majority of photographs are taken by laboratory staff with developing and printing performed by the specialist unit, provides for maximum versatility and efficiency. The specialist unit may also be used for more difficult photography requiring intricate lighting and optical systems.

## Camera

The majority of modern cameras are fully automatic and ensure reproducible exposures. It should be appreciated, however, that the greater the $f$ number, the greater the depth of field, i.e. the greater the depth of specimen that will be in focus, and it is necessary to set the $f$ number accordingly. In practice, with artificial lighting, there is often a trade-off between adequacy of illumination and depth of field since the higher the $f$ number, the smaller the lens aperture and less amount of light entering the camera. For specimens of substantial height/depth, the lens aperture should be as small as possible to increase the depth of field ($f$-stop of 16 or more).

Consideration should also be given to the lens type. Large specimens may require a wide angle lens whilst such a lens may not be suitable for smaller specimens. This can generally be overcome by using a single zoom lens rather than interchangeable lenses of differing field widths. Although close-up pictures can now be taken with most cameras, extension rings can be added to the lens system for very close work. Alternatively, photography of small specimens can be performed using a dissecting microscope fitted with a camera attachment. Such photography is capable of producing very detailed macroscopic pictures but is generally only used for research or teaching.

Cameras that have automatic film advance and rewind help to reduce any contamination of the camera back by blood, formalin and similar fluids. Similarly, a cable release for operation of the shutter not only prevents movement of a mounted camera but also helps prevent contamination, although with most models, it is still generally necessary to focus the camera manually and this necessitates consideration of health and safety procedures. With cameras having a manual rewind, care should be taken to ensure the film is rewound in the direction of the arrow. Rewinding in the opposite direction drags the film across the inside of the camera and may result in linear scratches throughout the length of the film.

Many laboratories use polaroid cameras for routine macrophotography. These produce colour or black-and-white prints. Polaroid cameras have the advantage of prints being produced immediately for inclusion in the report. The drawbacks are that reproduction is often not as good as with conventional negatives and it is generally more expensive.

## Illumination

Whilst flash units attached to the camera body provide for adequate exposures, the illumination is not always even across the specimen. Separately mounted flash lights synchronised with the camera shutter and evenly spaced over the work area provide the best illumination. It is often better not to direct the flash lights directly onto the specimen but to 'bounce' the light off a white surface for more even and diffuse illumination, preventing bright spots on the specimen. Bright spots are often due to reflection from the wet surface of a specimen and this can be a particular problem with fresh specimens, necessitating careful drying of the specimen surface. Reflection of light from chrome fittings on the front of the camera can also cause problems but may be overcome by placing a matt black cardboard sheet with a central hole through which only the camera lens can protrude, between the camera body and specimen. Further uneven illumination may result from nearby fluorescent lighting and extraneous natural light which should be avoided. Illumination for very close work may require either a ring flash unit attached to the camera or a flexible fibreoptic light source. Such intricate photography is better carried out by a specialist photographic unit.

## Background

The background is of equal importance but to some extent a matter of preference. A coloured background giving maximum contrast with the specimen is ideal for colour photography whereas a white background is best suited to black-and-white photography. The chosen background may be in the form of a coloured perspex sheet which is placed under the specimen or, preferably, some distance below a glass plate bearing the specimen. The latter method gives a greater three-dimensional appearance to the final picture, especially if there is even illumination below the perspex. Again, care should be taken to nullify any reflections from the surface. For this reason, a dampened cloth background can be used but it is essential to minimise diffusion of blood and other fluids from a fresh specimen and to ensure the cloth background is not wrinkled. The texture of the cloth can be a distraction in a magnified photograph. Special effects may be obtained with photography of a specimen immersed in water or with the use of polarising filters but these are generally more difficult to perform.

## Film

As with photomicroscopy, black-and-white prints are mostly used in publications and in

surgical pathology reports. Colour photography is generally used for the production of colour transparencies for use in oral and case presentations. Care should be taken in the selection of either daylight film or artificial light film depending on the illumination source. This is discussed in greater detail in Chapter 13. It should be remembered, however, that most flash units attached to the camera have colour temperatures similar to daylight and require daylight film, in contrast to photofloods which require artificial light film. Light balancing filters attached to the front of the camera lens allow daylight film to be used with artificial light and vice versa.

Film cassettes can be rolled from a bulk loader. This avoids wastage and is often less expensive, but the film can be easily scratched during the process of loading if performed without undue care.

## Photographic set-up

An ideal photographic set-up comprises a portable trolley incorporating fully adjustable camera mountings, two to four mounted flash units or photofloods for even illumination, a transparent glass plate on which the specimen can be placed and provision for different coloured backgrounds to be inserted under this plate. A camera mounting capable of accommodating two camera backs allows for easy interchange between black-and-white and coloured photography without the necessity of removing and replacing the camera backs from a single mounting. This avoids wastage of film and minimises handling and contamination of delicate and expensive equipment. Automatic cameras with automatic film advance and rewind facilities also help minimise contamination. Where photography is performed infrequently and the prints are to be included as part of the surgical report, a polaroid camera set-up is ideal.

## Taking good macrophotographs

Even with the most advanced photographic equipment, good pictures can only be obtained with attention to detail and picture composition. All too frequently photographs are marred by improper specimen orientation or inappropriate background conditions.

A major fault is the failure to utilise the whole of the picture field. Although an identification tag and ruler should generally be included in the picture, it is inappropriate for these to occupy a more prominent position than the specimen itself. They should be placed to one edge or corner and occupy as little of the picture field as possible. It may seem superfluous to state that the orientation of the specimen should be such that the pathology or feature of interest is best displayed and yet, all too often, this is not evident from the final picture. Inclusion of normal structures in the field serves as a frame of reference for the lesion. Some specimens require pinning out on a corkboard for appropriate demonstration and it is in this situation that a dampened clean cloth background covering the board can be very useful. Other specimens may require partial elevation to ensure all aspects of the specimen are in focus. Model plasticine can be used for this purpose as well as to support specimens and identification markers.

Needless to say, great care should be taken in any preliminary dissection that might be required. Preparation and trimming of the specimen such as removal of fat and other tissues from around a tumour and washing of a soiled specimen,

improves the photograph considerably. Solid organs should be sliced with a long sharp knife preferably with one stroke to avoid step marks across the cut surface which results from any sawing action. It is desirable to photograph one half rather than both halves of a partially cut specimen and the cut surface provides more information than the intact external surface of a tumour. The washing of bone dust from bony surfaces cut with a bandsaw results in a much better demonstration of the pathology. It may be desirable to pin out fresh specimens, e.g. bowel or stomach, and in some cases, perform photography after fixation. Photography should be done before sampling for histological examination, but if this is not possible, the specimen should be dissected in such a way to ensure that it is still presentable at a later date. It is seldom necessary to decimate a specimen in order to take adequate sections. Photography of fixed specimens often overcomes the glare that a fresh specimen produces but has the disadvantage of inaccurate colour rendition. This may be corrected by reducing the period of exposure to formalin which removes the sheen but does not destroy the colour. Alternatively, immersion of the fixed specimen in alcohol often restores the colour, particularly in haemorrhagic or congested specimens.

The other common faults in macrophotography, including bright spots from reflection of the camera front, overhead lights or wet surface of the specimen, inappropriate background contrast, wrinkling of a cloth background, blood or fluids surrounding the specimen and inappropriate picture framing or composition, can be overcome by the use of a little common sense, time, patience and attention to detail. It is for these reasons that the pathologist should have a major input into any macrophotography since it is the pathologist who will ultimately make use of the photograph. Probably the best advice that can be given to the trainee is to look down the camera viewfinder and consider not only the specimen but also the background and picture composition.

# 12 Microscope function, maintenance and special techniques

As with motoring, although it is not necessary to understand the workings of the car to be able to enjoy driving, the more one appreciates how the car works, the more one is able to obtain better performance. So with microscopy, whilst it is not absolutely necessary to understand the workings of the microscope to be able to interpret histological sections, the more one appreciates the principles of light energy and mechanics of the microscope, the more one is able to obtain the best results from the instrument.

## Principles of light energy

Diagrams illustrate the passage of light rays through a given medium as straight lines but light energy is more accurately represented by a sine curve indicating the pulsatile nature of the light source. The *amplitude* is the brightness of the light which decreases with increasing distance from the light source and is measured as the maximum deviation of the sine wave from zero. The *wavelength* is the distance between two apices of the sine wave whilst the *frequency* is the number of waves per second. Most light sources emit waves over a wide range of wavelengths but the frequency of any given wave remains constant. Rays of identical frequency are *coherent* and may combine or interfere with each other, a principle exploited in phase contrast and interference microscopy.

*Reflection* of a light ray occurs when the incident ray rebounds from the surface of a second medium. If an incident ray is not perpendicular to the surface of a second denser medium, it is refracted towards the normal and vice versa. The higher the density of the medium, the higher the *refractive index*, which is calculated as the ratio of the sines of the angles of incidence and refraction and is of use in the design and construction of lenses.

## Passage of light through lenses

The principal axis of a lens is perpendicular to its surface and passes through its middle, joining the centres of curvature of the two surfaces. A ray of light travelling along it, passes through the lens without deviation. Light rays incident on the lens other than along the principal axis will be refracted at the anterior surface and again at the posterior surface resulting in deviation of the ray as the ray emerges. A ray incident on the centre point of the lens emerges parallel to the incident ray but is only slightly deviated as the opposite surfaces of the lens near its middle are virtually parallel. Effectively, this means that for a thin lens a ray incident on the middle of the lens can be considered as passing through it without deviation. It is this principle that helps in the understanding of how an object is seen as an image in the lens. For a thin *convex* or convergent lens, a narrow beam of light rays parallel and close to the *principal axis* is brought to a focal point on the principal axis behind the lens. For a *concave* or divergent lens, the deviation of light rays is in the opposite direction away from the principal axis, the *focal point* being on the same side as the incident rays and from which the divergent rays appear to emanate.

### Images in lenses

For a convex lens, the image of an object perpendicular to the principal axis and further from the lens than the focal length, is formed behind the lens below the principal axis, i.e. it is real and inverted. The image of an object placed at twice the focal length from the lens appears real, inverted and the same size as the object at a similar distance behind the lens. If the object is moved nearer the lens the image appears further away and is enlarged. However, if the object is placed nearer to the lens than the focal length, the image appears on the same side as the object above the principal axis and is thus virtual, erect and always magnified. In the case of a concave lens, the image is always virtual, erect and diminished in size. Figure 12.1 illustrates these points.

## Defects of lenses

The image of an object formed by a single lens may be distorted by a number of causes.

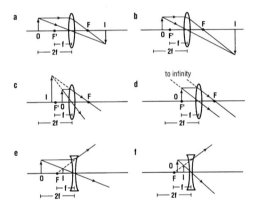

**Fig. 12.1**   Diagrams of images produced by convex and concave lenses. **a**, An object placed at twice the focal length from a convex lens produces a real, inverted image the same size as the object. **b**, An object placed nearer to the focal point of a convex lens produces a magnified, real, inverted image. **c**, An object placed inside the focal point of a convex lens produces a magnified, virtual, erect image. **d**, An object placed at the focal point of a convex lens produces an image which appears to come from infinity. **e**, **f**, Images produced by a concave lens are always virtual, erect and diminished in size regardless of their position along the principal axis. O = object, I = image, F = focal point, f = focal length

*Spherical aberration* occurs when a wide beam of light is incident on a lens. Parallel rays that are not close to the principal axis have a larger angle of incidence and are deviated to a greater degree than rays close to the principal axis, such that they are focused at points slightly closer to the lens than the focal point resulting in distortion of the image.

*Field curvature* makes a flat object appear curved and results from the image field focused by a lens being naturally curved so that when the centre of the field is in focus, the periphery appears blurred and vice versa.

*Coma* results from different magnifications occurring in the various lens zones leading to object points away from the principal axis appearing as short comet-like images.

*Distortion* also results from different magnifications occurring within different parts of the lens. If the magnification of a square object increases with distance from the centre, it appears to have concave sides. If it decreases with distance from the centre of the object, the image has bulging sides.

*Astigmatism* results from widely varying lens curvatures in different planes so that from an object, rays in one plane will be focused at a different place from rays in another plane.

*Chromatic* aberration is the colouring of the image produced by dispersion of white light through a lens due to the differing colours of the spectrum having different wavelengths. In axial chromatic aberration, for a convex lens, the red rays are brought to a focus on the principal axis slightly further away from the lens than blue rays, thus producing coloured images at slightly different positions on the principal axis. Lateral chromatic aberration is chromatic aberration transverse to the principal axis and arises when different wavelengths are magnified at different ratios leading to colour distortion around the periphery of any one image.

Advanced optical instruments utilise combinations of lenses with different refractive indices, curvatures and thicknesses to produce optimal images.

## The light microscope

The early or simple microscope was nothing more than a convex lens or magnifying glass. However, a lens of short focal length is required for high magnification and it becomes impracticable to decrease the focal length beyond a certain limit owing to the difficulties in manufacture of such a lens. This led to the production of a compound microscope which utilised two separate convex lenses of small focal lengths in order to obtain a high magnification. The lens nearer to the object is the objective and the lens through which the final image is viewed is called the eyepiece.

The ciliary muscles allow the eye to focus objects at different distances, a property known as accommodation. The most distant point the eye can focus is known as the far point and is at infinity for the normal eye. The ciliary muscles are completely relaxed and the eye is unaccommodated or at rest. However, an object is seen in greater detail when it is placed as near to the eye as possible whilst still remaining in focus. This is known as the near point and is about 25 cm for a normal eye. At this point the eye is fully accommodated and the ciliary muscles are fully strained. The microscope is an instrument used for viewing near objects and when in normal use, the image formed by the microscope is usually at the near point of the eye. As such, it is useful to rest the eyes

periodically by focusing on a distant image (infinity) after prolonged use of the microscope.

Modern microscopes are much more complex with many more components than merely the simple objective and eyepiece lenses outlined above.

## The modern day microscope

### Light source

A light source is an essential part of the system and has graduated over the years from sunlight through separate oil lamps and low voltage electric lamps to the powerful pre-centred in-built low voltage halogen filament lamps of today.

### Aperture

With simpler instruments, the light is directed through an aperture iris diaphragm situated at the front focal plane of the condenser lens into the substage condenser by reflection from a simple mirror or by refraction through a prism. The purpose of the aperture iris diaphragm is to control the diameter of the light beam and to maintain optimum conditions of image resolution, contrast and focal depth. In the fully open position, extraneous light interference leads to glare and lack of contrast, with poor resolution. If closed too much, the image appears refractile as a result of diffraction. The optimum image quality is achieved if the aperture diaphragm is adjusted to between 60 and 80% of the aperture and should be adjusted for each change in objective. Another method is to close the aperture iris diaphragm until there is diffraction of the image and then opening it slightly until the diffraction disappears. This adjustment of the aperture diaphragm is of utmost importance in photomicrography.

The purpose of the condenser is to focus the light onto the plane of the object since the more light at the specimen, the greater the resolution of the image. This is known as *critical* illumination. Most microscopes have adjustable condensers which may be centred or varied according to the height or thickness of the object and many condensers are fitted with a swing-out accessory lens for use with high power objectives. This additional lens situated above the condenser focuses the light into an area more suited to the smaller diameter high power objectives but will result in illumination of only the centre of the field when used with low power objectives.

## Field lens and iris diaphragm

With critical illumination and modern filament lamps, the image of the filament is seen and causes uneven illumination. This can be overcome by the insertion of a field lens complete with field iris diaphragm between the light source and the condenser. This is the basis of *Koehler illumination* which provides even illumination for the formation of an image against a uniformly bright background (Fig. 12.2).

## Objective lenses

There are many different designs of objective lenses which have endeavoured to correct the various lens defects described earlier. Since a concave lens, in contrast to a convex lens, deviates rays away from the principal axis, axial chromatic aberration or the dispersion between two colours produced by a convex lens can be annulled by placing it beside a suitable concave lens made of a different glass. This is the basis of *achromatic lenses* which correct for blue

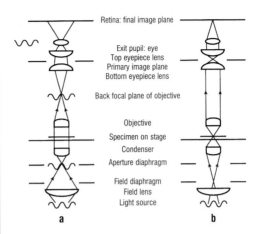

Retina: final image plane

Exit pupil: eye
Top eyepiece lens
Primary image plane
Bottom eyepiece lens

Back focal plane of objective

Objective
Specimen on stage
Condenser
Aperture diaphragm

Field diaphragm
Field lens
Light source

a                                    b

**Fig. 12.2**  Diagrammatic representation of the two simultaneous beam paths in a microscope set up for Koehler illumination. In **a**, the direct light beam path provides illumination. An image of the light source is formed by the field lens at the aperture iris diaphragm or front focal plane of the condenser. The emerging parallel rays of light from the condenser transilluminate the specimen and are focused at the objective's back focal plane where an image of the light filament is formed within the mechanical tube of the microscope. The bottom lens of the eyepiece illuminates the plane of the primary image whilst the top lens causes the light rays to converge on the exit plane (level of observer's eye) and illuminate the retina. Thus the source filament, aperture iris diaphragm, back focal plane of the objective and exit pupil of the microscope all appear in simultaneous focus. In **b**, a second image-forming beam leads to an image of the field iris diaphragm being focused through the condenser onto the specimen. Diffracted light is focused by the objective and bottom lens of the eyepiece at the primary image plane situated at the front focal plane of the top eyepiece lens. The beams leave the top lens of the eyepiece as parallel rays seemingly coming from infinity so that the observer's eye, which forms an image of the specimen on the retina, is adapted and relaxed. The field iris diaphragm, the specimen, the primary image and final image are all in simultaneous focus

and red chromatic aberration. Further correction of blue-violet aberration may be achieved by the addition of more lenses, such a combination being known as an *apochromatic lens*. Lateral chromatic aberration is usually greatest at the periphery of the visual field and may be corrected for in the design of the objective alone or in both objective and eyepiece. Spherical aberration may be reduced by excluding the peripheral rays and only allowing mainly those rays with a small angle of incidence to pass through the lens. This may be brought about by the use of a diaphragm with a small central hole but it will result in a reduction in brightness since it also reduces the amount of light energy passing through the lens. A practical method of reducing spherical aberration is to utilise two, usually plano-convex lenses which allow the deviation of light to be shared by four surfaces and the angles of incidence to be as small as possible.

Similarly, the other types of aberrations may be greatly improved by combinations of lenses having different refractive indices, curvatures and thicknesses. Objectives that correct for field curvature are known as plan, planar or flatfield objectives.

Theoretically, magnification can be increased to infinite levels but beyond a certain point, the image becomes indistinct. The resolving power of the objective depends on the wavelength of the light and the numerical aperture of the lens; the latter normally engraved on the objective housing. With a constant wavelength, the resolved distance between two points can be decreased by increasing the numerical aperture. Thus, the higher the numerical aperture, the greater the resolution. The numerical aperture is a product of the refractive index of the medium between the specimen and lens, and the sine of the angle between the optical axis of the lens

and the most oblique ray of light that can possibly enter the lens. Thus, the ability to increase the numerical aperture of a lens is limited and this in turn effectively limits the meaningful magnification of an objective. Since the refractive index of oil is higher than that of air, the numerical aperture of an oil immersion lens is greater than that for a dry objective, resulting in greater resolving power. Greater resolution may also be obtained by decreasing the wavelength of the energy source, a concept utilised in electron microscopy; the electron beam having a far shorter wavelength than that of light results in a resolving power of more than 1000 times that of the light microscope. However, one drawback to a high numerical aperture or magnification is that whilst it provides a greater resolving power, the depth of a specimen layer that can be held in focus at any one time is shorter, i.e. the shorter is the depth of focus.

The performance of high power objectives varies depending upon whether or not a coverslip is used. Most objectives are designed for use with coverslips of 0.17 mm thickness and are accordingly marked '0.17'. However, with high dry objectives having a large numerical aperture, slight variations of the coverglass thickness can increase the amount of spherical aberration. This can be overcome by a correction collar situated in the objective which allows the internal lens elements to be moved so that a sharp image can still be obtained for varying coverglass thickness. Such objectives may be marked '0.11–0.23'.

### Eyepiece lenses

The image produced by the objective is projected within the microscope tube to a point 10 mm from the eyepiece shoulder where it is further magnified by the eyepiece. As for objectives, sophisticated lens systems have been developed for the eyepiece to overcome lens aberrations not totally corrected by the objective and to accommodate measuring grids and graticules. These micrometer discs are inserted into the eyepiece lens system on the image forming plane. The visual field seen through the eyepiece is limited by the eyepiece diaphragm which may either be located between the lens elements (Huygens type) or outside the lens elements (Ramsden or Kellner type), depending on the type of eyepiece. The diameter of the diaphragm is known as the field number. On some eyepieces, the letter 'W' is used to described a widefield eyepiece (also known as periplan) whilst 'SW' describes a super widefield eyepiece. The eyepoint is the optimal position for the eye when looking through the eyepiece and varies depending on the magnification of the eyepiece system. Recently, high eyepoint lens systems designated 'H' with an eyepoint set slightly away from the eyepiece have been manufactured to allow observation through spectacles. In binocular microscopes, the interpupillary distance is important and can be adjusted. Often, such a binocular head also accommodates independent eyepiece focusing for one of the two eyepieces. This allows for slight variations in focusing between the eyes of the user. The same result can be achieved with focusing eyepieces. These eyepieces are indispensable in photomicrography when precise focusing on the eyepiece graticule ensures that the image is sharply focused on the film plane.

## Mechanical and optical tube length

The mechanical tube length of the microscope is the distance between the objective shoulder and the top of the sleeve housing of the eyepiece. Magnification, focus and optical corrections are dependent on the tube length. Microscopes manufactured for biological use have mechanical tube lengths of 160 or 170 mm depending on the manufacturer. For industrial microscopes the standards are 200 or 210 mm. The tube length is usually engraved on the objective and it is important that all objectives and eyepieces are designed for the same tube length to allow interchange between objectives and eyepieces with different magnification ratios. The microscope is also designed with a fixed parfocal distance, i.e. the distance from the objective shoulder to the specimen. This allows interchange between different objectives with the minimum of fine adjustment of focus. In contrast, the working distance is the distance between the front lens of the objective and the specimen and decreases with increasing magnification. For this reason, medium and high power objectives often have a front lens that is recessed into a spring-loaded central component to protect both the specimen and the front lens of the objective.

## Infinity corrected microscopes

Currently, microscopes are being designed to accommodate a universal infinity system whereby the lenses are infinity corrected. Such systems allow the increase of contrast and sharpness overcoming the restrictions of the mechanical tube length. The physics of such systems is complex and the details are often the manufacturer's closely guarded secret.

From the foregoing account, it can be appreciated that the modern day microscope is an exceedingly complex optical instrument which bears little resemblance to the models of yesteryear. It cannot be overemphasised that such an instrument is a carefully integrated system, the components of which have specifications that are calculated with integration in mind. It is unwise to mix different types of objectives and eyepieces on the same microscope and in some cases this practice will result in utter incompatibility and inability to obtain a suitable image of the specimen.

## Maintenance

Maintenance of the microscope by the pathologist is usually limited to keeping the instrument dust free and the optics clean. Periodically, it is advisable to have the instrument properly serviced to ensure smooth operation of the rack and pinion components of the stage and focus, and other moving parts such as the focusing collars on high power objectives. Covers should be used when the instrument is not in use, particularly for extended periods, to minimise the amount of dust contamination. Care should be taken to avoid contamination of dry objectives by oil left on the slide. Lenses contaminated in this way may take a long time to clean properly. Dirt and dust particles observed through the optics may be difficult to locate but this can often be overcome by rotating the various lenses and observing for movement of the particles. Dust can usually be removed by using an air gun or blower brush designed for this purpose. Persistent dust may become difficult to remove and, like fingerprints or perspiration marks on eyepieces, proper lens cleaning is required to move them. A cleaning mixture of seven parts ether and three parts alcohol or special lens cleaning fluid may be used. Xylene and other solvents should not be used as these can lead to partial dissolution of the lens cement. The use of special lens cleaning tissues wrapped around an orange

stick will avoid leaving small fragments of material behind on the lens. However, the use of 'cotton buds' soaked in lens cleaning fluid is ideal. Lens tissue paper is more appropriate for large glass surfaces such as filters. Care should be taken to clean all externally exposed glass or lens components since particles anywhere within the optical system may lead to image distortion. This is especially true when taking photomicrographs. After cleaning, uneven reflection of colour from the surface of a lens, when viewed through a magnifying glass or up-turned eyepiece, indicates residual dirt on the lens. Internal optics remain relatively clean and dust free but should they require attention, it is best to have this done professionally. It should be remembered that certain additional optic components, e.g. photo eyepieces and removable analysers for polarised microscopy, may predispose to the introduction of dirt into the internal optics. The microscope frame itself may be cleaned with neutral detergent if necessary. Again, organic solvents should not be used as they may damage plastic parts.

## Setting up the microscope

In setting up the microscope, two aspects require consideration – that concerned with the comfort of the user and the setting up of the optics to obtain the best possible image.

Today, most manufacturers have become aware of the need for ergometrically designed instruments. Long periods of use may lead to eye strain, fatigue, neck and back problems, and even neurological deficit, not only because of inappropriate posture but also from inadequate forearm support. While employers now accept the need for specifically designed workstations for clerical staff, they pay little attention to similar needs of the pathologist. However, this is fast becoming an issue of which every trainee pathologist must be aware. A full description of the ergonomic requirements is beyond the scope of this book. Suffice it to say that each pathologist will have individual needs and that the workstation should be adjustable. Fully adjustable chairs and work tops may be supplemented by padded and adjustable forearm rests that clamp onto the work top. Similarly, the microscope may be fitted with aids that help in combating fatigue. Stage and focusing controls may be remotely operated or automatic whilst a tilting binocular eyepiece head may help to combat neck and back problems.

Once the workstation and microscope have been ergometrically set up to suit the individual, it is necessary to adjust the optics of the instrument to ensure optimal illumination. Before the instrument can be adjusted for Koehler illumination, a number of conditions must prevail. All lenses and exposed glass surfaces must be spotlessly clean. The lamp source should be centred and focused with respect to the lamp condenser. In modern instruments, this is pre-set by the manufacturer and needs no further adjustment. The correct combination of sub-stage condenser lenses and auxiliary swing-in condenser lenses should be in use, and the objective and eyepiece lenses matched with regard to the mechanical tube length. Each eyepiece should be independently focused and the interpupillary distance of the eyepieces set for the user. Koehler illumination may now be achieved by the following steps:

1 Adjust the light intensity to a safe working level and half close the field diaphragm.
2 Using a $10\times$ objective, focus on the microscope slide of interest and swing in the auxiliary condenser lens.

3 Raise the substage condenser as far as possible, open the aperture diaphragm to its full extent and slowly close the field diaphragm.
4 Centre the image of the field diaphragm by manipulating the centring screws controlling the position of the substage condenser.
5 Lower the substage condenser until the edges of the field diaphragm are sharply focused, making sure the viewed specimen also remains sharply focused. The edges of the field diaphragm will be ringed by a magenta halo and the auxiliary swing-in lens will be very close to the bottom of the slide. If the substage condenser is raised too much, the halo appears orange; if lowered too far, it appears blue. If dust is brought into focus, the substage condenser may be slightly lowered until it disappears from view.
6 Open the field diaphragm until its edges just disappear from the field of view, adjust the aperture diaphragm until the best contrast is obtained and swing the auxiliary condenser lens out of place. Remember that the aperture diaphragm is used to produce maximum contrast and resolution and not to regulate light intensity. Optimal conditions are achieved with an aperture diaphragm of between 60 and 80% of the numerical aperture of the objective and this will of course change for the different objectives. To save time, the field diaphragm as set for the $10\times$ objective may be left open for the higher power objectives. However, this should also be adjusted to obtain the best results for photomicroscopy.
7 Correct setting for Koehler illumination may be checked by removing one eyepiece and observing the filament of the light source in the back focal plane

of the objective within the microscope tube. It should be noted that this can only be done in the absence of a frosted filter between the light source and field lens.

## Special techniques

The light microscope may be adapted in a number of ways to allow better visualisation of certain objects.

### Dissecting microscopy

The stereoscopic or dissecting microscope was designed for low power inspection, specimen dissection and manipulation of specimens at low power. Original instruments used two matched objectives, each with their own eyepiece. They were positioned to collect slightly different images of the same specimen approximately 7 degrees either side of the vertical axis from whence these images were reconstructed into a single three-dimensional image by the user's brain. Since the optical axis of each objective was not perpendicular to the plane of the specimen, the resulting image was not always in focus across the whole field. This lead to the development of instruments having a single objective lens and optics which allow the resulting image to be split, again 7 degrees from the vertical axis. Each split image is viewed simultaneously through separate eyepieces using parallel light path geometry and, once again, the brain is able to reconstruct a three-dimensional image. The objective lenses have a long working focal length and low numerical aperture to give images with good depth of focus. A zoom magnification lens is inserted between the objective and the eyepieces and a good illumination source is required. Care

should be taken to avoid drying out of the specimen and cold sources of light are preferred.

The dissecting microscope is only of limited use in routine surgical pathology but is a useful adjunct in the low power examination of fresh tissues. Its uses include the examination of the villous architecture of small bowel biopsies, renal biopsy cores for the presence of glomeruli, and the dissection and teasing out of nerve and muscle biopsy preparations. When used with a photomicroscopic attachment, it produces good images of macroscopic specimens at low magnification.

### Polarised microscopy

Polarised microscopy is an extremely useful technique for the identification of foreign material, crystals, certain pigments, lipids and protein-derived material such as amyloid in a histological section. It can also be used to identify certain tissue components such as collagen and is particularly useful in the examination of bone. Polarised light is obtained when natural randomly orientated light is passed through a filter which only allows the passage of light orientated in one particular plane. With polarising light microscopy, one polar filter, the polariser, is placed below the microscope stage and another, the analyser, above the tissue section. When the planes of the two polars are parallel, polarised light from the polariser will travel up through the analyser uninterrupted. When the planes of the polars are at right angles to each other, polarised light from the polariser will be completely blocked by the analyser so that the field appears dark. It is this arrangement of crossed polars that is commonly used in polarised microscopy. Substances through which light can pass in any direction at the same velocity are called isotropic and are not able to influence polarised light. Anisotropic substances such as crystals allow the passage of light at different speeds depending on the plane of the light path. In other words, they have different refractive indices which may be recognised by the optical properties of birefringence. A birefringent material placed on the microscope stage between crossed polars with its optical axis in the same plane as the polarised light will allow light to pass freely through it and be completely blocked by the analyser. When its optical axis is rotated to 45 degrees to the plane of polarised light, the light will be resolved into two components travelling at different speeds by the two relevant optical planes of the material being examined. The two components are recombined at the analyser and the material appears brightly visible against the dark background of the crossed polars. Since they are travelling at slightly different speeds, they will be out of phase when reunited giving rise to interference and frequency, or colour change. These two properties of birefringence, i.e. relationship of the dark position to the planes of the polars (angle of extinction) and type and extent of colour change, are typical for each birefringent material, and form the basis on which different crystals may be identified. In practice, for simple recognition of birefringence, the substage polariser is manually rotated in and out of the crossed polarised position whilst the specimen remains stationary on the stage itself. Polarising filters are easily obtained from the microscope manufacturer or made simply from two pieces of plastic polaroid sheets.

A tapered wedge of birefringent material placed between crossed polars and rotated to 45 degrees appears as a series of different colours similar in order of sequence to

Newton's rings. Further birefringent material superimposed on the wedge will shift the colours up or down the spectrum. In compensated polarised microscopy, a flat quartz plate, known as the compensator, manufactured to produce the red colour of the first order of a corresponding wedge (first order red), is inserted obliquely between the two polars with its slow component at 45 degrees to the planes of the two polars. The whole field now appears red and against this, a birefringent crystal will produce a colour change. A urate crystal, for example, will show strong negative birefringence turning yellow when the long axis of the crystal is parallel with the slow component of the first order red plate and blue at right angles to this position. In contrast, pyrophosphate crystals exhibit weak positive birefringence turning blue when the long axis of the crystal is parallel with the slow component of the first order red plate and yellow when at right angles to this position.

## Fluorescence microscopy

Fluorescence microscopy utilises the property of some substances which, when excited by relatively high energy of short wavelength, re-emit light of lower energy and longer wavelength (Stoke's law). A substance, or fluorspar, that contains a naturally occurring fluorophore, emits primary fluorescence or autofluorescence. Stains used in microscopy to produce secondary fluorescence are known as fluorochromes. Induced fluorescence refers to the emission from a substance which has been converted to a fluorspar by an appropriate chemical reaction, e.g. the production of fluorescent quinoline compounds by the treatment of catecholamines with formaldehyde vapour. In fluorescence microscopy, the exciting radiation is usually ultraviolet light although light of longer wavelengths may be used. The applications of fluorescence microscopy are numerous, being used both qualitatively and quantitatively, in microbiology, histopathology, immunology and protein chemistry.

Modern day instruments are standard microscopes modified for fluorescence with a reflected epi-illumination system rather than the transmitted illumination systems. Ultraviolet light from a mercury vapour or xenon gas lamp is passed through a series of heat filters, collector lenses and lamp condenser to the exciter filter which excludes light of unnecessary wavelengths. From here, the exciter beam is reflected down through the objective onto the specimen by a dichroic mirror placed at 45 degrees to the illumination source above the objective. The dichroic mirror allows reflection for excitation wavelengths but transmits fluorescent light emanating back from the specimen through the objective and thus onto the eyepiece. A barrier filter placed between the dichroic mirror and the eyepiece prevents the passage of any excitation light not absorbed by the specimen. This increases fluorescence observation and protects the observer's eyes from harmful ultraviolet light. Exciter and barrier filters must be matched for the specimen and fluorochrome under observation. A reflected epi-illumination exciter system allows transmitted techniques such as brightfield, darkfield and phase contrast to be used simultaneously if desired and produces a more efficient image than a transmitted exciter system. Fluorescence microscopy is generally performed in a dark room as most fluorescence is of low intensity.

Fluorescent microscopy as outlined is relatively infrequently used in routine diagnostic histopathology but the trainee pathologist should have knowledge, and expertise in the interpretation, of immunofluorescence microscopy. In immunofluorescence microscopy, specific antigens can be detected by fluorescent-labelled (fluorescein isothiocyanate) antibodies viewed under ultraviolet light. The principles of the technique are similar to those pertaining to the immunoperoxidase techniques described in Chapter 9. Despite the many advantages of immunoenzyme techniques, there are a few situations where immunofluorescence may still be preferred, e.g. the investigation of the glomerulonephritides and of bullous skin disorders. With time, fluorescence fades, necessitating the photography of the specimen for a permanent record and a further disadvantage is the requirement for frozen sections where the degree of resolution is considerably less than that of paraffin sections. However, fluorescence techniques can generally be performed far quicker than peroxidase techniques and are particularly useful when time is of the essence, e.g. the diagnosis of anti-glomerular basement membrane disease by positive linear immunofluorescence in a patient with acute renal failure. Immunofluorescence techniques are still widely used in immunology laboratories for the initial investigation of certain immune-based diseases and the identification of autoantibodies, e.g. anti-neutrophilic cytoplasmic antibody (ANCA), in certain types of vasculitis, although these too are gradually being replaced by techniques such as radioimmunoassay (RIA) and enzyme-linked immunoabsorbent assay (ELISA) techniques.

## Dark ground illumination microscopy

The examination of stained sections employs brightfield illumination whereby stained preparations are viewed against a bright background. Examination of some unstained specimens such as live micro-organisms is not satisfactory under brightfield illumination since such specimens have similar refractive indices to the media in which they are suspended, leading to lack of contrast between the specimen and its environment. Dark ground or darkfield illumination overcomes this problem by illuminating the specimen against a dark background. Most brightfield microscopes can be adapted for darkfield illumination by the inclusion of a simple patch stop of black paper placed on top of the condenser lens. This allows the passage of light from the periphery only and illuminates the specimen obliquely. The only light allowed to enter the objective is that which is reflected or diffracted from the specimen. This causes the contrast to be reversed and increased, and the specimen to appear as a bright object against the dark background. In contrast to brightfield illumination where optimum results are obtained when the numerical aperture of the objective matches the condenser, in darkfield illumination, the numerical aperture of the objective must be lower than that of the condenser. In order to accomplish this with high power objectives, the objective must be provided with a built-in iris diaphragm which can be stopped down until all direct rays of light are prevented from entering the image. This in turn reduces the numerical aperture and resolution, and is a compromise to the increased contrast. More specialised condensers such as the paraboloid or cardioid types may also be utilised to produce the required light paths. Since only light reflected and diffracted from the specimen enters the objective, a powerful light source is required.

## Phase contrast microscopy

Darkground illumination microscopy allows the examination of unstained and living specimens but often fails to reveal internal structure. Phase contrast microscopy overcomes this problem and allows detailed examination of internal unstained cell structure. Light rays diffracted from the specimen are displaced by up to one quarter of a wavelength shift in phase but this displacement results in no change in amplitude and is generally not visible. If the shift in phase is increased to one half of a wavelength and the amplitude of the light rays is the same, maximum interference occurs but the rays cancel each other out and no light is seen. If, however, one light ray is brighter than the other but still one half a wavelength out of phase, maximum interference is maintained and the difference in amplitudes of the rays can be visualised so that specimen details become visible.

In phase contrast microscopy, a hollow cone of light is produced by an aperture ring slit placed at the front focal plane below the substage condenser. Some of these light rays will be diffracted or retarded by approximately one quarter of a wavelength by the specimen whilst others will pass through unaltered. The light rays enter the objective and pass through a phase plate placed at its back focal plane. The phase plate is so designed to increase the phase difference of the direct and diffracted rays to one half of a wavelength and to reduce the intensity of the direct rays. Each objective requires a different sized ring slit aperture. A special focusing telescope in place of the eyepiece or a Bertrand lens situated in the body tube of the microscope ensures that the ring slit is centred and superimposed on the phase plate. When the diffracted rays are recombined with the direct rays of different amplitude, maximum interference will now occur and an image of contrast is obtained. Constructive interference is brought about by the diffracted rays having a greater amplitude than the direct rays and causes the specimen to appear as a bright object against a dark background whilst destructive interference occurs when the direct rays have a greater amplitude than the diffracted rays leading to a dark specimen against a light background.

## Interference microscopy

The major disadvantage of phase contrast microcopy is that it produces halos around the specimen which may be useful in viewing small objects, but decreases resolution in thick specimens or specimens with many structural details. The use of interference microscopy eliminates these sometimes confusing halos, allows optical sectioning whereby focusing of a thin plane of section within a thick specimen may be achieved and, in modified interference microscopes (differential interference contrast microscopes of the Nomarski type), allows optical staining whereby images can be viewed with a striking three-dimensional coloured shadow-like appearance.

Light passing through a narrow slit will fan out on either side due to diffraction at the edges. Fans of rays formed by light passing through two slits close together will cross each other and lead to interference if coherent. Phase conditions of increased amplitude and extinction occur at points where the waves of light cross and interfere, resulting in a series of alternating bright and dark paralleled bands across the field of view. In the interference microscope, a specimen introduced into one beam path will cause a shift in phase that will result in displacement of the parallel interference bands and visualisation of the specimen. In the Nomarski system, light first passes through a polarising filter that causes light waves to vibrate in the same plane perpendicular to the direction of travel. The polarised light is then split into two beams vibrating perpendicular to each other but in slightly different directions by a modified Wollaston prism positioned in the lower section of the substage condenser. A different prism is required for each objective magnification. The rays intersect at the front focal plane of the condenser and emerge from the condenser as two parallel beams so close to one another that the distance between the rays, known as the shear, is less than the resolving ability of the objective thus preventing any halo effect. Since the rays are still vibrating perpendicular to each other, they are unable to cause interference at this point. With passage of this split beam through the specimen, the wave paths are altered according to the varying thicknesses within the specimen. The parallel beams are focused at the back focal plane of the objective and enter a second modified Wollaston prism that removes the original shear created by the first prism and recombines the split beam. However, the paths of the parallel beams from throughout the specimen are not of the same length, i.e. there is an optical path difference. Thus, following recombination, they can interfere with each other provided that they are brought into the same plane no longer perpendicular to each other by passage through a further analysing polariser. With white light as the source, the optical path differences are seen as differences in intensity and colour (optical colour staining) through the eyepiece.

## Confocal microscopy

Tandem scanning reflected light microscopy or confocal microscopy is a relatively recent invention, first reported by Petran in 1968. It allows examination of a restricted optical slice within a given specimen and, through focusing, enables the specimen to be 'optically sectioned'. The thickness of the optical section can be varied with a resolution of half a micron being possible with modern instruments. Light from a carbon arc lamp is passed through one side of a rotating Nipkow disc and by a system of mirrors through the objective into the specimen. Reflected light from the specimen passes back into the objective and, with the use of a beam splitter, through the opposite side of the Nipkow disc. The Nipkow disc is a thin metal film with thousands of tiny square holes arranged in Archimedean spirals radiating from a central spindle. The apertures are so arranged that they are geometrically opposite one another with respect to the central spindle. The system is designed such that light from one aperture will only be imaged by its corresponding aperture in the other half of the disc if it is reflected from a narrow plane at the focal plane of the objective lens. Light reflected from above or below this plane will be focused in front of, or behind the disc respectively and not imaged.

Fresh intact tissue can be examined with no need for fixation, embedding, sectioning or staining. For example, relatively dense tissues such as bone can be examined at multiple optical sections up to a depth of 180 μm. Whilst its routine service applications are at present limited, it has immense research potential in that a three-dimensional stereological image can be obtained simply by examination of multiple optical sections through the one specimen. It can also be used as a fluorescence microscope and can be used to increase the resolution of renal immunofluorescence frozen sections in the interpretation of glomerulonephritis.

## Further reading

Bancroft JD, Stevens A 1995 Theory and practice of histological techniques, 4th edn. Churchill Livingstone, Edinburgh

Basics of the Optical Microscope. Produced by Olympus Optical Company Limited, Tokyo

Shotton DM 1989 Confocal scanning optical microscopy and its applications for biological specimens. Journal of Cell Science 94: 175–182

# 13 Photomicroscopy

The main ingredient of a good oral presentation is the quality of the transparencies used to illustrate the talk. This is true not only for photographs of macroscopic specimens (see Ch. 11) and text transparencies (see Ch. 19), but also for photomicroscopy. There is nothing more off-putting than a presentation which is illustrated by poorly composed macrophotographs, poorly edited text slides and photomicrographs that are out of focus and inappropriately illuminated. Similarly, black-and-white photomicrographs used in journal publications should be of the highest quality to complement the written word.

## Equipment

Although microscopes designed solely for photomicroscopy and possessing fully automated functions such as automatic focusing, automatic exposure and automatic calibration are available, photomicroscopy is mostly performed with a camera mounted on a standard microscope via a phototube attachment.

### Microscope

The ideal microscope for photomicroscopy is one with a pre-centred built-in light source which provides uniform Koehler illumination over the range of objective magnifications and sufficient light intensity to match the observation and photography conditions. There should be provision for the insertion of filters ideally between the light source and the field iris diaphragm as well as at the exit window of the field iris diaphragm. The microscope stand should be sufficiently robust and stable to bear the camera attachment and to resist external vibration. The microscope should have a field iris diaphragm as well as a condenser iris diaphragm and the condenser should have a centring device to allow correct alignment of the optical axis. A rotatable object stage is invaluable in the correct positioning of the field to be photographed. The objectives should have high resolution and flatness, ensuring a flat image to the periphery of the visual field. Microscopes that employ focusing by adjusting the height of the object stage rather than the height of the nosepiece bearing the objectives avoid problems that the additional weight of the camera attachment might have on focusing. High sensitivity of the fine focusing adjustment greatly facilitates accuracy in focusing. A triocular head combining the inclined binocular eyepieces and a vertical phototube allows the image to be viewed alternatively through the eyepieces and phototube. The majority of such heads have an optical path selector which allows the image to be viewed solely through the phototube, solely through the eyepieces or conjointly through both depending upon desired light intensity and specimen conditions. The phototube accepts the photomicrographic camera attachment.

### Photographic equipment

The photographic equipment comprises a camera attachment, a camera back, an exposure control unit and miscellaneous filters. Although the commonly used film in photomicroscopy is of 35 mm size, an ideal camera attachment is one that also accepts a large format film size. Some set-ups provide for two camera backs so that black and white and colour photography can be performed on the same field, otherwise it is necessary to manually change camera backs to achieve the same result or repeat the session with the different films. Most modern day camera backs have an automatic film advance. Automatic rewind functions are available on some instruments although the majority require manual rewinding of the film. With manual rewinding, care should be taken to rewind in the direction of the indicator arrow. If the film is rewound in the opposite direction, linear scratches may be produced throughout the length of the film as it is dragged across the inside of the camera back.

The camera attachment sits between the camera back and triocular head of the microscope. Modern instruments provide for adjustment of the colour temperature of the light source according to the type of film used. A focusing monocular telescope fitted with adjustable dioptre ring and a further optical path selector allows the light source to be directed to the colour temperature control module, the telescope or to the camera back. A focusing magnifier can be attached to the focusing telescope of the camera attachment to allow precise focusing, especially with low power objectives. On some photomicroscopes there is a further device which allows integrated metering or spot metering of the light according to the specimen area. The camera attachment is attached firmly to the phototube of the triocular head of the microscope. A photo eyepiece, which may be interchangeable to allow for different magnifications of the photographic image, is inserted in the phototube. These photo eyepieces permit the objective to deliver its full performance on the film plane.

An exposure control unit is coupled via a cable to the camera attachment. This unit allows for a wide range of ISO/ASA film speed sensitivities, compensation for film reciprocity, exposure adjustments and, usually, automatic, manual and time-lapse exposures.

## Films

Black-and-white photomicrographs are used in most publication illustrations and selection of the appropriate film depends on the specimen conditions. The key to obtaining good prints lies in selection of the right film for the job. Generally, a high contrast film with fine grain is used to document minute structures and to achieve sharp photographic reproduction. With high contrast films, however, the range of proper exposure is narrow and either over- or underexposure will occur unless the exposure is optimum. With instruments having automatic exposure facilities, this is not such a problem and slight differences in exposure can be nullified in the final printing. Fast films with high ISO/ASA numbers are used, with dark specimens requiring long exposure times. The use of contrast filters as described below depends on the colour of the specimen and the desired effect.

Colour photomicroscopy is rather more complex and requires a basic knowledge of film types. The colour temperature of a film refers to the properties of the light source and is determined by reference to the temperature of a blackbody which, when heated, emanates light of different colours. Daylight film is balanced for sunlight and will produce excessively red photomicrographs when used with an artificial light source. Tungsten film is designed for use with artificial light and will produce excessively blue photographs when used in daylight. Thus, the use of a daylight film having a colour temperature of 5500–6000 degrees Kelvin with a tungsten light source having a colour temperature of 2800–3400 degrees Kelvin, requires the use of a light balancing filter to convert the light source to daylight. Alternatively, if the camera attachment is fitted with a colour temperature control module, then this can be adjusted to automatically compensate for the differences in colour temperature depending on the type of colour film used. Generally, a colour film with a fine grain, good colour contrast and good colour rendition, having a film speed between 50 and 100 ISO/ASA, should be satisfactory for most needs. Photomicroscopy of specimens viewed under phase contrast, polarised light or fluorescence may require higher film speeds although this in turn may result in excessive grain.

For normal photographic emulsions, the reciprocity law states that the total exposure for a given film frame is the product of the amount of light striking the film surface (luminance) and the exposure time, but, for long exposure times this rule no longer holds true resulting in underexposure and changes in colour reproduction. Since in photomicroscopy, usually there is no camera aperture diaphragm, i.e. there is a fixed *f* number, exposure compensation can only be adjusted by altering the exposure time leading to reciprocity law failure for long exposures. Compensation can be carried out automatically with most modern instruments by setting the correct reciprocity compensation factor on the control box for the appropriate film in use. Alternatively, colour compensating filters must be used for long exposure times.

*Filters*

In black-and-white photomicroscopy, contrast filters can be used to control the contrast of the negative and thus final print. The choice of filter depends on the specimen, with red/yellow being enhanced by a green filter, yellow/orange by a blue filter and blue by an orange filter. Use of a filter of the same colour as the specimen

will reduce the contrast. The most common filter used is a green filter since stains such as H & E absorb green light well resulting in higher contrast. Furthermore, objective aberrations are most effectively compensated near the green wavelength and a green filter will avert loss of clarity due to chromatic aberration.

Selection of filters in colour photomicroscopy depends on the type of film used. Filters are available to convert the colour temperature of the microscope light source to the film in use as described above. A blue LBD filter is used for daylight films and a pink LBT filter for tungsten films. Colour compensating filters may be used to correct slight differences in colour hue or fading in developed photos. A didymium filter is used to enhance the red colour of a specimen or compensate for the insufficient red colour rendition of a film. These filters are generally placed at the exit window of the field iris diaphragm where they are protected from the heat of the lamp source. Heat absorbing filters placed between the lamp housing and the field iris diaphragm may be necessary to protect live specimens but often impart a blue hue so that additional use of a colour correction filter may be necessary. For instruments having a colour temperature control module attached to the camera, once the correct colour temperature has been set by adjusting the intensity of the light source, the brightness of illumination should only be further adjusted by the use of neutral density filters inserted between the lamp housing and the field iris diaphragm. These filters reduce the light intensity to a comfortable working level without affecting the colour temperature. Since the colour temperature is not critical for black-and-white photomicroscopy, the intensity of the light source can be controlled in the usual way and neutral density filters are usually not necessary.

## Taking good photomicrographs

A basic understanding of the necessary equipment and its different functions is essential for good photomicroscopy. However, a number of other factors should also be considered. The photomicroscope should be set on a stable base and not subject to vibrations from other mechanical appliances. The instrument should not be used near a window where bright light interferes with correct focusing or where extraneous light can enter the eyepiece and result in the production of flares on the photo. A relatively dust free atmosphere will help prevent annoying dust spots. It is surprising how often such spots are unnoticed until the final print or transparency is viewed.

Once the camera is set up, it is essential to make sure the optics are clean and the correct Koehler illumination obtained. A few minutes spent cleaning the lens surfaces and setting up the microscope, as described in Chapter 12, will often save hours of frustration.

The photographic requirements can then be set. Ensure that the film is correctly loaded into the camera back and that it winds on after each exposure by observing rotation of the film rewinding crank. It is surprising how often failure to observe this elementary rule leads to an unexposed film after many hours of work. Set the relevant film size format, the film ISO/ASA speed, the appropriate reciprocity compensation factor and any necessary exposure adjustments on the control module. This information normally accompanies the photomicrography equipment manual or the film being used. Place the appropriate

light balancing filters or contrast enhancing filters on the light exit window immediately above the field iris diaphragm. Set the correct colour temperature on the camera attachment module to match the type of colour film used and adjust the light source to give the correct measurement. This should be set for a blank area of the microscope slide not covered by the section. Once the light source and colour temperature have been correctly set, no further adjustment of the light source should be made. Any reduction in light intensity must then be made using a neutral density filter placed between the lamp housing and the field iris diaphragm. For black-and-white photography, colour temperature is not critical but the light source should be set above 6 volts.

Special attention should be made to focusing, particularly when using the low power objectives. The binocular tube of the microscope or focusing telescope of the camera attachment is normally fitted with a finder eyepiece having cross hairs in the centre and an outline of the photographic frame. This eyepiece is fitted with a locating pin that must be firmly inserted into the groove of the eyepiece sleeve. Unless this is done, correct focusing is impossible. The finder eyepiece should be focused so that the cross hairs are seen as clearly distinguishable separate lines. The specimen should then be brought into focus for that eyepiece using the main focusing knob and the second dioptre eyepiece of the binocular head adjusted accordingly. In theory, when the cross hairs of the binocular eyepiece and the specimen are focused in this way and the specimen is simultaneously in focus through the focusing telescope of the camera attachment, the cross hairs of the focusing telescope should also be in focus. In practice, however, there is often a subtle observer difference between the focusing of the cross hairs in the binocular and focusing telescope eyepieces, such that if the binocular eyepiece is used alone for focusing, the photographic results are not infrequently slightly out of focus. Thus it is better to rely on the monocular focusing telescope of the camera attachment for precise focusing of the eyepiece finder cross hairs, since this gives a true reflection of the image portrayed to the film. For low power objectives, a focusing magnifier should be attached to the focusing monocular telescope to allow precise focusing of the specimen whilst maintaining precise focusing of the cross hairs. Failure to use this focusing magnifier will often result in slightly blurred photographs even in the most experienced hands. Once again, time taken to ensure precise focusing is time well spent.

The field iris diaphragm is used to adjust the illuminated area of the specimen depending on the objective used and plays a crucial role in photomicroscopy. If the diaphragm is opened wider than necessary, reflected light is scattered irregularly over the specimen resulting in loss of image contrast. If the diaphragm is stopped down too close to the photographic frame, the image may be cut at the corners. Thus the diaphragm should be closed down to just beyond the frame reticle area to provide pictures of good contrast.

Similarly, the condenser iris aperture diaphragm is used to provide optimum resolution, contrast and depth of field by adjusting the numerical aperture of the illumination system to match the numerical aperture of the objective. Optimum image quality is obtained when the aperture diaphragm is between 60 and 80% of the numerical aperture of the objective. When the aperture diaphragm is stopped down too far, image resolution deteriorates as a result of diffraction. In the fully open position, overall contrast is low.

Once the microscopic and photographic equipment are fully set up, attention must be paid to picture composition. Obvious artefacts such as section chatter marks or scores should be avoided whenever possible. The area to be illustrated should form the centre point of the photograph and particular attention should be made to exclude any dust particles or dirt that might ruin the end result. A rotatable specimen stage provides the best possible orientation of the specimen. Care should be taken to avoid inclusion of vast areas of empty space. Calculation of the magnification of a specimen depends on the equipment used but generally is the product of the objective magnification and the photo eyepiece magnification multiplied by a coefficient factor quoted for the appropriate photomicroscope. In calculating final print magnifications, negative to print ratio must also be taken into account. Lastly, having spent considerable effort in obtaining the best possible photomicrographs, developed negatives and prints should be treated with the utmost care. Finger prints impregnate negatives and can seldom be effectively removed. For colour transparencies, glass-covered jacket mounts provide long lasting protection. More recently, anti-Newtonian glass jackets which help prevent the formation of Newton's rings on projection have become available.

## Trouble-shooting

Basic photomicroscopic faults can be listed under the headings of unexposed film, poor colour reproduction, blurring of the image, loss of sharpness despite the image being in focus, uneven illumination, the presence of objects other than the specimen appearing on the film and film scratches. Table 13.1 gives some of the more com-mon faults, their causes and corrections.

**Table 13.1**    Common photomicrographic faults and remedies

| Fault | Cause | Correction |
|---|---|---|
| *Unexposed film* | | |
| With film not winding on | Film improperly loaded | Reload and ensure rotation of rewind crank |
| With film winding on | Incorrect optical path selection | Set optical path to camera |
| *Poor colour reproduction* | | |
| Background is coloured | Incorrect colour temperature | Select correct temperature and filters |
| | Lamp voltage too low (too high) | Raise (lower) lamp voltage |
| | Blackening of lamp | Replace lamp |
| | Use of different film from usual | Use colour compensating filter |
| Incorrect colour rendition | Excessively long exposure | Adjust exposure, set reciprocity factor |
| | No automatic exposure adjustment | Set exposure adjustment |
| | Actual and stated film speed differ | Adjust ISO/ASA setting |
| *Blurred image* | | |
| Overall picture blurred | Cross hairs of focusing telescope not focused | Correctly focus cross hairs |
| | Vibrations | Use vibration-proof table |
| | With use of low power objective | Use focusing magnifier for fine focusing |
| Periphery uniformly blurred | Use of Achromat type objective | Use Plan Achromat type objective |
| | Objective and photo eyepiece unmatched | Use correct photo eyepiece for objective |
| *Objects other than specimen on film* | | |
| Shadow-like image | Optical path selector between positions | Engage optical path selector correctly |
| | Field iris diaphragm stopped down too far | Open up just beyond frame reticle |
| | Dirt in optics or on prism of photographic equipment | Clean appropriate optics |
| *Image focused but not sharp* | | |
| Inadequate resolving power | Use of low power objective and high power photo eyepiece | Use low power photo eyepiece |
| | Aperture iris diaphragm fully open | Stop down to 60–80% of objective NA |
| | Field iris diaphragm fully open | Stop down to just beyond frame reticle |
| | Use of thick coverglass | Use coverglass of 0.17 mm thickness |
| | Specimen stain too weak | Restain specimen or use contrast filters |
| | Use of low contrast film | Use film of high contrast or contrast filters |

**Table 13.1**  *Continued*

| Fault | Cause | Correction |
|---|---|---|
| Hazy images | Objective correction collar not adjusted | Adjust and focus for coverglass thickness |
| | Coverglass objective used without coverglass (or vice versa) | Use correct objective |
| | Fingerprints, dirt or oil film on optical lenses | Clean optics |
| | Use of oil immersion lens with incorrect or without oil | Use correct oil |
| | Section too thick | Cut thinner section |
| *Uneven brightness* | | |
| Uneven areas throughout frame | Microscope light source not centred | Adjust light source correctly |
| | Field iris diaphragm off axis | Adjust condenser to centre diaphragm |
| | Optical system contaminated by dirt | Clean optics |
| *Marks on negatives* | | |
| Scratches | During loading of film cassette from bulk loader | Align film correctly on cassette spool |
| | Rewinding film in wrong direction | Rewind film in correct direction |
| | During development of film | Align film correctly on developer spool |
| | Inappropriate care of negatives | Use protective jackets and glass mounts |
| Fingerprints | Carelessness during development | Use gloves when handling negatives |
| | Inappropriate care of negative | Use protective jackets and glass mounts |

## Photographs for publication

Journals have different requirements for the submission of photographs and these should be strictly adhered to. Generally, it is a good guide to produce print sizes identical to those that appear in the journal. Duplicate copies may be required and one set should be retained for personal records together with the negatives. Unless otherwise stated by the journal, glossy prints are often preferred. Prints should be cropped to show only the relevant fields before enlargement to the final size for publication.

## Further reading

How to improve photography through the microscope 1988 Olympus Optical, Tokyo

Photography through the microscope 1980 Eastman Kodak (P.2, Cat No 152–8371), Rochester

Smith RF 1994 Microscopy and photomicrography. A working manual. CRC Press, Boca Raton

# 14 The cytological specimen

# Introduction

An ever-increasing variety of cytological specimens is being examined and a knowledge of the preparatory techniques that can be applied and inherent limitations is essential for the material to be used optimally. Accurate diagnoses can now be made on cytological material with the aid of powerful ancillary techniques such as immunocytochemistry, electron microscopy, flow cytometry and molecular diagnostics. Automated cell analysis by computerised systems is an exciting recent development with great potential to increase the accuracy of screening and to reduce the frequency of manual screening, the latter a tedious and laborious procedure.

# Types of specimens and preparation

Cell preparations from a variety of body sites may be submitted for examination and a proportion may be prepared outside of the laboratory. Specimens may be obtained from the cervix, vagina, vulva, endometrium, skin, oral and nasal cavity; endoscopic brush and wash smears are taken from the respiratory, gastrointestinal and urinary tracts; and smears are prepared from nipple discharges, tissue imprints and fine needle aspirates.

## Cervical smears

The commonest cytological specimen received is the cervical smear and a vast array of scrapers and brushes are utilised, including the Ayre spatula, cotton tip swab, cytobrush and Unimar cervix-brush. Clinicians should be discouraged from using lubricated speculums as the lubricant interferes with cell staining. They should also avoid taking smear from menstruating patients because of the attendant blood, debris, and endometrial cell and histiocytic contaminants. A combination of the spatula and endocervical brush, smeared in a two-step procedure on one slide, is currently recommended, particularly in post-menopausal women or those with previously treated cervical dysplasia in whom the transformation zone may not be visible. Endocervical brushes are not recommended for use in pregnancy. Air-drying before fixation must be avoided. Cervical smears must be fixed immediately either by immersion in 95% alcohol for a minimum of 15 minutes followed by air-drying, or by spray fixation.

## Urine

For urine specimens, patients should be instructed to discard the first morning sample which contains degenerate cells. Three consecutive mid-morning voided specimens of 50–100 ml are collected for examination. Lowering urine pH by administrating 1 g of vitamin C on the preceding evening aids cell preservation. The addition of an equal volume of 50% ethanol improves morphological preservation.

## Sputum

Three early morning spontaneous deep expectorations or induced deep cough samples of sputum provide the best diagnostic samples. Unless delivery to the laboratory is immediate, the sputum is best collected into containers with equal volumes of 50% ethanol, alternatively, a 3-day sputum pool can be collected in Saccomannos' fixative. To avoid interpretive problems introduced by inflammation and reactive bronchial epithelial atypia, sputum samples within 2 weeks of bronchoscopy are best avoided. Nebulisers with hypertonic or isotonic saline, with or without propylene glycol, can be used to encourage sputum production.

## Effusions

The provision of 50 ml is optimal in the investigation of pleural, pericardial and peritoneal effusions. Specimens should be submitted promptly to the laboratory and refrigerated at 4°C if delays are anticipated. An equal volume of 50% ethanol may be added to the sample but alcohol can induce protein precipitation with cell trapping, hardening and decreased cell adhesion to slides. Unfixed fluids are easier to filter and their protein content and specific gravity can be measured. Anticoagulants such as 3.8% sodium citrate, EDTA or heparin (1 ml of 1 : 1000 heparin solution per 100 ml of fluid) are added to prevent clotting.

## Cerebrospinal fluid

Cells in cerebrospinal fluid rapidly degenerate and, if not transported promptly to the laboratory, should have an equal volume of Hank's balanced salt solution and 20% human serum albumin added. This allows cell preservation for up to 24 hours and longer durations of preservation are possible with Saccomannos' fixative and refrigeration but this interferes with Sudan black, acid phosphatase, esterase and Giemsa stains. Saccomannos' fixative is best avoided if leukaemia or lymphoma are suspected.

## Fixatives

Both air-dried and alcohol-fixed 'wet' smears are commonly used in cytology and the two methods are complementary and should be used whenever possible.

The four basic fixation methods in cytology are:

1 *Wet fixation*: the material is immersed into the fixative while still wet and prior to commencement of air-drying. Fixation is for at least 15 minutes.
2 *Wet fixation followed by air-drying*: the smears are subjected to wet fixation and are then air-dried. Immersion in 95% ethanol is needed prior to staining.
3 *Spray fixation*: the wet sample is spray-fixed then allowed to air-dry. The coating requires removal with 95% ethanol prior to staining.
4 *Post-fixation after air-drying*: this technique is employed to kill micro-organisms, continue cell fixation and assist in subsequent staining.

## Wet and spray fixation

The alcohols in general use for 'wet' and spray fixation include 95% and 95% ethanol, 80% isopropanol, 100% methanol, 95% denatured alcohol and a multiplicity of commercial spray coating fixatives. Ninety-five per cent ethanol is favoured as it gives excellent nuclear detail. The slides are stained with Papanicolaou (Pap) and fixation has to be immediate, and if air-drying has supervened, staining is suboptimal. Three per cent glacial acetic acid added to 95% alcohol has been claimed to improve nuclear protein fixation. One hundred per cent methanol is mainly used to fix air-dried smears prior to Giemsa staining. Between 15 and 20 minutes is required for adequate fixation. Ethanol generates greater cell shrinkage and is not an appropriate substitute.

Spray fixatives such as Cytofix are an alternative for immersion fixatives and are supplied as high pressure aerosol sprays or finger-operated spray pumps. They are particularly useful for cervical smears and comprise a waxy material (polyethylene glycol) in an alcohol base. The smears must be spray coated before air-drying ensues, and from a 25–30 cm distance to avoid material loss from too close application. The polyethylene glycol precipitates in and around the cells as the alcohol evaporates, resulting in less shrinkage.

## Saccomannos' fixative (Carbowax)

Saccomannos' fixative (Carbowax) is a fixative comprising 50% alcohol with 2% polyethylene glycol 1540. Its main use is for fluid specimens that may benefit from pre-fixing such as sputum and urine. The polyethylene glycol must be removed prior to staining by soaking in 95% alcohol for 10 minutes.

## 10% phosphate buffered formalin (Millonig's fluid)

This fixative is used for the preparation of cell blocks, small tissue fragments and fibrin clots from fluids and fine needle aspiration (FNA) biopsy specimens. Fixative penetration is slow but the cell blocks are suitable for special stains and immunocytochemistry.

## Lysing fixatives

These include Carnoy's fixative (absolute alcohol : chloroform: glacial acetic acid, in a ratio of 6 : 3 : 1) and Clarke's fixative (absolute alcohol and glacial acetic acid, mixed 3 : 1). They are used on heavily blood-stained smears to lyse red blood cells through the action of acetic acid but fixation for more than 5 minutes gives coarse chromatin clumping, cell shrinkage and overstaining by haematoxylin unless stain times are reduced.

## Other fixatives

One hundred per cent acetone has been employed to post-fix air-dried smears for immunocytochemical staining of lympho-cyte surface antigens, while cells fixed in 10% formol phosphate-buffered saline are assayed for steroid hormone receptors. Formol saline fixation of air-dried smears followed by 100% ethanol is useful for immunostaining of most other cellular antigens. The presence of lipids can be assessed in smears fixed with formalin vapour in a sealed Coplin jar, whilst glutaraldehyde is used in cases requiring ultrastructural examination and occasional-ly for enzyme histochemistry.

# Transport media/cell suspension solutions

Although not fixatives, these solutions support maintenance of cell morphology. They include balanced electrolyte and salt solutions such as Hank's solution and RPMI 1640, and normal saline. The solutions are commonly used to rinse needles following fine needle aspiration and the cell suspension can be centrifuged and smeared, submitted for flow cytometric analysis or made into a cell block. Balanced salt solutions maintain cell osmotic pres-sure, optimise the pH range and provide water, inorganic ions and glucose for cell metabolism and energy.

# Coated slides

Slides coated with Poly-L-lysine, Gelatin-chrome alum or Mayer's albumin are used for specimens of low cellularity and/or a low protein content, to enhance cell adhesion. Poly-L-lysine is a polymer of lysine that utilises positive amino acid charges to stick the cell preparations to the glass slide. Gelatin-chrome alum is heated prior to coating the slides whilst albumin can be added to fluid prior to centrifugation and smearing.

# Fine needle aspiration biopsy

The use of fine needles with or without aspiration to obtain cells and microtissue fragments for cytopathologic diagnosis has enjoyed a meteoric rise in acceptance by both pathologists and clinicians since its resurgence in the 1950s. Its diagnostic accuracy approaches that of the traditional haematoxylin and eosin stained tissue section in many instances and sophisticated radiological imaging methods have taken the fine needle from its traditional role in investigating superficial masses to many deeply placed lesions.

Fine needle aspiration can be learnt relatively quickly and requires, at least for the superficial palpable lesions, no expensive equipment. The technique is relatively painless for patients with minimal morbidity, and local anaesthetic is not generally required. The ability to provide rapid diagnoses has undeniable economic savings, reduces patient anxiety and can be the method of choice for patients who are anaesthetic risks.

Needling does not generally hamper subsequent histopathological examination of the excised lesion, does not interfere with surgical planes, and may allow a specific diagnosis to be made. For cysts and abscesses, the technique can be both diagnostic and therapeutic.

Common sites for fine needle aspiration biopsy (FNAB) include lymph nodes, thyroid and salivary glands, breast, subcutaneous nodules and prostate. Radiology has enabled directed sampling of organs and tissues such as lung, mediastinum, pancreas, kidneys, adrenals, liver, bone, retroperitoneal masses and even spleen.

Contraindications to FNAB are few. Haemorrhagic diathesis has been associated with fatal haemorrhage following aspiration of liver, kidney lung and spleen but the procedure is usually performed without incident in superficial sites where direct pressure can be applied or in those patients whose diathesis is mild or correctable. FNAB should not be performed on known or suspected aneurysm, vascular malformation or paraganglioma. The prostate gland should not be needled if extremely tender, or if the patient is febrile or has active epididymo-orchitis. Contraindications to FNAB include a clinical suspicion of malignancy in the testis, phaeochromocytoma of the adrenal, primary melanocytic lesions of skin, solid/cystic ovarian neoplasms in the absence of peritoneal or wider dissemination, and most primary bone neoplasms. Severe jaundice and hydatid disease are contraindications to hepatic FNAB, whilst for the lung, FNAB is best avoided in bullous emphysema, severe cough, absent cough reflex, pulmonary hypertension, unconscious state, respiratory failure, suspected hydatid disease and some perihilar lesions.

Serious complications from FNAB are rare. Haemorrhage may occur but other adverse effects include biliary peritonitis after liver aspiration, septicaemia following prostate aspiration, anaphylactic shock after aspiration of hydatid cysts, hypertensive crises precipitated by needling phaeochromocytomas, tension pneumothorax following lung or axillary/supraclavicular lymph node or breast aspiration, spinal cord injury after vertebral bone aspiration and acute pancreatitis complicating needling of the pancreas. If aseptic techniques are employed, there is minimal risk of developing infection at the aspiration site. Knowledge of local anatomy is essential to avoid damage to nerves and larger vessels such as the carotid artery or jugular vein. Vasovagal episodes can occur during FNAB. Implantation of tumour cells along the needle tract is extremely rare and unless needles larger than 19 G are used.

## Equipment requirements

The following materials are required for FNAB and are conveniently contained in a 'FNAB tool box' which can be carried to the bedside.

### Needles

The standard needle used in superficial FNAB is 22 or 23 G, disposable and between 30 and 50 mm in length. Twenty-five gauge needles are sufficient for most head and neck lesions, including the vascular thyroid, and in children. Apart from fibrous lesions, larger calibre needles do not improve cellular yield.

The 23 G 210 mm Franzen needle inserted into the Franzen needle guide is used for prostatic aspiration and 22 G 90 mm lumbar puncture needles are useful for deeper lesions as the trocar prevents needle blockage during passage to the lesion. Other needles used largely by radiologists in the sampling of deep lesions include the 22 G 200 mm Chiba, Shiva, perforated and the Rotex II. The latter is useful for sclerotic lesions of the mediastinum.

### Syringes and holders

Standard 10–20 ml disposable plastic syringes are used. Syringes can be attached to any one of a number of commercially available syringe holders such as the Cameco, which can be used for 100 aspiration procedures. Intravenous extension tubing between the syringe and needle allows the pathologist to use both hands to place the needle and may be useful in agitated or young patients.

### Slides, coverslips, mounting media, plastic slide mailers/containers and metal trays

### Fixatives and stains

The FNAB kit should contain 95% alcohol in plastic Coplin jars and/or spray fixatives for wet fixation. A Diff-Quik staining kit is useful, particularly for radiologically guided aspirates, and a portable microscope with ×4, ×10, ×20 and ×40 objectives should be available. An extension cord/lead is invaluable as most radiology departments have not been designed with the cytopathologist in mind. Ten per cent buffered formalin and glutaraldehyde in containers should be on hand for difficult cases. Carnoy's fixative may be carried to lyse red blood cells in bloody smears.

### Sterile containers

These are carried for aspirates of infective material to be submitted for culture. Small containers with balanced salt solutions such as Hank's are useful for rinsing needles.

### Infection control

Superficial aspirates require only simple skin disinfection with pre-packaged alcohol or iodine swabs whilst the deep organ biopsies require surgical skin disinfection and drapes. Wear latex gloves routinely and with suspected infection such as tuberculosis, hepatitis B and C, or HIV, use double gloves, gowns, splash-proof glasses and masks. Plastic guards designed to fit over the metal trays reduce the creation of aerosol during the expulsion of aspirated material onto the slides. Plastic bags to contain soiled clothing and a sharps container must be accessible.

### Anaesthesia

Pre-biopsy sedation is rarely required unless the patient is extremely anxious and aspiration from a deep-seated lesion is planned. Local anaesthesia is not necessary in superficial aspirations involving needles finer than 22 G. Furthermore, the anaesthetic damages cell preservation, distorts tissue planes and the injection is painful. Xylocaine sprays have a role as a local anaesthetic in sampling lesions of the oral cavity and 1% lignocaine injection is acceptable in tender sites such as the nipple and around the genitals. Emlar anaesthetic gel can be applied to skin, particularly in children, but takes at least 30 minutes to become effective. Local anaesthesia is used to reduce pain and patient movement in transperiosteal, transpleural and transperitoneal biopsies.

### Other equipment

These include sterile scalpel blades, pencils and glass slide etching pens, lubrication gel for prostatic biopsies, sterile gauze dressings, bandaids, a ruler for measurement, and specimen request and patient consent forms.

## Biopsy techniques for superficial lesions

Prior to any aspiration procedure, the indication for the test should be reviewed, informed consent is required and the patient must be co-operative.

Three basic methods are involved in fine needle biopsy of superficial lesions. All are preceded by local skin disinfection. If local anaesthetic is required, it is best injected adjacent to the nodule with gentle massage into the region of needle passage.

The needle, attached to a 10 or 20 ml disposable syringe contained within a holder, is passed through the skin into the target lesion or tissue. The lesion is immobilised between two fingers or pushed with one finger along its tissue plane until it is fixed against an immobile anatomical structure such as bone. Needle passes should be directed at an angle close to the vertical. Having entered the lesion, the syringe plunger is withdrawn at least two-thirds to apply a negative pressure to the barrel and the needle is advanced several times back and forth quickly along the same track within the lesion. The negative pressure is released with the needle still in the lesion. The needle is then withdrawn and detached. Air is drawn into the syringe and the aspirating needle reconnected and the needle contents are expelled in 1–2 drop aliquots on one or several glass slides.

The principle of creating negative pressure is not to suck cells but to apply tissue against the cutting edge of the needle, the tissue collecting in the lumen as the needle is advanced. Multiple passes may be needed in fibrous lesions of the breast and soft tissues as well as solid/cystic lesions to minimise the chance of a false-negative result. Two to three passes are the norm, apart from highly vascular organs such as the spleen. Releasing the negative pressure before withdrawing the needle minimises contaminant material entering the needle. In large tumours, direct the passes at the edge of the lesion in order to reduce sampling from areas of necrosis, haemorrhage or cystic degeneration. The aspiration should be repeated if a palpable lesion remains after evacuation of a cystic lesion.

Needle biopsy without aspiration is helpful to sample superficial vascular lesions as it reduces dilution of material by blood and enables the pathologist to more accurately appreciate the consistency of the lesion. A 22 or 25 G needle held between the index finger and thumb, is inserted into the lesion and rotated whilst advancing and withdrawing in different planes to cut and scrape cells into the needle lumen. The cell yield is generally less than for aspiration and the technique is not suitable for fibrous lesions, e.g. in the breast. A syringe needs to be handy in the event of needling an unsuspected cyst.

It is outside the scope of this chapter to detail extensively all the radiological organ imaging techniques that can be used to guide FNAB. The simplest and safest technique should be employed. Methods currently in use include plain radiography or fluoroscopy, fluoroscopy plus contrast radiography, radionuclide scanning, ultrasound, computerised tomography and magnetic resonance imaging.

## Smear preparation

The ideal smear creates a cell layer on the slide with abundant cells suspended in a minimum of background tissue fluid.

Place a drop or two of the aspirate at one end of a clean slide and draw the material towards the other end with the flat of another slide or coverslip, exerting just enough pressure to produce a thin film. Excess pressure will produce crush arte-facts. A slightly thicker smear is preferable. Wet aspirates are best smeared in a two-step process. A slide or coverslip orientated at an angle to the material-containing slide is moved to the centre of the slide, causing the cells to be dragged along and leaving the fluid behind. The concentrated cells in the centre of the slide are then smeared

with the same slide or coverslip over the rest of the slide, using the technique for a dry aspirate described above. An alternative is to tilt the slide after smearing to allow gravity to move the unwanted fluid to one end prior to smearing the cell-concentrated material. Dabbing off excess material onto other clean slides allows transfer of suitable amounts of specimen.

Bloody specimens can be left to clot on the slide and together with added thrombin converted into a cell block for formalin fixation and histological processing. Cyst fluid and cell aspiration needles and syringes should be rinsed out with Hank's solution for cytospin preparations.

For most aspirates it is advantageous to prepare air-dried Giemsa-stained smears as well as 95% alcohol wet-fixed smears for staining by the Papanicolaou method. Direct smears are usually superior to rinsed material for cytospins but cell suspensions can be useful for further investigations such as flow cytometry, special stains and immunocytochemistry. Air-drying artefact is avoided by immediate transfer to alcohol. If only air-dried smears are made, it is possible within 2 hours of sampling, to wet-fix smears by rehydrating the slides in normal saline for 1 minute before fixing in 95% alcohol. Cell blocks are very useful for ancillary investigations and may retain histological architecture. They are best stained with haematoxylin and eosin.

In infection, transfer the entire contents of one needle pass into a sterile container, rinsing with sterile normal saline if neces-sary or keep the material in the needle which is resheathed and submitted for culture. Submitting only a portion of the aspirate for culture is rarely satisfactory. If electron microscopy is required, eject the material from one needle pass into a small plastic tube containing glutaraldehyde. This is subsequently centrifuged.

# Specimen preparation

## Mucoid specimens

These are predominantly sputum samples but also include nasopharyngeal, gastric and bronchial aspirates. Many specimens can be smeared directly onto slides due to the adhesiveness of mucin. Watery and mucopurulent specimens can be fixed in 95% alcohol for 20–30 minutes and heavily bloodstained specimens should be initially fixed in Carnoy's for 3–5 minutes followed by post-fixation in 95% alcohol.

The 'pick and smear technique' for sputum should be undertaken in a safety hood. Wooden applicator sticks are used to tease the specimen contained in a petri dish, and solid, discoloured or bloody particles are selected for smearing. Malignant cells are more likely to be found in the translucent threads within clear sputum. Pea-sized particles are transferred to slides, and using a second clean slide, the specimen is spread evenly using a rotating motion before fixing in alcohol. Residual material can be stored in the fridge. This technique cannot be employed if the specimen arrives prefixed in Saccomannos' fixative (Carbowax) or 50% alcohol.

Saccomannos' method was developed to concentrate atypical cells in sputum. The specimen is placed in the fixative and the container is inverted several times to mix the contents. It can be stored for up to 48 hours in the fridge. The sample is blended at high speed in a commercial blender until there are no visible flecks or fine threads. It is then centrifuged for 10 minutes at 500 $g$; the supernatant is decanted and the sediment resuspended in the residual fluid using a vortex mixer. Sediment drops are placed on glass slides, air-dried and immersed in 95% alcohol for 10 minutes to remove the Carbowax coating prior to Pap staining.

Saccomannos' fixation produces a high cell yield and a background clear of most mucous strands. It is claimed to result in more diagnostic cells and a lower false-negative rate compared to the 'pick and smear' method.

Specimens obtained by bronchial trap are often mucoid and arrive in glass or plastic containers with attached rubber tubing. The tubing is rinsed with Hank's into the container, mixed and poured or pipetted into centrifuge tubes and spun for 10 minutes at 500 $g$. The smears obtained are alcohol fixed. Thick mucoid specimens may necessitate pre-digestion with a mucolytic agent such as Sputasol or overnight incubation in 8% hydrochloric acid prior to centrifugation. The vacuolation of adenocarcinoma cells may disappear after the use of mucolytic agents.

## Fluid specimens

Effusions are arbitrarily subdivided into transudates and exudates. Transudates which result from congestive cardiac failure, hypoalbuminaemia or vascular obstruction are clear, have a specific gravity of less than 1.015, a total protein of less than 3 g/dl, LDH which is lower than the serum LDH and are paucicellular. Exudates, mostly commonly post-inflammatory or associated with malignancy, are often blood-stained or turbid with fibrin clots and abundant cells. They are characterised by a specific gravity of greater than 1.015, a total protein level greater than 3 g/dl and LDH which is greater than serum LDH level. Carcinoembryonic antigen (CEA) levels may be elevated in some effusions from metastatic adenocarcinoma.

### Centrifugation

Centrifugation is ideal for concentrating cells in fluid specimens (serous effusions, urine, washings) with a volume of more than 5 ml. Fibrin clots are best removed and processed separately as a cell block in formalin. The volume, colour, any blood-staining, texture and turbidity should be recorded prior to centrifugation. A highly viscous effusion may contain hyaluronic acid and is suggestive of mesothelioma.

The fluid is centrifuged at 600 $g$ for 10 minutes in a pair of plastic screw-top centrifuge tubes. Plastic tubes are preferred as they are less breakable, disposable, inexpensive and cause less cell adhesion than glass. The cellular buffy coat is pipetted and smeared directly. Centrifuged sediment may be resuspended in 50% alcohol and used to make smears and cell blocks. Blood lysing solutions may be used to treat blood-stained material either prior to centrifugation or after smears have been made, and crystalline material may need to be removed in some urine specimens. For specimens collected into heparinised tubes, the centrifuged sediment requires washing with Hank's solution to enable cell block formation with the plasma/thrombin method. Addition of albumin to watery specimens aids cell attachment to the slides.

## Cytocentrifugation

The cytocentrifuge processes small volumes of fluid and directly centrifuges the specimen onto a glass slide. The cells are deposited into a circumscribed 6 mm diameter circle on the slide making it ideal for ancillary studies. Both air-dried and alcohol-fixed slides can be produced. A few drops of Saccomannos' fixative can be added to the cytocentrifuge chamber to reduce air-drying artefact in 95% alcohol-fixed specimens.

Typical specimens for cytocentrifugation include cerebrospinal fluid, ureteric catheter urine specimens, ovarian cyst fluid,

cell suspensions in Hank's solution and bronchiolar lavage specimens. Advantages of the technique include rapid specimen preparation, increased screening speed and safety, as many models enable specimen loading in a biohazard cabinet. The main disadvantages include some cell loss due to filter absorption, partial air-drying of watery specimens prior to alcohol fixation and inhibition of effective filtration in some mucous specimens.

## Membrane filtration

This process concentrates the cell sample by trapping the cells against a membrane filter composed of either cellulose acetate (Millipore, Gelman) or polycarbonate (Nucleopore). Fixation, staining, clearing and mounting are all carried out on the membrane and a cell monolayer with minimal cell overlap is produced. Filter pore sizes range from 5 to 8 $\mu$m with a filter diameter of 47 mm.

The fluid specimens are initially centrifuged at 2000 rpm for 10 minutes to remove protein, fibrin and debris which clog the filter pores, although this step is often omitted with small volumes of clear fluids such as CSF and urine specimens.

The nucleopore filters are moistened with saline and placed on the filter base with the shiny side up. Contamination is reduced by handling filters with forceps. The filter is held in position with metal clamps and an aliquot of the cell suspension pipetted into the normal saline solution on the filter and is slowly filtered with the aid of negative pressure created in the filter flask. Air should not pass through the filter but 95% alcohol can be drawn through the filter for fixation. After passage of alcohol, the filter membrane is placed on a glass slide, cell side down, blotted with paper, and dried in a vacuum desiccator. The filter is then dissolved by adding chloroform and the slide mounted.

Membrane filtration allows the recovery of cells from large volume samples which can be sparsely cellular. It also enables direct filtration without centrifugation, and unfixed as well as some pre-fixed specimens can be handled directly, reducing infectious risks and processing delays.

Disadvantages of the technique include easy blocking of filters by high protein fluids such as effusions, and pre-fixed specimens such as urine which contain dissolved salts. Other problems include unsuitability for staining with Giemsa, and the expense and relative lengthiness of the procedure which also has a tendency to produce cell distortion and fragmentation.

## Blood-stained fluids and smears

Microscopic examination of blood-stained smears is difficult as diagnostic cells may be obscured. Fixed red blood cells may be lysed with glacial acetic acid, 2 M urea or Carnoy's. Slides can be placed in 5% glacial acetic acid for 10 minutes or 2 M urea for 30 seconds if unfixed, or for 1 minute if previously fixed or stained. Following treatment, the slides are placed in 95% alcohol for 5 minutes to complete fixation and halt haemolysis prior to staining with Pap methods. 2 M urea is stable and does not need to be prepared fresh like Carnoy's solution.

Red blood cells may be removed from fluids using density gradient columns, acid or enzyme haemolysis or the buffy coat technique on centrifuged specimens. The first of these procedures is best for heavily blood-stained specimens. Density gradient solutions include Ficoll-Hypaque and Histopaque 1077. Centrifugation at 1200 rpm for 20 minutes in the gradient separates the red blood cells from the nucleated cells on the basis of density differences, the latter being collected at the Ficoll and the fluid supernatant interface. Red cells are pelleted at the bottom of the tube. The cellular band of white cells is removed, and placed in another tube. It is washed with isotonic saline by filling the tube and inverting several times. This is then centrifuged at 1500 rpm for 5–7 minutes. The supernatant is discarded and the pellet resuspended in 1–2 ml of saline. Cytospin smears are prepared. Cell preservation is not always ideal. Acid haemolysis is conducted by applying 1 ml of glacial acetic acid to 50 ml of the bloody specimen and 0.1 M hydrochloric acid is added to obtain a uniformly brown colour. Enzymatic haemolysis is performed with Saponin solution or Zap-oglobin. Excess Saponin will destroy cells and can be reversed with calcium gluconate. Zap-oglobin functions through a detergent action and inhibits clotting and thus cell deposits must be washed in Hank's to enable formation of plasmathrombin cell blocks.

## Synovial fluid examination

The optimum amount for examination is 10 ml and it is best collected in a heparinised container. A drop of spun fluid is placed on a clean non-albuminised slide for crystal examination under polarised light (albumin contains cholesterol). Differential cell counts are best performed on 200–300 cells along the edge of the smeared fluid film. Specimens can also be filtered or cytocentrifuged and fluid can be sent for determination of pH, uric acid levels, total protein, enzymes and bacterial culture.

## Cell blocks

Cell blocks can be made from effusions, cyst fluid, fine needle aspirate cell suspensions in Hank's solution, specimens with small clots and tissue fragments, urinary sediment and even sputum. Solid blood and fibrin clots can be placed directly into fixative. Cell blocks retain histological architecture and are suitable for special staining techniques including immunocytochemistry. Although 10% buffered formalin is the most common fixative, others such as Bouin's solution, picric acid and mercuric chloride-based fixatives may be used.

The plasma thrombin clot method entails addition of two drops of plasma (INR 1) and two drops of thrombin to the centrifuged sediment. This is followed by 5–10 ml of fixative for 1 hour to harden the cell block before processing and paraffin-embedding. Fluid specimens collected in heparin, EDTA or pre-fixed in formalin must be washed in Hank's solution before subjecting to the plasmathrombin method.

An alternative method uses warmed agar which is added to a centrifuged sediment button contained in fixative for up to 1 hour. Two to three drops of agar are added after draining the fixative, and the specimen is subjected to further centrifugation. The tube with cell block are cooled in a refrigerator until the agar sets. The block is then pried from the tube, excess agar trimmed and the cell block placed in fixative prior to processing and paraffin-embedding.

# Staining, mounting and coverslipping

The routine stains employed in cytology are the Papanicolaou stain and one of the Romanowsky methods. Haematoxylin and eosin may be used but it does not give good cytological detail and is best restricted to staining cell blocks. The important stains are discussed.

## The Papanicolaou stain

This is the standard stain for alcohol or wet-fixed material. It is a polychrome stain consisting of a nuclear stain (haematoxylin) and two counter stains (eosinazure (EA) and orange G (OG). This stain gives good nuclear chromatin detail, differential cytoplasmic counterstaining and cytoplasmic transparency. Progressive and regressive methods are available.

The solutions used in the Papanicolaou (Pap) stain include haematoxylin (Harris and Lillie-Mayer's haematoxylin for regressive staining, Gill's for progressive staining), acid alcohol (0.6 and 0.25 solutions of hydrochloric acid in 50 or 70% alcohol), blueing solutions (Scott's blue, lithium bicarbonate, ammonium hydroxide), modified Orange G6 stain (OG6) (aqueous orange G, phosphotungstic acid, 95% alcohol) and modified eosin-azure stain (EA). The latter is available in three formulations: 36, 50 and 65. EA36 was originally developed for gynaecological smears whilst EA65 has been used for thicker cell samples. EA50 is a commercial formulation similar to EA36. The stain is a mix of 95% alcohol, absolute methanol, glacial acetic acid, light green SF (3% aqueous), eosin Y (20% aqueous) and phosphotungstic acid.

The Pap stain can be performed manually or automated, with staining times individualised for each laboratory. The stain decorates nuclei purple/dark blue, the cytoplasm of metabolically active cells blue green, keratin orange and the cytoplasm of superficial squamous cells pink. The modified eosin azure stain needs to be applied for at least 5 minutes and the reagents should be regularly filtered.

## The Romanowsky stain

These stains, originally developed for blood films, are performed on air-dried smears. Air-dried cells are larger compared to alcohol-fixed and formalin-fixed cells.

The three most commonly used Romanowsky stains are the May–Grünwald–Giemsa, Giemsa and Diff-Quik. The smears must be post-fixed in methanol to reduce the risk of infection. These stains label nuclei purple-blue, cell cytoplasm blue shades, eosinophil granules red and basophil granules dark blue. Stromal features such as mucin are highlighted.

The May–Grünwald–Giemsa (MGG) stain comprises MGG (BDH product no. 00360), Giemsa (BDH product no. 35014), buffer pH 6.8 (GURR product no. 33199) and absolute methanol. The Giemsa stain components are Giemsa stain and buffer, whilst the Diff-Quik stain is a proprietary product and comprises a fixative and two dyes. The Diff-Quik stain can be performed in under 60 seconds and its principal use is with fine needle aspiration specimens to assess on site specimen adequacy, the need for auxiliary investigations and rapid diagnosis. The stain quality is usually somewhat inferior to the aforementioned and does not tend to penetrate thick cell clusters. The Diff-Quik system fixative comprises methanol and triarylmethane dye (0.002 g/l); solution 1 is a buffer and xanthene dye (1.25 g/l) and solution 2 is a buffer and a thiazine dye mix (1.25 g/l). To perform the Diff-Quik stain, slides are placed in fixative for 60 seconds and then dipped 15 times each in solution 1 and solution 2, followed by two water rinses, before mounting and coverslipping. Rapid Pap and H & E stains have also been developed.

## Special stains

Many of the special stains used on tissue sections can be used on both alcohol-fixed and air-dried smears. Examples include: PAS with or without diastase and Alcian blue for mucins and glycogen; Perls' stain for iron; oil red O for fat; Gram stain; methenamine silver; Ziehl–Neelsen and PAS for microorganisms; Grimelius for argyrophilic granules; Masson-Fontana for melanin; and Congo red for amyloid. Enzyme histochemistry can be performed on air-dried smears. Esterase and peroxidase can be used for lineage typing of malignant haematopoietic/lymphoid neoplasms, and acid phosphatase may help diagnose metastatic prostatic adenocarcinoma.

The hyaluronic acid test may be used in the study of malignant mesothelioma. Fifty per cent glacial acetic acid is added to effusion fluid diluted with distilled water. In the presence of hyaluronic acid, a clot forms quickly on the end of a wooden spatula dipped in the specimen. Absent clotting in a control tube to which hyaluronidase has been added suggests the presence of hyaluronic acid.

## Stains for wet sediment

These rapidly performed stains (2–5 minutes) include methylene blue, toluidine blue and thionine blue. They have a role in: (1) assessing cell preservation; (2) determining the degree of specimen cellularity; (3) detecting crystals in urinary sediment; (4) identifying malignant samples for separate staining to avoid contaminants; and (5) as a diagnostic technique.

## Destaining of smears

Often, the material available is sparse and necessitates, on occasion, re-use of the slides for different stains or special investigations. Coverslips can be removed by warming slides on a heating plate for 4 hours, placing slides in a freezer for 15 minutes, or soaking the slides in xylol or a substitute. After removal of the coverslip, residual mountant is removed with xylol and then the slides are taken back through grades of alcohol to water. To remove the nuclear haematoxylin stain in Pap smears, 0.25% acid alcohol is used, whilst for Giemsa, 0.25% acid methanol is effective. Smears for immunoperoxidase staining do not need destaining if a hydrogen peroxide blocking step is used.

## Mounting and coverslipping

Suitable mountants are optically clear, with a refractive index close to glass. The coverslips generally employed for smears and cytocentrifuged slides are 50 × 22 mm and 22 × 22 mm respectively.

## Artefacts and contaminants in cytology

Air-drying prior to alcohol fixation induces cellular eosinophilia, loss of chromatin detail and a distortion of the nuclear/cytoplasmic ratio. Rough smearing causes nuclear streaking and aggregation, potentially causing confusion in the separation of lymphocytes and cells of small cell carcinoma. Air pockets result from drying before coverslipping and cryogenic artefacts may result from spraying of aerosol fixatives at too close a distance. If the coating fixative of Carbowax is not removed prior to staining, a golden brown pigment results.

Light green in the EA stain of the Pap smear fades quickly if exposed to light.

Contaminants in cytology include fungi such as *Alternaria sporidium* which have brown snow-shoe-shaped conidium, fibres from many sources and birefringent cellulose fibres from cytocentrifuge filter cards. Glove powder crystals and mites can be observed on Pap smears, as may pollen grains on smears prepared near open windows. Empty spaces on cervical smears may reflect gynaecological lubricant gels, and water-borne contaminants such as diatoms and round worms can be transferred to the slides during staining. Meat fibres and vegetable cells, the latter sometimes confused with squamous cell carcinoma, may be seen in sputum samples.

Cellular malignant effusions can contaminate the staining reagents and thus other smears during staining, a problem reduced by filtering the reagents, changing rinse baths frequently, and staining effusions separately.

## Special techniques in cytology

These include immunocytochemistry, in situ hybridisation, the polymerase chain reaction, cytogenetics, morphometry and image analysis, flow cytometry and electron microscopy. The techniques and applications are discussed elsewhere. All these techniques are applicable to cytological specimens. Only a few issues relevant to cytological specimens are discussed.

Cell smears, cell blocks, imprints and cytocentrifuge preparations can all be used successfully for immunocytochemistry. Membrane filter preparations generally suffer from background staining which is also a nuisance in smears of necrotic tumours and effusions with high protein content. Centrifuged cell sediments of effusions or cell blocks washed in Hank's reagent are best for immunostaining. Previous Pap stained smears can also be utilised. Most cytoplasmic antigens such as the intermediate filaments, hormones and peptides are retained following alcohol fixation but many surface antigens are either lost or the reactivity decreased. The reaction for S100 and most lymphoid markers is poor in alcohol-fixed specimens. Air-dried smears give inconsistent results. Cytospin preparations can be post-fixed in acetone, methanol–acetone (1 : 1) or buffered formol-acetone (1 : 1) for analysis of lymphocyte markers. A universal fixative for cell preparations is yet to be found and the fixative needs to be varied with the antigen to be demonstrated. Generally, fixation of air-dried smears in formol saline for 14 hours followed by 10 minutes in 100% ethanol allows good preservation of immunoreactivity. Centrifuged aspirates should be washed in buffer to reduce background staining. Fine needle aspiration can be used to collect cells for oestrogen and progesterone receptor assays in breast carcinoma. The aspirated material can be directly smeared, air-dried and fixed in formol saline for 10 minutes. Following microwave epitope retrieval, oestrogen and progesterone receptors can be demonstrated with the antibody clones 1D5 and PgR-ICA respectively (Dako, California and Abbott Lab., North Chicago, USA).

It is critical to ensure that the cells showing positive staining are the tumour or cells in question and not contaminants. False-positive staining is not uncommon in thick, poorly smeared cellular clumps and haemosiderin pigment in macrophages may appear as a positive reaction. Background staining is also a problem. False-negative reactions are more common in smears compared to histological sections.

Alcohol-fixed, stained or unstained smears, centrifuge specimens, imprints and cell blocks can be used for molecular studies but the slides must have an adhesive coating. Smears and cytocentrifuged cell suspensions can be fixed with ethanol, ethanol-acetic acid or periodate-lysine-paraformaldehyde-glutaraldehyde (PLPG). One slide is generally used for each probe but the advent of fluorescence in situ hybridisation (FISH) and flow cytometry enables simultaneous multiprobe analysis.

The main application of in situ hybridisation in cytology has been viral detection such as CMV and herpes in bronchoalveolar lavage fluid, but other uses include assessment of oncogene expression in neoplasia and neuroendocrine gene expression. Polymerase chain reaction (PCR) has been employed on cytology specimens to detect gene rearrangements in lymphoma, identify human papilloma virus (HPV) infection in cervical smears, genetic mutations, polymorphisms and oncogenes. The ability of PCR to render an unequivocal diagnosis of lymphoma on limited cytological material, such as finding *bcl*-2 in lymphocytes in the cerebrospinal fluid, makes this technology a powerful tool for the cytopathologist.

Two to three passes are generally needed to provide adequate material for cytogenetic studies. These are collected in a sterile fashion and placed into cell culture media. Cost has precluded the routine use of cytogenetics in cytology.

Cell image analysis is usually undertaken on 95% alcohol-fixed material and measurements of nuclear size, shape, density, nuclear condensation and a variety of cytoplasmic parameters can be assessed and immunocytochemical staining can be quantitated. Image cytometry with ploidy analysis has been used to distinguish benign, malignant mesothelial cells and carcinoma cells in pleural fluid, increase the detection of low-grade papillary neoplasms in urine and identify patients with low-grade cervical squamous dysplasias which have greater potential for progression.

Flow cytometry (FC) can assess hundreds and thousands of cells for morphological parameters, DNA content, S-phase fraction and cytochemical composition. The single cell suspensions needed for FC may be derived from body cavity fluids, FNA material or cell blocks which have been mechanically disaggregated or enzyme digested. Examples of applications include the detection of monoclonal lymphoid populations and subtyping in effusion fluid, and ploidy assessment on urine of patients with bladder carcinoma. DNA abnormalities can precede cystoscopically visible tumour. Human germinal epithelium has a unique DNA distribution and FC on testis FNA samples has been used to evaluate male infertility and follow cases of radiation-induced in situ carcinoma.

Material for transmission electron microscopy (TEM) usually derives from effusions and fine needle aspirations. If an unusual or poorly differentiated neoplasm is suspected prior to or following Diff-Quik staining, aspirate from a pass can be ejected into a plastic container with 2.5% glutaraldehyde, the specimen centrifuged and the sediment processed. An alternative method entails ejection of a few drops of aspirate onto a glass slide which is placed into glutaraldehyde and processed from the slide.

Effusions are centrifuged and the pellet is fixed with 2.5% glutaraldehyde, made into a thrombin clot and diced into 1–2 mm cubes for processing and resin embedding. Ethanol fixation is not satisfactory for TEM. Fluid can be passed through nucleopore filters with secondary gluteraldehyde fixation, osmium tetroxide and, following dehydration, the filter is cut and placed in resin moulds. Retrieval of cells from the surface of glass slides is possible when cytological material is sparse.

Scanning electron microscopy has a role in evaluating cell surface changes and junctions, and variations in surface microvilli have been used to diagnose low-grade urothelial tumours.

## Automation

### Monolayer smear preparations

The Cytyc Thin Prep processor (Beckman Instruments, Carisbad, California, USA) was developed in response to demands for an instrument that will produce high quality cell monolayers that overcome the problems of uneven smearing, cell clumping and air-drying. The arrival of the ancillary specialised cytology techniques outlined earlier, particularly morphometry has also created an increased need for standardisation of cell preparation, fixation and staining to improve data collection and enable interlaboratory comparison. The Cytyc Thin Prep processor produces cell monolayers with enhanced cell detail, little overlap and removal of much of the potentially obscuring background debris, red blood cells and mucus.

While Thin-Prep preparation may have many potential advantages with cost savings from reductions in screening time of up to 60%, they must be balanced against increased processing time, machine cost and expense of approximately A $4 per slide. All solutions need to be obtained from the machine manufacturer.

### Automated coverslipping

These machines are expensive, easily operated and use a thin Tri-cellulose acetate film which is rolled onto the slide. Xylene activates the dry coverslipping resin on the film which adheres to the slide. Problems may be encountered with thick uneven gynaecological and sputum smears.

## Automated cervical smear screeners

Manual screening of cervical smears has a false-negative rate of between 10 and 15%. This error rate has led to the design of automated screeners which overcomes the human error factor in screening.

Current screening systems are algorithmic systems such as AutoPap 300 (Neopath Inc, Redmond, Washington, USA) or artificial neural network systems such as PAPNET (PAPNET Neuromedical Systems, Suffern, New York, USA).

Both systems can evaluate conventionally prepared and stained cervical Pap smears. In the AutoPap system, bar-coded smears are loaded onto special trays into the device which has a computer-controlled microscope with a scanning stage, autofocus and a imaging camera capable of generating 25 images per second. Imaging electronics digitise, process and perform feature extraction with cell discrimination. An analysis score between 0 and 100 is generated and a threshold score is determined and set at a level where normal smears are detected with a zero false-negative rate.

Up to 12 slides per hour continuous unattended operation throughout the day is possible. The machine has been intended for operation as a primary screener although most laboratories with this device are using it as a rescreener of negative slides. It is currently not licensed as a primary screening device by the Federal Drug Administration (FDA) in the USA. Manufacturers of the AutoPap 300 claim the system can determine specimen adequacy (staining, squamous cellularity and an endocervical component), level of inflammation, presence of normal endometrial cells and classification of smears as either normal or requiring review. Approximately 50% of smears screened by AutoPap 300 are safely regarded as normal and can be signed out without technologist/pathologist viewing. The AutoPap 300 QC has been specially designed for quality assurance rescreening of manually screened negative cases and the system has at least 80% sensitivity and 80% specificity for detecting squamous and glandular abnormalities.

The PAPNET screening system can learn from 'experience' due to its artificial neural network. Pap smear slides are transferred from a loaded cassette holder to an automated microscope stage via a robotic arm with slide recognition facilitated by bar codes. The area delineated by the coverslip is first scanned at low power then high power, with a primary algorithmic classifier which screens out normal cells, using morphological criteria before passing the remaining smears onto the neural network-based secondary classifier. One hundred and twenty-eight video images of abnormal cells (single and groups) are created per slide and the system can screen 100 slides every 16 hours. The images are stored on cartridge and this is analysed by the cytotechnologist on a colour monitor. Training is required to interpret these video images and determine which smears require closer scrutiny. PAPNET has been claimed to be excellent at finding small numbers of abnormal cells on a smear and it can be used by laboratories as a quality control measure to rescreen negative smears. The machines are not for purchase and slides have to be mailed to a regional machine for screening, with the video image returned to the laboratory for examination. The machine has screening as well as diagnosis capabilities.

## Further reading

Koss LG 1992 Diagnostic cytology and its histologic basis, 4th edn. Lippincott, Philadelphia

Koss LG, Woyke S, Olszawski W 1992 Aspiration biopsy: cytologic interpretation and histologic basis. Igaku-Shoin, New York

Linder J, Rennard SI 1988 Bronchoalveolar lavage. ASCP Press, Chicago

Meisels A, Morin C 1990 Cytopathology of the uterine cervix. ASCP Press, Chicago

Orell S, Sterrett GF, Walters MN-I, Whitaker D 1992 An atlas of fine needle aspiration cytology, 2nd edn. Churchill Livingstone, London

Suen KC 1990 Atlas and text of aspiration biopsy cytology. Williams & Wilkins, Baltimore

Wied GL, Keebler CM, Koss LG, Reagan JW 1990 Compendium on diagnostic cytology, 6th edn. International Academy of Cytology, Chicago

# 15 Technical problems, mishaps, artefacts and quality assurance

## Introduction

There would be few, if any, laboratories that have not made errors in diagnostic reporting as a result of technical problems and artefacts. Such diverse situations from a simple clerical mistake through technical mishaps in producing a histological section to the misinterpretation of a section as a result of an introduced artefact may all lead to disastrous consequences for the patient. Fortunately, the majority of artefacts are readily recognised and of little consequence, but the trainee pathologist must be aware of the possible pitfalls so that potentially serious errors can be avoided. As with motor vehicle accidents, it is usually a combination of errors that leads to the final mistake. Technical problems and artefacts may be introduced prior to receipt of a specimen in the laboratory or more commonly within the laboratory itself, and can occur during accessioning of a specimen, at the cut-up stage, during processing, embedding, sectioning or staining of the tissue, at the diagnostic stage, and at the time of generating the final report.

## Mishaps and artefacts prior to receipt by the laboratory

### Errors in specimen labelling

Mislabelling or inappropriate labelling of specimens before receipt by the laboratory is commonplace. Quite often, these situations can be easily resolved but, occasionally, serious errors such as the wrong patient's name can go undetected. Unfortunately, the laboratory has little control over these mishaps but the trainee pathologist should be wary whenever the clinical history or stated nature of the

specimen provided on the request form does not match the specimen. If there is any doubt, the clinician must be contacted. The same situation applies to unlabelled specimens which should not be processed until properly identified by the relevant clinician. Laboratory staff should be particularly careful when the number of specimens received does not match the information on the request form. It is not uncommon for multiple specimens to be separated and for some to be left in the operating theatre overnight.

### Specimens for disposal

Occasionally, specimens intended for histopathological examination are disposed of prior to receipt by the laboratory. We have witnessed a leg amputation for osteosarcoma being disposed of by portering staff in the misbelief that it was yet another ischaemic limb. A tissue audit requirement that all specimens be examined by a pathologist would eliminate this potentially disastrous event.

### Contamination, diathermy and crush artefact

Carry over relates to the contamination of tissue from one case to another. Whilst uncommon, this problem may be introduced by clinical staff. Endoscopic biopsy forceps that are inadequately cleaned between cases may, for example, introduce tumour from the biopsy of one patient into the specimen container of another. Carry over, however, is more commonly introduced at the laboratory level. More common problems encountered with endoscopic biopsy procedures are the crushing of tissue leading to the well-recognised crush artefact in histological sections, and the heat coagulation and eosinophilia of diathermy artefact which may appear as coagulative necrosis without inflammation. These artefacts may make interpretation, particularly of a suspected tumour, impossible. Needle biopsies may occasionally result in the unusual juxtaposition of tissues which may appear strange to the unwary, e.g. hair may be introduced into prostatic tissue when the biopsy is taken transrectally.

## Introduced foreign materials

Foreign material may be introduced prior to receipt of the tissue in the laboratory and may result from contamination of the specimen at the current surgical procedure or from previous surgery. Unlike previously introduced foreign material, starch particles from surgical gloves, suture material and fibres from gauze swabs introduced during the current procedure will not be associated with any inflammatory reaction or giant cell response. Carbon particles, fragments of metal and polythene from hip prostheses, Gortex and fabrics from vascular prostheses, and silicone from implants may all be recognised in histological sections. Rather than being artefacts, many of these foreign materials form an integral part of the pathology and require recognition by the trainee pathologist.

## Artefacts related to disease

In some cases, the disease process or interventional therapy may lead to an artefactual appearance in tissue sections. Patients with overwhelming sepsis who have been maintained on a respirator may show 'autolysis' of various organs during life. The interpretation of the significance of such change in the absence of inflammation may be difficult. Linear cracking of tissue sections (parched-earth effect) in tissues from patients maintained on artificial respirators may resemble artefacts produced by faulty tissue sectioning.

## Mishaps during reception and accessioning

By far the commonest source of error in the laboratory resides in the transfer of data, whether this be by clerical, technical or medical staff. Incorrect data entry at the time of accessioning may lead to reports being issued under a different patient's name. It is wise to cross reference patients' names with unit record numbers, dates of birth, age and sex. Mismatches at this stage may result in previous histology not being found or reviewed. Any discrepancy between specimen and accompanying request form should immediately be brought to the attention of laboratory and medical staff.

## Mishaps and artefacts during cut-up

### Identification and mislabelling

Full concentration during the cut-up procedure is essential. Specimens should be religiously checked against request forms and tissue cassettes to ensure that the specimen is placed in the appropriately labelled cassette. The specimen should be identified by at least two of the following parameters: name, unit record number and site of biopsy. Only the specimen designation on the container should be accepted as the correct one. If no designation is provided on the container, this should be noted in the macroscopic description.

## Contamination, carry over and specimen loss

Instruments and work surfaces should be thoroughly cleaned between the handling of each specimen to ensure against carry over of one specimen to another. Ideally, in order to minimise unrecognisable carry over, two similar specimens, e.g. uterine curettings, should not be cut up consecutively. Friable tissues should be wrapped in paper or encased in foam to prevent contamination of other specimens as should small specimens that are capable of falling out of the cassette. Care should be taken to accurately describe numbers of tissue fragments so that any later mishandling of specimens can be identified more easily. Particular care is required with small specimens and biopsies to prevent loss on the work bench, loss down the sink or from the tissue cassette. Very small specimens can be difficult to see following processing and can be highlighted by brief immersion of the tissue or cassette in eosin, methylene blue or any similar stain.

In addition to carry over, contamination of tissue blocks may result from excessive use of ink to mark excision margins, starch granules from surgical gloves, and tissue debris such as may be introduced through the sawing of a bony specimen. Less commonly, post-fixation washing of specimens may introduce foreign material from perished rubber hoses or minerals, particularly iron, if the water source has a high mineral content. Micro-organisms such as acid fast organisms may be contaminants from tap water. These are recognised by the absence of an accompanying inflammatory response.

## Selection of blocks

Selection of appropriate blocks is obviously of utmost importance. Wrong diagnoses may be due to the wrong or incomplete sampling of tissues. This does not necessarily mean examination of an inordinate number of blocks routinely. There is no substitute for careful macroscopic examination and description. If in doubt, ink excision margins to enable assessment of true margins in histological sections. It is all too easy to assume that a tumour involves the deep excision margin as a result of taking an incomplete section at cut-up. It must be remembered that different tissue planes often move against each other as a section is taken so that unwittingly, although labelled as such, the deep margin may not be included in the block. Accurate block keys are essential and must accompany the macroscopic report in every case.

## Fixation artefacts

Poor fixation of specimens may result in poor and even uninterpretable sections. Large specimens such as a uterus or bowel left unopened, fix poorly despite immersion in adequate volumes of formalin. The resulting autolysis may prevent accurate diagnosis. Saprophytic organisms continue to multiply, often appearing to 'invade' the poorly fixed tissue and may lead to the formation of gas bubbles resulting in difficulties in diagnostic interpretation. There is poor penetration of fixative into solid organs such as the spleen when placed in formalin unsliced. This results in autolysis of all but a peripheral rim of tissue producing a characteristic pattern of staining. Some tissues may require special fixatives for optimum results. Urate crystals are water soluble and leach out when placed in 10% buffered formalin. Their demonstration in tissue sections requires fixation in absolute alcohol. On the other hand, fixation in absolute alcohol causes rapid dehydration of tissue and denatures protein by coagulation. This can lead to extensive shrinking and distortion which is often more marked at the periphery of the section.

## Freezing and refrigeration artefacts

Freezing artefact is seen in specimens that are frozen prior to fixation or that undergo freezing within the fixative. This artefact appears as interstitial and intracellular vacuoles due to the formation of ice crystals within the tissue section. Ice crystals that form over a longer period of time tend to be larger than those formed when freezing is rapid. For this reason, tissue for cryostat sectioning should be snap frozen, preferably using an isopentane slurry which is surrounded by liquid nitrogen. This allows more rapid freezing to take place in a liquid/solid interface medium rather than a gas/liquid interface medium such as with liquid nitrogen alone. Ice crystal artefact is normally easy to recognise but may cause diagnostic problems for the unwary particularly if the specimen has unknowingly frozen in the fixative during transportation. Lengthy refrigeration of unfixed specimens, whilst not as disastrous as freezing artefact, may lead to crenation of cells in tissue sections.

## Pigment artefacts

Formalin pigment (acid formalin haematin pigment) is produced by the reaction of formic acid in unbuffered formalin with the haem moiety of haemoglobin. It appears in tissue sections as deposits of black birefringent pigment around red cells and wherever the haem moiety is found. Unbuffered formalin should not be used for fixation since it leads to artefactual pigment formation, its prolonged use may alter or remove some pathological tissue pigments and minerals such as copper, iron and calcium,

and it may lead to adverse staining reactions. In some instances, the use of calcium salts in neutral buffered formalin as a neutralising or preservative agent, may produce pseudocalcification in tissue sections which may be mistaken for true calcification. Acid haematin is a dark brown, anisotropic, microcrystalline pigment which is similar to acid formalin haematin and may be formed in blood-rich tissues that have been fixed in Bouin's fixative.

# Mishaps and artefacts during tissue processing

## Carry over and specimen loss

Inadequate care when placing friable tissues such as products of conception into cassettes may lead to fragments of tissue being carried over from one cassette to another during processing. This can generally be overcome by wrapping such specimens in tissue paper or foam. Care must also be taken to ensure that cassette lids are firmly snapped shut. There is seldom a more embarrassing moment than finding three or four empty tissue cassettes and tissue lying free at the bottom of the processing container. Such mishaps can also occur with cassettes with plastic lids which buckle as they pass through the processing reagents, particularly xylene. Unfortunately, there are occasions where minute fragments of tissue do not survive the processing schedule but such losses should be minimised by the wrapping and staining of such specimens as outlined above.

## Artefacts due to faulty processing

### Inadequate processing

Artefacts due to inadequate tissue processing are generally the result of tissue blocks that are too thick or processing schedules that are too short. Large blocks which completely fill the tissue cassette can prevent access of processing fluids into the tissue. This may result in a tissue block that is poorly penetrated by wax and difficult, if not impossible, to section. Similarly, the more recent use of foam to prevent small pieces of tissue from escaping from the tissue cassette may prevent access of processing fluids to the tissue if used dry. A simple solution is to store the foam pads in alcohol. Another artefact seen with the use of foam is the result of focal compression of, usually poorly fixed, tissue by the foam. This produces characteristic, often triangular or star-shaped holes where the foam spicules have indented the tissue. In some instances, these spaces may resemble cholesterol clefts and be mistaken for atheromatous cholesterol emboli. However, careful examination shows that, unlike cholesterol emboli, there is a narrow rim of compressed tissue around the hole.

## Machine faults

Occasionally, a machine fault will result in inadequate processing or interruption of the process in mid-cycle. Most modern day processors are fitted with alarm systems which are triggered in the event of malfunction and, in the majority of cases, the deficiencies can be salvaged by reprocessing. With older histokinettes, mechanical and electrical faults can result in a basket full of tissue blocks becoming suspended in mid air during transfer from one fluid to another. However, with modern hypercentres, fluid levels and machines still require regular maintenance to ensure that all tissue blocks are fully immersed in processing fluids. Prolonged exposure to air brought about by incomplete immersion causes the tissues to become over dehydrated. The use of more complex automated

processors requires greater attention to programming and this should ideally be checked by a second person.

## Excessive tissue shrinkage

Inadequately fixed specimens undergo excessive shrinkage of the tissue components during clearing and this is more noticeable with the use of xylene than chloroform. Some degree of specimen shrinkage during processing is inevitable but is more pronounced with certain tissues such as bone marrow and tissue containing inflammatory infiltrates. This may cause problems in interpretation and lead to an erroneous diagnosis of undifferentiated malignancy. In squamous epithelium, the resulting vacuolisation of the cell cytoplasm may erroneously be interpreted as koilocytosis. Improper fixation may also lead to denaturisation which produces poor uptake of haematoxylin and eosin and indistinct staining. Denaturisation generally takes place during clearing or infiltration with paraffin wax.

## Excessive dehydration

Excessive dehydration of tissues during processing may also produce vacuolation of cells, an appearance not dissimilar to diathermy artefact, or result in tissue which is harder than the impregnating paraffin wax. The passage of the microtome knife through excessively hard tissue produced in this way can result in a moth-eaten appearance to the tissue sections. Alternatively, a 'venetian-blind' chatter appearance may be seen at the periphery of the specimen and is due to the hard tissue vibrating within the paraffin block during sectioning. The appearance is similar to that produced by a loose knife or tissue block. Lengthwise scratches produced by fragments of hard tissue being dragged through the specimen by the microtome knife may also be seen.

## *Insufficient dehydration and faulty paraffin wax impregnation*

Inadequate dehydration is usually due to reduced concentration of alcohols. This may be due to contamination of the alcohols with water during processing as a result of infrequent changes of alcohol or absorption from the atmosphere. Inadequate dehydration prevents effective impregnation by the hydrophobic paraffin wax. When the tissue is embedded, residues of the clearing agents may ooze from the specimen and cause increased crystallinity of the solidified paraffin and a halo effect which stains poorly. Residues of clearing fluids may also allow focal imbibition of water and tissue swelling. Such foci, when surrounded by tissue fully impregnated with hydrophobic wax, are prevented from even expansion and lead to wrinkling or folding of tissue sections when floated out on the water-bath. Wrinkles which run in various directions are generally due to poor impregnation by paraffin, whereas a dull microtome knife will produce wrinkling aligned parallel to the knife edge. Such artefacts caused by faulty processing cannot be corrected. Inadequate infiltration with paraffin may also cause the tissue section to spread rapidly when floated out leading to artificial clefts within the tissue that may be mistaken for a pathological process. Immersion of the specimen in excessively hot paraffin wax during processing will lead to burning of the tissue with poor uptake of stains and suboptimal morphology.

## Mishaps and artefacts during embedding

### Carry over and mislabelling

Contamination of a specimen by tissue fragments of another specimen may occur at the embedding stage if the forceps used to transfer tissue from cassette to block are not flamed in between the embedding of each specimen. At this stage, care is also required to ensure that the tissue is transferred from the cassette to the correctly labelled block. With the use of modern Tissue Tek stations, whereby the cassette also forms the base of the block, such errors are now uncommon.

### Artefacts due to faulty embedding

The sole purpose of embedding specimens in paraffin or plastic is to support the tissue so that it may be sectioned on a microtome. Any factor which reduces the ability of the media to support the tissue may result in artefacts being produced during microtomy.

When multiple portions of relatively hard tissues such as myometrium are embedded in the one tissue block, the supporting wax may be insufficient to prevent movement of some of the tissue portions within the block during sectioning. This is another cause of the 'venetian blind' effect whereby alternating thick and thin zones are produced in the tissue section, often making interpretation difficult. Entrapped air within the tissue block brought about by failure to use vacuum procedures or by the slow transfer from the molten wax to the embedding mould may have a similar effect or produce crevices within the section.

Embedding of multiple different tissues within the one block, as commonly occurs with veterinary specimens, may lead to inadequate support due to the variable consistency of the tissues and results in wrinkles in the tissue section. This can be compounded by linear nicks throughout the section produced by the edge of the microtome knife through vibration of the denser tissues in the block. Wrinkling of sections may also be due to the embedding medium being harder than the specimen as a result of the inherent nature of the embedding medium or the temperature at which sectioning is performed. Cracks parallel to the edge of the knife, pin cushion distortion, the rolling up of sections and the inability to form ribbons of sections may all be due to this cause.

Proper orientation of specimens during embedding is important for ease of sectioning and for accurate interpretation. Multiple portions of skin in the same block when not embedded in the same plane will result in an incomplete face of each portion appearing in the section with erroneous interpretation of excision margins. From a technical point of view, to prevent mutilation during sectioning, it is important to orientate the specimen so that any resistance to the knife from different components within the tissue is spread evenly over the edge of the knife. Thus, skin should be orientated so that the surface is horizontal to the knife edge with the epidermis being presented to the knife last.

Prolonged exposure to hot molten wax, as may occur with the embedding of multiple portions of tissue within the one block, can lead to heat dehydration and 'cooking' of tissue with dire consequences on staining.

## Mishaps and artefacts during sectioning and mounting

### Floaters and mislabelling

Tissue contamination from one case to another can occur during sectioning, as a result of fragments becoming stuck to the edge of the microtome knife, and during floating-out on the water-bath whereby fragments of one case are left behind on the water to be picked up during slide mounting of subsequent cases. Such contamination is usually termed a 'floater', in that subsequent investigation with multiple levels and examination of the tissue block will reveal that, unlike true carry-over contamination, the misplaced tissue is not contained within the paraffin block. Most floaters are identified through their incongruence but their presence should always be investigated and brought to the attention of the histotechnologist. More difficult to identify are floaters consisting of similar tissues and for this reason particular care is needed if similar tissues are floated out after one another without cleaning the water surface of the water-bath. Worse still is the complete transposition of cases that may occur through the floating out of multiple cases together. We have witnessed such transposition involving three separate cases of uterine curettings that were floated out together on the one water-bath. Whilst this may sound a dangerous practice, it is done to ensure that adequate flotation time is provided in order to obtain perfectly flat sections without undue delay. Strict protocols must be adhered to in order to minimise mistakes. One method is to attach one end of the ribbon of sections to the edge of the water-bath and place the cut block adjacent to it. Sections must then be checked against the block and labelled slide before the section is picked up from the water. Just as utmost care and attention is required of the pathologist at the time of cut-up, so the same care and attention is required of the technologist at the time of sectioning, slide mounting and labelling. Mislabelling of slides at this stage is, again, normally a serious problem only if similar cases are transposed. The trainee pathologist must at all times be wary of any inconsistency between clinical history, macroscopic description and histological appearance and must investigate such discrepancies fully.

## Contamination

Contamination of sections may also be caused by extraneous debris and organisms introduced at the time of sectioning and mounting. Squames from the technologist's hands and arms or as dandruff, may be picked up from the knife surface, water-bath or glass slide and recognised as such in final sections. Dust particles may be particularly bothersome when taking photomicrographs of the tissue sections. Cigarette ash should no longer be seen as a contaminant in present day laboratories. Microscope slides stored in damp or humid conditions may be contaminated by fungal organisms whilst bacterial contamination may result from proteins such as albumen and gelatin, which are good growth media, employed as section adhesives. These organisms may be confused with pathogens, but on careful examination will be seen to beout of the tissue plane of focus and not confined to the tissue itself. Excessive use of section adhesives may lead to clumps of gelatin adhering to the tissue and appearing as basophilic or eosinophilic strands or splotches in stained sections. Some bacterial water-bath contaminants may simulate acid-fast bacilli in both morphology and staining reactions. Every effort should be made to avoid contaminants of this type. Water-baths should, ideally, be changed daily and demineralised water should be used. The use of tap water may result in unwanted minerals and iron deposits being artefactually introduced into the tissue section. In some laboratories, a few grains of thymol are added to the water to prevent bacterial growth.

## Artefacts due to faulty sectioning and mounting

Paraffin blocks are often chilled on ice to facilitate sectioning. If a chilling aerosol spray is used instead of ice, prolonged exposure of the surface of the block may lead to surface dehydration and result in the formation of fissures along anatomical lines of cleavage. Alternatively, due to differences between the hardness of the paraffin and the tissue, and to a blunt microtome knife edge, the tissue sections may become wrinkled as they are sectioned. Frequently, such sections may be flattened out on the water-bath.

Dull knife distortions may also produce compression artefacts, cracks which are parallel to the knife edge, streaks or corrugations, focal compressed areas which stain more intensely than the surrounding tissue, thick and thin zones and increased shrinkage of tissue. This shrinkage may be significant and influence accurate measurement such as assessment of the depth of invasion of a malignant melanoma.

Alternate thick and thin zones may also be seen when the section is thick and the knife too thin, or when the knife is loose within the microtome. In each case, the knife has a tendency to vibrate leading to irregular sectioning. Alternatively, a loose knife may lead to the 'venetian blind' effect whereby the compressed zones of tissue are separated by open spaces. A focal venetian blind appearance or scoring of the section is not uncommon and is usually due to contamination of the knife edge by foreign material, a fragment of hard tissue or a nick in the knife. Focal compression of tissue within a section may also be seen when the angle of the cutting knife is set at too acute an angle.

If the water-bath temperature is not sufficiently high, the tissue will not spread out sufficiently when floated out producing tissue wrinkling when the section is picked up on the glass slide. If the water-bath temperature is too hot, the tissue expands excessively and shrinks when dried out on the glass slide. This may result in the section falling off the slide, artefactual separation of tissue planes within the section or a parched-earth cracking effect. Bubbles of air may become trapped under the tissue section as it is floated out on the water-bath. These should be removed before the section is picked up on the glass slide but occasionally they can go undetected. When the section is stained, the bubble may burst and shatter the overlying tissue which stains more intensely than the surrounding tissue. Once the section has been picked up on the glass slide, it must be adequately dried before staining. Failure to dry a section results in erratic staining.

## Mishaps and artefacts during staining, coverslipping and labelling

### Staining

It is beyond the scope of this book to describe the artefacts that may be encountered with the multitude of different staining techniques available in histopathology. A few general comments regarding such artefacts follow but the reader is referred to specialised texts on staining techniques for greater detail.

#### Effects of storage of wet specimens, tissue blocks and slides

The effect of prolonged storage of a specimen in formalin prior to embedding often leads to altered staining properties whereby the tinctorial quality is very light.

In contrast, formalin-fixed paraffin-embedded tissues and their deparaffinised unstained sections are well preserved throughout prolonged storage. However, this is not so for all tissue fixatives and, generally, the sooner the embedded tissue can be sectioned and stained, the better. Stained sections, on the other hand, may deteriorate markedly with prolonged storage. This depends to a great extent on whether they are exposed to light or kept in the dark. Sections faded by daylight may be satisfactorily re-stained after removal of the coverslip.

#### Deceration

Deceration refers to the removal of the paraffin-embedding medium by solvents such as xylene prior to staining with water-based stains. Xylene that is saturated with paraffin wax prevents adequate deceration and results in areas of the section failing to take up the stain. This may also happen if the mounted sections are not fully immersed in the solvent or stain.

#### Clearing

Following staining, the section is dehydrated in alcohols and cleared in xylene prior to coverslipping. With use of contaminated xylene, the water and alcohols are not adequately removed and their retention appears as refractile globules when viewed through the microscope. If the dehydrated section is exposed to xylene for too long, it will become dried out and, after being coverslipped, will have a parched earth effect. Automatic staining machines should be regularly checked to ensure that the levels of xylene, alcohols and stains are sufficient to fully cover the glass slides. Xylene and alcohols must be regularly replaced.

## Blueing artefact

One specific artefact that has been described throughout the world over many years is worthy of specific mention: the blueing artefact. This is characterised by a peculiar and sometimes hazy blue hue in haematoxylin and eosin stained sections, particularly in the periphery of certain specimens such as uterine curettings and small biopsies. Few laboratories appear immune from this artefact but it is extremely spasmodic in its presentation. There will often be short periods where the artefact is observed followed by long intervening periods where it is absent. It has been the subject of several publications with several theories of causation being put forward including problems with fixation, problems with processing, use of contaminated tap water and variations in the quality of haematoxylin used. Our own investigations of this artefact have failed to identify a specific cause and we have been unable to reproduce it consistently under controlled conditions.

## Coverslipping

Contamination of sections with dust, fibres or carbon particles from slide labelling pencils may occur at the time of coverslipping or be introduced by the use of contaminated mounting medium. Such extraneous foreign material is usually sited above the plane of section and easily distinguished from particulate matter within the tissue section itself.

Coverslips should be large enough to cover all the tissue section and should be correctly positioned. Tissue close to the edge or not covered by the coverslip may loose its tinctorial staining properties. It is all too easy to ignore fragments of tissue not covered and yet, in specimens such as

uterine curettings or prostatic reamings, these fragments may be the only tissue involved by tumour, resulting in a false-negative report.

Air bubbles may be entrapped under the coverslip through faulty technique. If the stained section is allowed to dry out before applying the mounting medium and coverslip, tiny air bubbles may be dispersed throughout the section, and with certain stains, can be confused with finely refractile brown pigment. Sections should be moist with xylene prior to coverslipping. Some types of mounting media may crystallise and appear as anisotropic crystals above the plane of tissue section.

## Labelling

It cannot be sufficiently stressed that attention to labelling is of the utmost importance at all stages in the production of a histological slide. Normally glass slides are labelled by pencil or indelible ink prior to picking up of the tissue section from the water-bath. They are then labelled with sticky labels following staining and coverslipping. The trainee pathologist should routinely check the slide label against the request form and patient demographics prior to inspection through the microscope. Whenever there is an apparent discrepancy between histology and clinical history or between histology and macroscopic description, the slide label and request form should again be matched. If necessary, the sticky label should be removed and the pencilled label checked. The block should then be checked against the microscope slide for labelling and content and further sections cut if necessary. Finally, if all labelling appears correct and the discrepancy is serious enough, the possibility of a complete switch in tissue blocks should be considered and thoroughly investigated.

## Mishaps involving reports

Although many of the artefacts described are readily detected, some, as outlined, may give rise to false-negatives, false-positives and otherwise erroneous interpretation of tissue sections. The trainee pathologist must be aware of these possible pitfalls.

Besides differences of opinion leading to wrongful diagnoses, further errors may be introduced through inappropriate technique by the pathologist at the time of microscopy. It is easy to miss some tissue fragments unless the entire slide is examined systematically. Encircling all tissue fragments with black Texta pen prior to microscopy will ensure examination of the entire section. The trainee should also be careful not to cut corners in order to accomplish a fast turnaround time. The value of examining multiple levels in some cases cannot be overstressed and special stains may be of the utmost importance. The old adage of 'sleep on it overnight' for difficult cases often pays dividends.

One of the commonest sources of error in reporting is in the proof reading of typed reports. It is easy to be scrupulous about the microscopy report and yet cursory with regard to the macroscopic report and to neglect the patient demographics and nature of the specimen. At best, it is embarrassing to see a microscopic description of a uterine curetting accompanying a male gender. Far worse is the transposition of the two patients' names on two breast reports, one of which is benign and the other malignant.

One should be just as careful with the signing of reports generated by another pathologist. If necessary, it is advisable to hold back any report that does not quite make sense. In the prolonged absence of a colleague, the alternative is to examine and report the case oneself.

Delays in issuing reports may result from conflict of other duties, excessive repeated corrections and typed copies being temporarily 'lost' amongst paper work either in the typing pool, or more commonly on the pathologist's desk. Trainees must above all be organised in their approach to the discipline being fully conscious of the need to report the case as soon as possible. With computerisation and central dictation facilities, many of these delays may be overcome but computerisation in its own right may introduce delays and errors. It is not uncommon for computers to crash and require expert maintenance. Other sources of error may be encountered by the sending of reports to the wrong destination. Special attention must be paid to general practitioners and clinicians with similar names and every effort made to ensure that the report is issued to the correct clinician.

## Quality control and quality assurance

Although the majority of laboratories have always practised some degree of internal quality control (QC), recent emphasis on quality assurance (QA) has necessitated the participation in programmes nationally or internationally organised for accreditation. Each department should have a QC/QA committee chaired by a senior pathologist with representative members from the principal sections or divisions of the department. The committee should meet regularly and be responsible for updating the departmental QC/QA plan for surgical pathology. This plan should take into account performance indicators at every level within the department and should form part of the departmental accreditation manual.

## Processing and sectioning

Specimens submitted to the laboratory should be assessed in terms of adequacy of tissue submitted, specimen identification, fixation and safety requirements. Each stage of specimen preparation including, accessioning, fixation, processing, sectioning, mounting and staining should be regularly monitored and a record of time of delivery of slides should be kept. Evaluation of the quality of slides is the responsibility of both the technical and medical staff. A lost specimen may be defined as an irretrievable loss from whatever cause, that has occurred after the case has been accessioned within the laboratory. An acceptable number for lost specimens has been estimated as 1 in 3000 cases.

## Intra- and interdepartmental consultation

Intradepartmental case reviews may be carried out through review of selected cases by diagnostic staff as a group or individually by a staff pathologist. Often, second opinions from within the department are sought on difficult cases as a matter of routine and it is appropriate that this information is included in the report either by acknowledgment or by a double signatory. If a second pathologist's opinion is included, care should be taken that it accurately reflects what was said. The consulted pathologist must be allowed to sight the report or to be a co-signatory. There are a number of ways in which reviews may be carried out. Random case review should include not less than 1% of surgical cases or 25 cases per month, whichever is the larger. In addition, some departments review all cases in which a diagnosis of cancer has been made whilst others regularly review on the basis of an organ, lesion or procedure, e.g. endometrial carcinoma or TURP. It is desirable to review all cases on which a frozen section examination has been made and to analyse the accuracy of frozen section diagnosis and, if frozen section diagnosis was deferred, whether this was justified. An acceptable level for major disagreements between reports on frozen and paraffin sections has been given as 3% and for inappropriate deferral of frozen section diagnosis as 10%.

Such reviews should include all aspects relating to the case, e.g. final report, quality of sections, turnaround time and any special procedures. Acceptable turnaround times have been given as 1 working day for a verbal report and 2 days for a written report on any urgent case, and a verbal report of 2 working days and written report of 3 days for biopsy specimens and surgical specimens. An acceptable level for these turnaround times is 80% but in reality, in many laboratories in Australia, turnaround times are often shorter. Naturally, extra time should be allowed for overnight fixation, decalcification, special stains, special procedures and intradepartmental consultation where necessary.

Cases presented at interdepartmental meetings and clinico-pathological conferences are generally reviewed by the presenter. Should there be major disagreement between the written report and the presenter, the case must be discussed with the reporting pathologist whenever possible, and preferably before the presentation. Presentation of such discrepancies often requires tact and experience which is sometimes lacking even with senior pathologists.

## Interinstitutional review and quality assurance programmes

Review by outside institutions can be initiated at the request of the patient, clinician or pathologist as part of a co-operative study or as an individual opinion case. Assuming that the outside opinion is correct, it has been estimated that the level for significant disagreement is around 2%.

Many laboratories participate in externally run quality assurance programmes whereby circulated slides are sent out for 'routine' reporting. Care should be taken that these cases are dealt with in the same manner as routine cases from within the department. In many programmes, it is difficult to mimic the routine exactly. Representative slides of small portions of tissue pose a problem, as do isolated haematoxylin and eosin stains of a soft tissue tumour without access to specialised procedures. However, these programmes can monitor staining procedures and reporting formats in addition to diagnostic interpretation, and participation is becoming essential for reaccreditation.

## Further reading

Association of Directors of Anatomic and Surgical Pathology 1991 Recommendations on quality control and quality assurance in anatomic pathology. American Journal of Surgical Pathology 15: 1007–1009

Bancroft JD, Stevens A, Turner DR 1995 Theory and practice of histological techniques, 4th edn. Churchill Livingstone, Edinburgh

# 16 The surgical pathology report

# The role of the surgical pathologist

The surgical pathologist is the unique link between the patient and his/her clinician on the one hand, and the laboratory on the other. The role of the surgical pathologist has become even more indispensable with the increasing sophistication of diagnostic procedures which can be applied to small biopsies to provide prognostic information, often determining the choice of optimal therapy. The surgical pathologist is provided with diseased tissue which can be subjected to critical structural and functional analyses. The several modalities of morphological examination include gross, microscopic and ultrastructural examination which can be coupled with enzyme cytochemistry and immunohistochemistry to provide a detailed means of identifying cellular products, extracellular deposits and foreign material. Specific gene products can be examined by antibody probes and specific DNA and RNA sequences can be identified with corresponding probes in tissue sections. Objective quantitation assessment of cellular characteristics in reactive and neoplastic tissues and measurement of host response to the disease process are also possible. Importantly, as diseased tissue usually is accompanied by a border of interaction in which host responses are already visible, an opportunity to study the host's response to changes that may occur therein is available.

With his/her knowledge of the biology of the disease and its consequences, and the information learned from study at the autopsy table, the surgical pathologist is able to correlate histological changes in the biopsy with the clinical presentation. Thus, the surgical pathologist must not only be an expert in his/her own subject, but must also have a rich background in clinical medicine.

Diagnosis of the biopsy is not his/her only function. Pure diagnostic labelling of specimens represents no more than classification of diseases and can be likened to stamp collecting in which the stamp is identified and filed according to the country of origin. The surgical pathologist must be able to understand the significance of the diagnosis and to be able to communicate this to the clinicians both through a written report and orally, as well as at interdepartmental conferences. He/she should have insight into the clinicians' needs and respond to them accordingly. As such, he/she should be able to advise clinicians about the biopsy examined and must be able to discuss the extent of the disease, the adequacy of the excision, as well as providing other pertinent information such as behaviour and prognosis of the disease, and comment on appropriate therapy. In addition, the surgical pathologist should be discriminatory and be able to determine when such comments are appropriate. For example, it is often inappropriate to comment that 'careful follow-up is necessary', as this may not be well received by the specialist clinician who is likely to be sufficiently well-informed about the disease process to feel that the comment is unwarranted. However, if it is anticipated that the recipient of the report may not be conversant with the diagnosis, such as in the case of a general practitioner who receives a report of 'skin biopsy: epithelioid sarcoma, involving margins of excision', a comment on the behaviour of such tumours would be very appropriate. Pathologists also often develop a close working relationship with radiologists who deal with shadows and can frequently benefit from correlation of these shadows with the macroscopic and microscopic tissue pathology. Such correlations strengthen the diagnostic skills of the radiologists and explain errors in radiological interpretation. The pathological study of specimens removed after treatment also provides medical and radiation oncologists with valuable information about the susceptibility of normal and abnormal tissues to the effects of chemotherapy and radiotherapy. Because pathologists examine a large volume of material by way of biopsies and autopsies, and because they perform a uniform and precise classification of diseases, they are ideally situated to study the epidemiology of disease, to identify the emergence of novel diseases or unexpected changes in disease patterns and incidence, as well as to monitor the effects of newer forms of therapy and changes in lifestyle. Pathologists provide the best form of quality control in the hospital, as their relative clinical independence favours their role to monitor allegedly superfluous surgical procedures and to police and audit hospital mortality.

While there is considerable merit in exchanging information with clinical specialists at clinico-pathological conferences where the biopsies are presented and discussed, the assessment of biopsies should be performed objectively and in an unbiased fashion. It is impossible for clinicians who are familiar with a particular patient to be absolutely impartial. With strong clinical conviction, it is easy to introduce bias or to read into a biopsy an interpretation that may not be supported by objective evidence. As such, it is potentially hazardous for clinical specialists who have primary responsibilities for patient care to perform diagnostic surgical pathology. It is unfortunate that in some specialised areas of pathology, individuals who are fundamentally clinicians are still responsible for making histopathological diagnoses. Such individuals, who are not trained pathologists, may have some knowledge of pathology but it is difficult, if not impossible, to be both a competent clinician and a skilful pathologist. We are not aware of surgical pathologists who believe themselves to be capable of performing operations as a sideline and, while pathologists may well be conversant with the optimal forms of therapy for specific diseases, they do not themselves treat patients.

## The surgical pathology consultation

While the concept of a surgical pathology consultation is commonly accepted in North America, it is not generally embraced in some other parts of the world where clinicians sometimes forget that, as with clinical consultations, it is also a consultative process to solicit an opinion based on histological examination; it is not a request for laboratory results. Indeed, all too often, young clinical residents ring surgical pathologists for 'results'. We are often tempted to retort 'the renal biopsy contains no protein' or 'the biopsy contains 20 ± 2 g albumin'!

In the text of a surgical pathology report, the pathologist conveys to the clinician his/her findings and opinions as a consultant. Surgical pathologists provide opinions and interpretations of microscopic morphology which represent a distillate of clinical and laboratory data, accumulated knowledge of the disease process, and their experience and wisdom. While many experienced surgical pathologists can render accurate diagnoses without any clinical information, it completely defeats the purpose of surgical pathology reporting. Undoubtedly, many simple diagnoses such as cutaneous epidermal cysts do not require a clinico-pathological correlation. On the other hand, a biopsy showing chronic dermatitis will require clinical input for proper interpretation.

Clinicians sometimes fail to appreciate that microscopic diagnosis is a subjective evaluation that attains its full potential only when the pathologist is fully informed of the essential clinical data, surgical findings, and the type or nature of surgery performed. Incomplete communication between the clinician and pathologist may make diagnosis difficult or impossible. Interestingly, a request for consultation between clinicians is always accompanied by a detailed history and clinical work-up, but sadly, this is not so for pathology consultations. To perform his/her tasks intelligently, a pathologist must know all the facts that have any bearing on the case. To render a diagnosis on an inherently puzzling bit of tissue with only a vague knowledge of its source and with no concept of the clinical problem can be considered as foolhardy as undertaking a lobectomy on the hearsay that the patient may have a lung tumour. For example, a discussion between the surgeon and pathologist prior to a planned frozen section examination may facilitate matters for both, and, in many instances, the pathologist can offer valuable advice about the clinical nature of a lesion and where best to sample when he/she is called into the operating theatre or to the patient's bedside. With his/her knowledge of the pathology and precise orientation of anatomical relationships, and awareness of the limitations of different biopsy procedures, the pathologist is in the best position to advise on how to obtain the optimal tissue sample for microscopic examination and what adjunctive investigations may be helpful.

## The surgical pathology report

The surgical pathology report is an important medical document which contains, in a concise and thorough manner, all the relevant macroscopic and microscopic features of the tissue removed from the patient, as well as an interpretation of their significance. It is an important responsibility of the reporting pathologist that the recipient of the surgical pathology report fully understands the report and is able to act on it appropriately. To this end, the report should not only be clear and without controversy, but should also contain a comment elaborating on the diagnosis and predicting the behaviour of the disease and, when appropriate, a comment on therapeutic response. While the ability to recognise cytological and histological features is an essential component of training, it is the ability to integrate microscopic findings into a meaningful interpretation which characterises the ability of the surgical pathologist and his/her role as a consultant. The components of the surgical pathology report are: demographic data, clinical history, macroscopic description including a block key, microscopic description, diagnosis, comments if relevant and SNOMED (systematised nomenclature of medicine) coding and circulation list.

### Demographic data

All surgical pathology reports contain patient demographic data which should include the surname including previous names such as maiden name, initials or complete forenames, date of birth, sex, ward or address, hospital registration number and insurance status. The responsible clinician's name and address should be legibly printed and the date of the biopsy should be stated.

### Clinical history

The component of the report contains essential clinical data provided to the pathologist in the requisition form. Sometimes, additional information is available as a result of direct communication between clinician and pathologist. This information is dictated at the time of 'cut-up' or examination of the gross specimen. It is included with the dictation of the patient's demographic information and should include the clinical presentation, surgical findings and type of surgical procedure performed. In addition, if a frozen section has been performed, the diagnosis and relevant accession number should also be included as part of the history. The 'Clinical history' section is an important component of the report and, no matter how brief, it provides the reader of the report with an immediate orientation as to the nature of the problem that is being addressed in the histological examination and in the context of the patient's overall disease.

## Macroscopic description

The 'Macroscopic description' contains a gross description of the specimen or specimens received. This section of the report should indicate how many and what specimens were received and how they were individually identified by the requesting clinician. In addition, it should be documented whether the specimens were received fresh or fixed, intact or open. It is important to be precise and thorough because once the specimen is discarded, this description remains the only document by which the macroscopic features of the specimen can be evaluated. Documentation by way of photographs is an excellent method and should be used as frequently as possible. With improvements in technology, it may be possible to replace or supplement macroscopic descriptions with multiple digital images of the specimen stored on computer disks and reproduced in colour when desired.

The specimen should be described in a logical and sequential fashion, providing a clear documentation of the abnormalities and their location. The size, colour and location of all abnormalities should be recorded and it is important to avoid lengthy anatomical descriptions of normal structures. In describing location, it is useful to employ reference landmarks. For example, '20 mm from *the distal margin* is an annular constricting tumour extending over 30 mm of colon', and 'the 15 × 10 × 10 mm mass lies *5 mm from the deep surface* in the upper outer quadrant'. Do not provide comparisons with objects such as fruits or vegetables but provide specific dimensions and descriptions, using primary or other common colours. Remember that measurements, at best, can only be approximate as the specimen undergoes a variable degree of shrinkage with fixation, it may be stretched or compressed, and it may retract. Avoid using 'approximately' in your descriptions. Small pieces of tissue such as endometrial curettings, when measured in toto, will have different dimensions depending on how the fragments are arranged. Weights are more consistent and meaningful parameters. The weight of the entire specimen and sometimes the weight of individual organs or lesions in a specimen should be recorded whenever possible. Employ accurate, factual and non-committal descriptive terms, avoiding subjective interpretations and conclusions as much as possible. For example, 'milky' or 'creamy' is a preferred descriptive term for the colour of a secretion rather than 'pus', which is an interpretation which may well be incorrect. Do not employ unconventional terms and abbreviations as they may not be universally understood.

The other portion of 'Macroscopic description' is the key to the samples taken. In this 'Block key' employ letters of the English alphabet sequentially to identify tissue blocks taken from different sites. This is an important part of the gross examination as it provides a key to important sites of sampling such as surgical margins, which would not be otherwise identifiable. Use line diagrams to indicate the sites of sampling or mark these sites on a photograph of the specimen.

The macroscopic description should be concluded by a note whether sampling was representative or in toto and whether photographs were taken, and if other procedures were performed such as electron microscopy, karyotyping and molecular analysis. Lastly, the name of the pathologist performing the macroscopic examination should be recorded, particularly if the histological sections will be examined and reported by another pathologist.

## Microscopic description

The 'Microscopic description' should be succinct. It is important to remember that clinicians are often not particularly interested in the microscopic description. The description should include the histological features which justify or support the diagnosis and only relevant features are described. Do not describe normal tissue and it is superfluous to give a detailed description of straightforward lesions such as a simple pigmented naevus or lipoma. However, atypical hyperplastic lymph nodes and liver biopsies are examples which demand a detailed description of the histology. Often, if the histology is sufficiently unusual to be of interest to other pathologists, it is likely they would wish to examine the section themselves.

The other important aspect of the microscopic description is the recording of relevant prognostic parameters which allow staging of tumours and other therapeutic decisions to be made. It is important to have a checklist for the more complex specimens such as mastectomies, prostectomies, hysterectomies and colectomies for cancer where specific prognostic parameters have to be assessed microscopically. These parameters, such as surgical margins, histological grade, depth of extension and vascular invasion, should be clearly commented on in the microscopic description. Surgical pathologists come under increasing pressure from clinicians to assess an expanding number of purported prognostic parameters but a clear distinction should be made between established parameters and those which are yet to be proven and are largely of research interest.

## Diagnosis

The fourth component of the report is the 'Diagnosis'. Each specimen received should have a separate diagnosis or diagnoses and numbered accordingly in the order of their receipt. The diagnosis should be short and clear. It is good practice to present the diagnosis in two parts, incorporating the topography of the specimen and the morphology, separated by a dash or a colon. The topography may be that which is identified histologically or, more appropriately, that provided by the referring clinician. While it is easy to identify squamous mucosa, it may be impossible to distinguish mucosa from the mouth, palate, pharynx and even oesophagus. Under such circumstances, the topography should be as stated by the referring clinician and recorded in parenthesis. In some instances this designation may be of great relevance to the diagnosis, for example, 'intra-abdominal testis' would be of significance to a testis which shows histological features of atrophy. Its intra-abdominal site would not have been recognisable by macroscopic or microscopic examination alone. The morphological diagnosis, however, is strictly the responsibility of the pathologist and derived from histological examination. The nature of the surgical procedure performed can also be included in the diagnosis, for example, 'bone, neck of femur, needle biopsy: metastatic adenocarcinoma'. This approach provides the reader with all the essential information on the specimen and allows easy coding.

With the increasing demands for information for cancer prognosis, it now becomes necessary to incorporate important prognostic parameters in the diagnosis. While these may be clearly listed and identified in the microscopic description, some clinicians request that such information be provided in the bottom line diagnosis. Synoptic reporting is an alternative way of presenting such information (see below).

On occasion, it may be necessary to include qualifiers to your diagnosis, e.g. 'Diagnosis – skin biopsy, site not designated: squamous cell carcinoma, well-differentiated'; 'Diagnosis – ovarian tumour, excision, side not designated: serous cystadenocarcinoma, well-differentiated'.

Under appropriate circumstances, it is also correct to state 'soft tissue, right thigh, incisional biopsy: spindle cell malignancy, definitive typing pending immunohistochemical and ultrastructural findings'.

The term 'Diagnosis' is sometimes substituted by 'Interpretation' or 'Conclusion'. One of the reasons for the use of such alternative terms is to indicate that the bottom line label assigned to the specimen is only an interpretation and avoids the veneer of infallibility associated with the term 'Diagnosis' (see below).

## Comment

The final part of the report which is applicable only to some cases is a 'Comment'. Unlike 'Diagnosis' which is intended to be as objective a statement as possible, the 'Comment' portion of the report allows the pathologist to discuss the diagnosis or to expand on it. The pathologist may mention the differential diagnosis or diagnoses, discuss the features supporting one diagnosis over another, make some suggestions for appropriate management, prognosticate, and include appropriate references. If a comment is appropriate, the phrase 'see comments' should be added as a qualifier to the 'Diagnosis', i.e. 'Diagnosis – right cervical lymph node: metastatic spindle cell tumour (see Comments)'.

The report ends up with a distribution list which should include the attending physician, clinic or ward, and tumour registry. Also included at the bottom of the report is the SNOMED code for the case.

It is worthwhile mentioning that although current coding systems, including SNOMED, allow a five-digit code to be used, it is generally unnecessary to use all five digits. Three digits followed by '00' provide a sufficiently workable system to allow collation of related diagnoses, except in some situations, such as with metastatic tumours, when the fifth digit distinguishes a secondary from a primary tumour. SNOMED codes are most accurate when entered by the reporting pathologist but current anatomical pathology computer programs have provision for automatic SNOMED entries which are highly accurate and expedient.

It is important to document on the final report any discussion which may have been conducted on a given case, and also, all outside opinions should be recorded both in summary and verbatim. Each remark of importance given verbally should be incorporated into the final pathology report. In particular, frozen section diagnoses, if provided, should be incorporated in the microscopic description and followed up with examination of the paraffin section of the material submitted to frozen section. It is important to report all cases in an expedient manner. If avoidable, do not hold back reports because of pending special investigations such as electron microscopy or immunohistochemistry. These can be documented as supplementary reports. It is often possible to provide a preliminary report based on the gross and routine microscopic examination which is sufficiently useful for initiating clinical management, e.g. 'Right cervical node – malignant spindle cell tumour, definitive typing awaiting electron microscopy and immunohistochemistry'.

## Fallibility of histological diagnosis

The term 'tissue diagnosis' is associated with a ring of unquestionable veracity, but, like other diagnostic procedures and clinical disciplines, it has an appreciable measure of fallibility. It has been said that a mystic perversion 'prevails among those clinicians who believe that the pathologist, given only a piece of a patient's tissue, has all of the other ingredients necessary to produce a statement of absolute truth at the end of his report. More dangerous to mankind is a pathologist with the same concept...' (Oscar N. Rambo 1962). Dr Rambo also wrote 'pathologists are physicians and human beings. They have as great a capacity for error and susceptibility

to subjective distractions as other practitioners of the art of medicine.'

Dr Juan Rosai (1989) wisely stated:

recognisation of one's limitations is as great an asset as the sharpest diagnostic eye. There is a chain of command for handling serious and unfamiliar problems. Colleagues immediately available may offer a rapid solution from past experience or from lack of obsessive preconception. The community may be polled. Among the members may be one who has perfect and documented recall of an entity not previously encountered. Such a survey may yield only confusion, but from it one can usually salvage a list of experts with series of entities, ones that may come to the average pathologist only once or twice in his lifetime.

While it is true that world renowned experts are human and fallible and that there is an almost irreducible percentage of undiagnosable tumours, it is every physician's obligation to submit his insoluble problems to the highest court of appeal.

There are many well documented studies examining the diagnostic reproducibility and variability in the interpretation of radiographs, electrocardiographs, clinical assessments as well as histological interpretation of various disorders. For example, in one study of the reproducibility of lung tumour classification, each one of five pathologists was given one section from each of 50 lung tumours which were consecutively numbered. They were asked to describe and interpret the appearances free from the constraints of any particular classification and were told to expect sections from a second set of 50 tumours after they had completed their assessment of the first set. However, they were not told that the second set of slides was simply the first set re-numbered at random. The results analysed for inter-observer and intra-observer variability showed few inconsistencies in the diagnosis of well-differentiated tumours; however, the disagreement rate with poorly differentiated tumours was as high as 40% and intra-observer inconsistency ranged from 2% for the most consistent to 20% for the least consistent. In another study, when the diagnostic consistency of three pathologists was tested by challenging them with 51 liver biopsies, identical diagnoses were reached in only 21 instances and the three pathologists offered a total of three different diagnoses on 13 of the biopsies. Paradoxically, while they agreed on only 27% of the larger wedge biopsies, they were unanimous in their assessment in 52% of the 29 needle biopsies. The reasons for this paradoxical and anomalous result were uncertain. Perhaps theoretically, the larger sample provided a larger quantity of evidence on which to make a judgement, whereas fewer observations could be made on small biopsies which in turn raised fewer diagnostic possibilities. Another similar study found 80% agreement between two experienced histopathologists, but the consensus rate dropped to 56.7% when a trainee was included in the panel.

It is obvious that observer variability and diagnostic fallibility are real problems, and, to date, there have been few attempts to elucidate those factors which cause variations in the interpretation of a single sample by the same observer. Consensus diagnoses among a group of pathologists tend to be more reliable and reproducible than those made by individuals, but this approach is quite impractical for routine use. The increasingly widespread use of newer technologies such as electron microscopy and immunohistochemistry may allow a more objective diagnosis. They provide additional information to help resolve a diagnostic problem but the identification of the problem has still to be made by the pathologist as a first step, and the final step of interpreting the information provided by these new techniques is still subjective. Some have sought a solution in greater objectivity through the application of logic and mathematical analysis but this is contrary to the basis of histopathological examination of a specimen which is a subjective assessment of one or more perceived abnormalities which are then subconsciously compared with a memory store of knowledge and experience. The raw data obtained from the macroscopic and microscopic examination is incredibly complex and it has been suggested that objectivity can be improved by recording specific features according to a set of standardised criteria which then can be analysed statistically with the degree of significance ascribed to each feature. While some experiments along these lines have been performed with computers, the diversity of morphological patterns prohibits universal application so that histopathological diagnosis remains a fallible process.

## Synoptic reporting and checklists

The increasing sophistication of therapeutic options for various diseases is a result of the careful delineation of various histological parameters which have been established to be of prognostic relevance after correlation with the clinical course of the disease. This is particularly so for many types of neoplasms so that the pathologist has the responsibility of not only providing the tissue diagnosis but also information obtained from the pathological examination of specimens which are pertinent to patient care. In oncological surgical pathology, the required items of information are usually numerous and increasing. They include not only histopathological classification of the tumour and the status of the lymph nodes, but often the tumour grade as determined by proven grading criteria, stage, status of margins, size of tumour, depth of invasion, the presence of vascular invasion and other morphological parameters depending on the tumour type and its location. The importance of these parameters cannot be over-emphasised as they are frequently employed in making therapeutic decisions, provide the data on which prognosis is derived and are also used in the evaluation of treatment response. While many biological and molecular parameters are now employed to supplement morphological predictors of outcome, few of these parameters have surpassed the predictive power of morphological variables. The constantly increasing individualisation of therapeutic regimes, and the strict requirements for quality assurance regulations and clinical protocols, have resulted in the need to record an ever increasing amount of information on surgical pathology reports. It is often impossible to remember all these requirements and even more difficult to report them in a consistent and systematic fashion without the aid of checklists. This was clearly shown in a study sponsored by the College of American Pathologists on the adequacy of the surgical pathology report for colorectal carcinoma. The study, conducted among 532 laboratories in the USA and Canada, reported by Dr Richard J. Zarbo (1992), involved a review of 15 940 reports. It showed a wide discrepancy in the frequency of reporting morphological items as obvious as tumour size and degree of differentiation. The Association of Directors of Anatomic and Surgical Pathology of the United States of America recently concluded that a more standardised surgical pathology report may contribute positively to patient care and recommended the use of a checklist

approach for recording information needed for patient treatment and prognosis as well as all information needed to formulate the pathological state of a cancer. The Cancer Committee of the College of American Pathologists has developed protocols for data to be included in routine consultation reports from patients with a variety of carcinomas, including those of the breast, urinary bladder, colon and prostate and in Hodgkin's disease. They emphasised that the protocols are not a mandate, but a guide for pathologists who would like assistance and are meant to serve as a basis for the development of checklists and as outlines for full narrative reporting or a basis for research protocols or as a guide for other types of synoptic or reporting formats. It has also been argued that such synoptic reports are well received by clinicians as they tabulate specific information that documents appropriate examination of the specimen, as well as the anatomical extent of tissue removed, the anatomical extent of carcinoma in the specimen, histological type and other information that may be employed by the clinician to select primary or adjuvant treatment, evaluate new types of therapy, estimate prognosis and analyse outcome. Obviously, additional information not specified by these protocols may be included or the protocol may be modified to suit individual institutional needs.

A major problem in developing such checklists is the selection of morphological features that are proven to be valid predictors of outcome. This is not an inconsequential task because the necessary information is widely scattered in the literature and the validity of this information often depends on statistical analysis. The pathologist is often pressured into examining parameters which have yet to carry proven significance. While such parameters may be part of a research protocol, they should be clearly identified as such. There is little utility in continuing to report morphological parameters that have been proven not to be valid predictors, and new predictors should be added when their utility has been proven. When it becomes clear that parameters which appeared promising in pilot studies are, in fact, not useful predictors, they should be eliminated. Other objections to standardisation of reporting in surgical pathology include arguments that it inhibits thoughtful evaluation of a case, eliminates stylistic preferences and nuances and there is the danger of such forms and checklists becoming an education substitute for reading by trainees.

Because of the large numbers of tumours encountered in surgical pathology practice and because the amount of information required in the pathology report is often extensive, we usually cannot consistently remember all of the information required for each tumour and each tumour site. It is, therefore, helpful to develop checklists containing those parameters that should be evaluated and such lists should be readily available to pathologists and in laboratory manuals and regularly updated. The compulsive use of such checklists and adherence to established criteria when evaluating such parameters will have a major impact on the care of patients with malignant neoplasms.

Synoptic reporting and checklists should be clearly distinguished from pre-formatted reports. Although there is a strong temptation to have simple common specimens and diagnoses such as cholecystitis and appendicitis preformatted, it has been eloquently argued by Dr Bernard M. Wagner in an editorial in *Human Pathology* (1984) that while some specimens may be common or familiar, none is 'routine'. The pathologist conveys his/her opinion as a consultant and a pre-formatted report will not conform to this practice of individualisation but would be a component of an assembly-line practice, 'relegating pathologists as substitutes for computerised slide-readers'.

## The surgical pathologist as an educator and information specialist

Pathology is the basis of medicine and is so even today. A considerable segment of the pathologist's time is spent imparting his/her knowledge to others, not only to fellow clinicians but also to other members of the medical profession, including residents and students, nurses, medical scientists and technologists, and the lay public. Just by discussing his/her cases and explaining diagnoses reached, the pathologist plays a role as a teacher. He/she also has a central role in the dissemination of new information. This role is formally fulfilled through the careful documentation of pathological changes observed in biopsy samples and through thoughtful comments and carefully chosen references provided in the written surgical pathology report. In addition, clinico-pathological conferences provide another venue for the teaching and dissemination of new information to clinicians at all levels of experience as well as to medical students and other paramedical personnel. In addition, pathologists are responsible for the accessioning, maintenance and proper catalogue of all tissue biopsy samples which form an important repository for research. Critical attention to the appropriate means of tissue preservation and tissue storage is extraordinarily important and opportunities are missed if tissue is not retained, improperly preserved, or, even worse, exposed to some of the materials we seek to identify, particularly in the case of environmental, occupational and lifestyle diseases. Besides the diagnosis of cancer, the surgical pathologist is also concerned with the diagnosis and cataloguing of other conditions such as complex congenital anomalies, inflammatory diseases of all types from all locations, problems of skin disease, and the end results of trauma. The versatility of various biopsy instruments has lead to the diagnosis and study of many medical diseases prior to a patient's death, thus saving the lives of many patients who might otherwise have died. Small bits of tissue are now removed from thyroids, lungs, hearts, livers, bone marrows, kidneys, intestines, and from everywhere else in the body for the examination by surgical pathologists.

It is, therefore, important that the pathologist plays an important leadership role in the hospital, particularly with his/her central contributions in various hospital committees such as 'Tissue Committees', 'Tumour Boards', 'Infectious Disease Control' and 'Finance Committees'. In the present climate of burgeoning health costs, the pathologist is in an ideal position to advise on appropriate laboratory tests and the cost-effective use of laboratory facilities.

Pathologists were among the first in the medical profession to use computers for the storage and retrieval of patient data and laboratory results, assist in billing and financial planning, catalogue diseases, assist in research and for storage of information.

Image-intensive disciplines such as surgical pathology are unique in that the intellectual problems posed to the pathologist include image recall and interpretation, a process which is readily apprehended, but poorly understood. The objective criteria which operate during the analytical process of rendering a diagnosis from a histo-

pathology slide often differ from one observer to another. As such, computers have been employed to analyse these processes as well as to aid in the recall of images and the correlation of information that will assist in diagnosis. While the transfer of established and new information traditionally has been through the use of words and diagrams which are spoken, written or projected, the computer can now be used extensively in the communication of verbal and graphic information. Such systems such as the Intellipath (Intellipath, Pasadena, California, USA) have been configured as a pathologist's workstation, consisting of an analogue videodisc and computer expert-system program, designed and produced to allow instantaneous and random accession of text information and up to 3000 video pictures to illustrate the spectrum of disease in a comprehensive database of organised knowledge. Such systems allow information on lesions with similar histological features to be accessed and provide an excellent basis for differential diagnosis and clarification of diagnostic criteria. The text includes discussion of similar histological features, illustrating a wide spectrum for each disease entity and, finally, allows morphological and clinical information to be customised and integrated into a traditional lecture format by the user.

Computers and related electronic technologies have an increasing role in modern day industrial societies and John Naisbitt, in his book *Megatrends*, described the restructuring of America from an industrial society to an information society and outlined the profound implications of this shift for managers and professionals in various industries, including that of health care. He pointed out that the pyramid structure of organisation and management in industry is giving way to a new paradigm, networking. Networks are people talking to each other, sharing ideas, information and resources, and Naisbitt predicted that the new leaders in such an information society will be facilitators, not order givers.

All hospitals, both large and small, have embraced the use of computers and related electronic technologies in patient care, and as the financial management-orientated hospital information systems are replaced by computer systems that provide tools to network health care information among multiple patient databases, information managers are required. Such managers are required to optimise the quality and recovery of health care information generated from diagnostic and clinical services, facilitating the flow of medical information within networks, and, most importantly, extracting value-added information from clinical databases. Such information includes institutional outcomes of the treatment for specific diseases and assessments of the relative effectiveness of individual medical staff members in delivering health care services. This information will be required for purposes of resource allocation and it is becoming apparent that the performance of such medical information managers will have an impact on the level of competitiveness and financial viability of their respective hospitals. Up to now, medical information database managers have been appointed from the ranks of the technocrats and computer experts but the job will require a blending of expertise derived from several different fields, including medicine, computer science and management. The pathologist with his/her central role in the collation and cataloguing of diagnosis and skills in management and financial planning, foundation in the medical sciences and familiarity with computers is the ideal

information specialist. A person with a background in medicine rather than a PhD or MBA is more suited to the role of medical information specialist and many pathologists have more experience with computers and information services than other medical specialists. Furthermore, pathologists appreciate the value of information and the need for information management. Pathologists are already in charge of managing huge amounts of health care information and often are responsible for large departmental budgets. It is for these reasons that the discipline as a whole should have an increasing interest in the area of medical informatics and provide adequate training in this field so that pathologists will play a central role in data management.

The magnitude of growth in the laboratory information system was estimated to be about 800% during the 1980s in the USA, and currently more than 2000 of the 5433 acute care community hospitals in the USA employ laboratory computer systems. This growth can be attributed to the hardware advances of the 1980s which allowed substantial price reductions and faster and easier development. Hospital information systems have lagged behind those of laboratory information systems but the two are evolving on much the same course. The interconnection of all modules will allow the interaction between the laboratory and pharmacy, the laboratory and patient status, and many other areas within health care institutions. Office management, billing and electronic medical record systems can now be created, resulting in a demand for all laboratories to be able to transmit results electronically to physicians' offices, clinics and hospital wards.

The pathologist's workstation which will become common in the future will comprise an extremely powerful personal computer with full graphics capability and a variety of programs to assist with data manipulation, linked to a larger system on which resides a large database of information. Accompanying such a system will be items such as compact disk read only memory (CD ROM), literature search capability, image retrieval, and electronic mail so that pathologists with the appropriate skills will become masters of information.

Literature retrieval is already available on the National Library of Medicine's 'Medline' and programs such as 'Grateful Med' have also become available for microcomputers to assist with the search process.

Linking video-cameras to computers is a simple process and current systems are inexpensive and allow good resolution. In the near future, the routine capture, storage and retrieval of X-ray images will be available and such technology would also allow similar storage of pathology microscopic images. For example, Cell Analysis Systems (CAS) Incorporated markets the CAS200 system, which provides image analysis for DNA analysis, receptor assays, proliferation index, oncogene expression and cell morphology. The system can quantitate specified areas of microscopic image and subject the data to a variety of algorithms. Image transfer is another area of development and telepathology, which emerged during the 1980s, allows microscopic images to be transmitted to distant sites, where they can be reviewed, perhaps by persons with greater expertise.

The bar-code technology came into existence during the 1980s and is now widely used for patient demographic entry and in some analytical instruments. Portable readers, higher quality labels printers and standards for bar-codes have been developed and will permit this technology to be used even more widely.

Audiostorage and voice recognition can be achieved by computers but requires large amounts of memory. Voice recognition has evolved dramatically but still has a 5–20% error rate, depending upon the extent of the vocabulary required. Systems rely on being trained to recognise specific voices, and the speaker must dictate using brief unnatural pauses. Nonetheless, the technology can be used as an alternative to the keyboard and soon should be practical to employ for direct dictation to word processors.

Microprocessors have had an astounding impact on the laboratory equipment industry and today there is hardly a device that does not have a microprocessor built into it. They have allowed miniaturisation and automation of instruments that can be used in the home by patients as well as in the laboratory. They have been responsible for the rapid growth of robotics which, well established in industry, are being introduced to the clinical laboratory. In surgical pathology, they have been adapted for automated immunostainers and cytology screeners.

Computer-aided training decision support systems are another area of major development. Videodiscs allow 54 000 independent pictures to be stored on each side and each picture can be displayed on a television screen in 1 second, or less. The combination of a computer, videodisc, and television monitor and possibly a compact disk reader for text, provides an environment in which entire textbooks and photo collections can be linked in a variety of interactive ways. Systems like the Intellipath combine an artificial intelligence expert system with a videodisc and television monitor to lead the user through a vast spectrum of disorders of each organ system.

Decision analysis uses Bayesian logic to discover the impact of specific choices made in the course of diagnosis and treatment. Fully automated or interactive expert systems which are programs that attempt to emulate the expertise of a specialist in some narrow field are being developed and in the area of cytology, several such systems are available in the form of automated screening programs. While many of these employ an algorithm approach with the necessity for monolayer smears, some use a combination of algorithmic and neural network systems and can directly screen cytological smears without special preparation.

Lastly, computers allow the passage of information from one system to another in a fluid, accurate and rapid fashion. For this, a variety of terminology and transmission standards have been or are being developed with SNOP and later SNOMED and, ICD9 representing examples of standardised terminology. With such standards and terminology in place, the complex task of passing information from one system to another is facilitated and the possibility of an open network of medical information comes closer to reality.

## Surgical pathology report turnaround time

Besides the aim of generating surgical pathology reports which are clear, accurate and informative, there is also the consideration of speed of turnaround. Financial constraints on hospital costs throughout the world impose the need for speed in diagnosis so that the patient's period of hospitalisation is kept to a minimum. The turnaround time for a surgical pathology report is the time between removal of the specimen and the clinician's receipt of the written report. When examining turnaround times in surgical pathology, three areas require consideration – specimen collection, section preparation and reporting, and report delivery. It is interesting that an Audit Commission in the UK, looking into pathology services, 'found that slow turnaround times for specimens and reports were not uncommon, but were rarely the result of slow work in the laboratory. They were usually caused by poor arrangements for collecting specimens or returning results. Often these arrangements were not managed by laboratories themselves but they were invariably blamed when things went wrong' (Audit Commission 1993).

It is beyond the scope of this text to discuss specimen collection and report delivery except to say that there is almost always room for improvement in these areas in any laboratory set-up. In particular, report delivery can be easily improved with the use of facsimile transmissions which are inexpensive. Improvements in laboratory turnaround in tissue preparation and reporting have been brought about by the introduction of several procedures. The advent of microwave fixation, microwave-assisted tissue processing and vacuum-assisted automated processing schedules have resulted in significant reductions in tissue processing times. Reporting of surgical pathology is greatly expedited by use of dictaphones. In teaching institutions, checking out with pathology trainees and residents is an unavoidable step which delays reporting. In many institutions, the introduction of a 'hot seat' pathologist who handles all biopsy specimens for the day contributes to the reduction in turnaround times. This pathologist provides a preliminary report, without description, often in the form of a diagnosis constituting specimen topography and morphology only, and makes requests for deeper levels, additional blocks and special stains as appropriate. Relevant important features such as adequacy of clearance may be included but the formal full descriptive report is made later by a trainee and checked-out accordingly by another pathologist. In this manner, in selected cases, the clinicians can be directly notified as soon as the histological sections are prepared. The telephoning of the diagnosis bypasses any potential delays in the delivery of a formal written descriptive report. While some clinicians find the one-line preliminary diagnosis unsatisfactory, many others feel that it is sufficient for management planning.

It is important for the trainee to appreciate that surgical pathology reporting must be treated with a sense of urgency. While it is easy to be caught up with the many other activities of a pathology laboratory, surgical pathology reporting must be given priority.

## Further reading

Audit Commission 1993 Working with users. In: Critical pathology: an analysis of pathology services. HMSO, London

Henson DE, Hutter RVP, Farrow G 1994 Practice protocol for the examination of specimens removed from patients with carcinoma of the prostate gland. Archives of Pathology and Laboratory Medicine 118: 779–783

Henson DE, Hutter RVP, Sobin LH, Bowman HE 1994 Protocol for the examination of specimens removed from patients with colorectal carcinoma. A basis for checklists. Archives of Pathology and Laboratory Medicine 118: 122–125

Leslie KO, Rosai J 1994 Standardisation of the surgical pathology report: formats, templates and synoptic reporting. Seminars in Diagnostic Pathology 11: 253–257

Morris JA 1994 Information and observer disagreement in histopathology. Histopathology 25: 123–128

Robboy SJ, Bentley RC, Krigman H 1994 Synoptic reports in gynecologic pathology. International Journal of Gynecological Pathology 13: 161–174

Rosai J 1993 Standardised reporting of surgical pathology diagnoses for the major tumour types: a proposal. American Journal of Clinical Pathology 100: 240–255

Schwartz WB, Wolfe HJ, Pauker SG 1981 Pathology and probabilities. A new approach to interpreting and reporting biopsies. New England Journal of Medicine 305: 917–923

# 17 Telephoned reports

The surgical pathologist is, *a priori*, a clinician and, as such, should be prepared to liaise directly with clinical colleagues when the need arises. All too often, the pathologist is seen merely as an interpreter of laboratory tests and as someone who has very little patient contact. One has to admit that, very often, this situation is brought about by the inability or lack of desire on the part of the pathologist to relate to clinical colleagues. The trainee pathologist should interact with clinicians whenever possible. Clinical meetings, clinicopathological conferences and even attendance at ward rounds, when time permits, are invaluable for optimal patient care. Where this proves to be an impracticable approach, the pathologist should not hesitate to talk to the clinician by telephone, and should not be put off by the difficulty sometimes experienced in contacting the appropriate surgeon or physician. Besides using the telephone to obtain additional clinical information or to discuss or explain aspects of the diagnosis, there are a number of situations in which the pathologist will need to telephone his/her report through to the attending clinician.

## Which reports require to be telephoned?

There are a number of situations in which the pathologist will need to initiate the telephoned report. These include diagnoses which have immediate therapeutic implications such as giant cell temporal arteritis, Arias-Stella and decidual change in endometrial curettings which suggest ectopic pregnancy, and certain unexpected findings such as the presence of adipose tissue in a curettage specimen raising the possibility of uterine perforation. For

medico-legal purposes, it is wise to record the time and date of the telephoned report on the final typed report. Whilst it is not always practicable to telephone every unexpected result, there are certain situations where it may be prudent so to do, e.g. the findings of unexpected malignancy, or where there is a marked discrepancy between the clinical diagnosis and the pathological diagnosis which necessitates different clinical management such as the findings of tuberculoid granulomas in clinically suspected peritoneal carcinomatosis. The decision to phone such reports requires more than a passing knowledge of clinical medicine, but if there is any doubt, it is better to telephone through the report.

The other main situation requiring a preliminary telephoned report is when a delay is envisaged in the issuing of the final report. This may be due to an intervening weekend or public holiday, or the need to perform special stains or techniques such as immunohistochemistry or electron microscopy. With the latter situation, it is preferable to issue a typed preliminary report followed by a supplementary report when the additional investigations become available. It is often possible to provide a limited diagnosis based on the gross and microscopic findings on H & E sections. Such a preliminary diagnosis is sufficient to formulate a clinical management strategy so that treatment is not delayed. If appropriate, it is also useful to speak to the attending clinician, explaining the reason for the preliminary report. This contact will also provide the opportunity of obtaining more clinical information which may be helpful in elucidating the diagnosis. In such circumstances, there is often a great deal of pressure on the trainee to provide a definitive diagnosis and this must be resisted. State the differential diagnoses and explain the reasons for the special investigations being undertaken but do not commit to a definite diagnosis.

## Telephoned reports initiated by the clinician

Obviously, the pathologist has no control over the selection of reports to be telephoned when they are initiated by the clinician. Such cases are usually identified through specific instructions on the accompanying request form or by a direct telephoned request. Such requests may have management implications, e.g. organisation of operation lists or arrangement of patient's discharge. Often the request is generated by the need to make bed management decisions or to allay the patient's anxiety. These, too, are valid reasons for an urgent telephoned report with which the pathologist should comply.

While it is ideal that the pathologist speaks directly to the attending clinician, this may not always be possible. If the report is straightforward, it can be left with the receptionist or secretarial staff or any other individual nominated by the clinician. Whenever possible, limit telephoned reports to the diagnosis only, keeping it concise and simple. In the case of non-medical staff receiving the report, always ask that the report be read back to you.

In all circumstances, note the name and station of the recipient and the time and date of reporting, preferably on the laboratory's copy of the report.

The laboratory may be called up for biopsy reports. This seemingly simple request can be fraught with controversy concerning patient confidentiality, as it may be difficult to verify the identity of the caller over the telephone. However, with familiarity, laboratory reception staff may be able to screen out unauthorised callers. In reports read out by non-medical personnel, it is important that they are kept brief and simple, limited only to the diagnosis if possible. The diagnosis should be spelt out in full and a record made of the time, date of reporting and the name and station of the recipient.

Only pathologist-validated reports can be read over the telephone and facsimile transmissions of such reports should be encouraged.

In all circumstances, the reporting pathologist should be accessible for discussions with the clinician.

# 18 Seeking a second opinion

All pathologists will, on occasion, require the input of another colleague's opinion although the reasons for consultation are varied. Assuming the consultation is not used to abdicate responsibility, the second opinion is a cornerstone of quality assurance and a method of improving the pathologist's database and patient care.

Second opinions or 'consultations' should be distinguished from 'reviews'. In the former, a diagnosis or opinion is sought on a difficult case, whereas in the latter situation, pathological material accompanies the patient transferred to another institution for further evaluation and/or treatment.

Although consultation in pathology generally entails the transfer of slides and/or paraffin blocks, it also applies to all other aspects of the specimen including the macroscopic examination. The macroscopic findings, particularly those of larger and more complex specimens, are often vital to the final opinion generated. It is unfortunate that trainee pathologists in particular, who are quite at ease asking for an opinion on a slide, feel constrained to follow this course of action with difficult macroscopic specimens. In some institutions this is fostered by the delegation of cut-up duties to trainees who come to believe macroscopic examination is not particularly important. This is regrettable, as in many instances difficulties in slide interpretation are a direct result of failure to appreciate complexities at the time of gross examination and cut-up. With declining autopsy rates limiting the exposure of trainees to macroscopic specimens, these problems have the potential to increase.

## Reasons for referral

The permanent nature of microscopic slides and paraffin blocks, and their ready trans-portability, makes consultation in pathology easier than many other specialities in medicine. This ability to review material at different periods in time or refer to other pathologists for opinions should be regarded as an advantage to our profession, although for some it represents an execration.

The Association of Directors of Anatomic and Surgical Pathology in the USA (1993) recently listed the following reasons for pathological consultation:

1  Uncertainty of the referring pathologist about the diagnosis.
2  An internal disagreement between two or more pathologists in a practice group about the diagnosis.
3  The patient's request for a second opinion.
4  A clinician's request for a second opinion.
5  Quality assurance documentation.
6  Transfer of the patient to a different institution, with a need for diagnosis by a pathologist at the new institution.

## Intradepartmental consultations

The majority of pathological consultations occur between pathologists, and in a review of 300 cases in which second opinions were sought, 226 were of this type. Less commonly, consultations are received from clinicians, patients, patient's families and other sources, including lawyers, scientists and veterinary surgeons. In large departments, it is possible to obtain a second opinion from colleagues but in a small department consultation usually means either a visit to colleagues at another centre, or sending the material away to someone at a distance.

Intradepartmental consultations are common, particularly in departments with trainees. In most instances, the opinion of a colleague whose judgement is trusted and/or who is acknowledged to have expertise or a special interest in the area of difficulty is sought. The opinion provided may be verbal or written. Histopathologists are one of the few true generalists in medical practice, and no individual pathologist can keep abreast of all the developments in a specialty with an exponential knowledge growth curve. Even if the slides are shown only for confirmation of a favoured diagnosis, the nod of reassurance from a more experienced colleague is helpful towards the expansion of ones own database of experience and knowledge. It clearly also performs a role in quality assurance and patient care as intradepartmental uniformity in diagnostic criteria and classification ensues. However, consultation should not be a substitute for a thorough work-up of the case, otherwise many of the aforementioned benefits will not be attained.

There is no magic formula to determine the number of opinions which should be sought for a given case although, undoubtedly, the number will increase if there are major difficulties with categorisation of the lesion, or if the first opinion rendered is opposed to the favoured diagnosis of the accessioning pathologist, or there are special circumstances such as potential litigation. With the use of independent techniques to confirm a histological diagnosis, such as electron microscopy and immunohistochemistry, the frequency of consultations may decrease. The interpretation of these ancillary techniques, however, is in itself a common reason for consultation.

Certain areas of pathology such as melanocytic lesions and lymphomas can be a frequent cause of diagnostic difficulty. As there are associated major therapeutic and prognostic implications, it is sound practice to have diagnoses of malignant melanoma and lymphoma confirmed by another pathologist. Indeed, a recent study suggested that all surgical pathology cases requiring microscopic sections be routinely reviewed by a second pathologist. This procedure added US$7 to the cost of each case and picked up 14 discrepancies of potential clinical significance in a study of 5397 cases (0.26% error rate).

Not wishing to take up too much time of the departmental 'expert', there is a tendency to 'flash' one H & E slide with the expectation of an accurate consultation. Quality opinions can only be given when all representative material, including the clinical history and macroscopic findings, are available and an impression imparted on the examination of one slide can be misleading. This is not to say the entire tray of slides with multiple levels and special stains, electron micrographs, macroscopic photographs and patient case notes should be dumped on the desk of the consultant for opinion in every case, although in more difficult cases this may well be appropriate. The judgement on what to show clearly improves with experience and confidence, but the trainee should always err on the side of excess. It is important to bear in mind that opinions, at least intradepartmental, are provided largely as a professional courtesy.

Judgement is required on what to do with a verbal opinion. The verbal opinion may be adequate for the reporting pathologist to sign-out the case without mentioning the source of the opinion. On the other hand, the opinion may be formally recorded as a single line 'case shown to Dr "x" who concurs with the diagnosis' or the report may be countersigned by the expert. It is essential that in the former circumstance, the report, even though not bearing the expert's signature, is sighted and approved by the consulted pathologist before it is released.

## Interdepartmental consultations

The pathologist sending a case for consultation has obligations to both the expert whose opinion is sought and the patient. The opinion sought should be assumed to carry medico-legal implications and, as such, the expert has the right to refuse to provide an opinion if he or she believes there are no clear patient benefits to be obtained. It is important to note that in some countries such as the USA, consultants may be found negligent if they make errors judged to be below the standard of care for consultants. More importantly, the referring pathologist may assume liability for a consultant's error under the legal doctrine of vicarious liability. This means that you can be held responsible for choosing a negligent consultant.

The outcome of the consultation process is largely dependent on the provision of appropriately fixed and processed *representative* tissue for analysis. Adequate sampling and fixation depends largely on the clinician who takes the biopsy, although in special cases, discussion between pathologist and clinician will determine the optimum methods of tissue handling, viz. fresh, formalin, Bouin's or gluteraldehyde, and can have a tremendous bearing on the likelihood of a definitive diagnostic outcome.

A referral letter should be included with the pathological material and it should contain basic demographic data on the patient for identification and to enable billing which is becoming more frequent with consultation cases. There is usually no charge if the material submitted is for research. The transmittal letter should include the relevant clinical data, specimen gross description, source of biopsy and nature of surgery performed. The reason for seeking the consultation should be stated as should any specific problems that need to be addressed. Some pathologists do not state their diagnosis or diagnoses, one suspects largely out of ego preservation, although the concept of introducing bias is often rationalised. We feel that the proffered diagnosis should be clearly stated as it enables the expert to write a more informative reply, its omission amounting to the withholding of information. A common approach to a consultation case is to assess the slide first and then to formulate a viewpoint based on consideration of the clinical data and the macroscopic description provided. Although time constraints may truncate this approach, many consultants adopt such a sequence in generating an opinion. There is no place for the omission of clinical data to offset perceived bias in the seeking of a second opinion. While some referring pathologists do not include a copy of the original surgical pathology report with the transmittal letter, for reasons already mentioned, we feel that it is a worthwhile addition. Previous reports, if relevant to the problem at hand, should also be enclosed.

The material submitted for second opinion must include all the information and tissue that is required to resolve the diagnostic problem. Generally this will comprise duplicate H & E stained slides. Original diagnostic tissue sections should not be sent unless it is unavoidable because the area of difficulty is not represented in recuts or in the case of cytology preparations. Material anticipated to require extra investigations such as special stains and immunohistochemistry, should be submitted as either additional unstained sections or paraffin blocks. Radiological information, particularly in the examination of bone neoplasms, may be needed, macroscopic photographs can be included when necessary, and for poorly differentiated neoplasms, electron micrographs, flow cytometric data and frozen tissue may be required. It is the practice of some pathologists to routinely send unstained sections so that the consulted pathologist can stain the sections in his laboratory to obviate problems imposed by idiosyncrasies of local stains. Previous pathology specimens need inclusion if deemed relevant and it may be advantageous to identify the area of interest to ensure that the consultant addresses the specific problem which should also be clearly stated in the transmittal letter. Duplicate slides must be checked to ensure technical quality and confirm the presence of lesional tissue.

All material needs to be packaged so as to minimise the chance of breakage. Duplicate slide copies may be retained by the consultant whose opinion is sought but all original material must be returned and this needs to be specified in the referral letter. We do not recommend sending immunohistochemical stains. These are originals and they are best interpreted by a pathologist familiar with the staining procedures of the laboratory, the controls, antibody panels and reagents employed. If immunostains are necessary, it is best to send unstained sections or the relevant paraffin block.

In urgent cases, it is appropriate for the referring pathologist to request a quick response but common courtesy in these situations necessitates a forewarning telephone call or fax to notify the recipient pathologist. Express mail services should be utilised and the telephone/fax number of the referring pathologist should be available. It would also be courteous to state if the case has or is being referred for other outside opinions. The Association of Directors of Anatomic and Surgical Pathology (1993) has recommended that a preliminary second opinion should be provided within one week of receipt as a reasonable turnaround time.

Whose and how many opinions should be sought are entirely matters of personal choice. Mostly, opinions are sought from individuals generally accepted to have expertise in the field and usually known to provide good opinions and promptly. Often, they are recommended by senior members of the department who have used such individuals before. It may be necessary, in some cases, to seek the opinion of more than one such expert, and rarely, because of the controversial nature of the diagnoses obtained, a third opinion may be sought.

## Institutional reviews

Pathology departments serving tertiary referral hospitals are often required to review biopsy material from patients transferred for further evaluation or treatment. The review serves a number of important functions:

1   Confirms the diagnosis before definitive treatment is instituted.
2   Allows the documentation of baseline pathology in the patient prior to commencement of therapy.
3   Serves an important role in quality assurance and pathologist education.

Slides for review in such situations are generated in the following manner:

1   The slides are sent directly to a specific pathologist or the department by the former attending clinician.
2   Slides are transferred with the patient's case notes and other clinical records.
3   The slides are sent in by the pathologist who made the initial examination at the request of the former attending clinician.
4   At the request of the attending clinician, the reviewing pathologist requests for appropriate slides from the pathologist who made the initial examination.

In the latter situation, it is proper that a copy of the reviewing pathologist's report be sent to the original pathologist. In the other situations, it would be courteous that the reviewer's report be sent to the accessioning pathologist if his/her name and address are available. In all the situations, the report must be available to the attending clinician, the patient's case notes and other relevant clinics.

## Tumour registries

A variant of the interdepartmental consultation is provided by tumour registries and consultative panels. Such registries and panels are set-up for a variety of reasons, including the collection of epidemiological data, pooling of uncommon pathological material for research and teaching, and standardisation of diagnosis and treatment. They offer the referring pathologist multiple opinions from a body of expert pathologists. Although some of these panels have proforma sheets for submission, others can be consulted in much the same way as described previously. However, more unstained sections or the paraffin block needs to be sent. Some of the registries provide individual written views

of the members of the panel whilst others formulate a consensus view.

## What to do with an expert opinion

An opinion from an expert pathologist is just that, a viewpoint of the diagnosis by an accepted expert in a specific field. Although the opinion should be regarded as having considerable credibility it cannot be regarded as fact in all cases. The referring pathologist may be held liable for the consultant's error so that the former ultimately has the responsibility for the final diagnosis.

The preliminary report by the accessioning pathologist should document that further opinions are being sought and when these become available they should be encompassed in a supplementary report. It is best to include the entire report of the expert to avoid any interpretative bias, with an appropriate comment by the accessioning pathologist. The consulted expert should not send a report directly to the attending clinician especially if the consultation was initiated by the pathologist. There are other issues of protocol and etiquette in the consultation and referral process that are likely to have local or regional differences. The College of American Pathologist's Professional Relations Manual (1993) addresses many of these issues.

## Medico-legal consultations

It is very unlikely that a trainee is involved in seeking an expert's opinion for a case involved in litigation. In the unfortunate event that this situation arises, the trainee should seek professional legal advice.

# Consultations of the future

Thus far, this chapter has addressed the typical intra- and interdepartmental consultation with transfer of pathological material generally taking place via the mail. Already operating, particularly in the more remote regions of Scandinavia, is telepathology which is technology utilising the telephone to transfer digitalised video images of pathological specimens including histology and cytology. The transfer of one image takes approximately 2 minutes by use of ordinary telephone lines and this can be compressed to 12–15 seconds by use of the digitalised telephone network. While its use for frozen section consultations is controversial, telepathology has a more established role in cytology consultations, including providing second opinions from video images. At present, the major drawbacks of this technology include the inability, in most cases, to scan the slides, and the images transmitted are generally too few in number due to the time lag, making this technology unsuitable for difficult cases. Image resolution is limited by the spatial resolution of the TV cameras and is thus useful only for medium or high microscopic magnifications. Since the quality of the video television image is generally inferior to the direct microscopic image there is increased risk of misdiagnosis, however, this will be influenced by experience with video image interpretation. The legal issues related to diagnosis made on transmitted images are currently unclear, but there is little doubt that the pathologist of the future will be expected to make diagnoses on transmitted images.

# Further reading

Association of Directors of Anatomic and Surgical Pathology 1993 Consultations in surgical pathology. American Journal of Surgical Pathology 17: 743–745

College of American Pathologists Professional Affairs Committee 1993 Professional relations manual, 10th edn. College of American Pathologists, Northfield, pp 5–9

Safrin RE, Bark CJ 1993 Surgical pathology signout. Routine review of every case by a second pathologist. American Journal of Surgical Pathology 17: 1190–1192

# 19 Clinico-pathological conferences and clinical audits

# Introduction

The surgical pathologist is a physician and a medical specialist. While his/her immediate function is the diagnosis of disease through the examination of tissue samples and organs, he/she also has an integral role in the management of the patient's disease. 'Pathology' is the study of diseases and although the practice of medicine today has evolved much further than the two basic disciplines of pathology and therapeutics, the surgical pathologist still retains a major responsibility to ensure that as a result of his/her pathological diagnosis, the appropriate management is imparted to the patient. This is done formally through the written report as well as through oral communication with the attending clinicians and discussions at clinico-pathological conferences.

# The clinico-pathological conference

The clinico-pathological conference is one of the major areas of contact between pathologist and clinician and is a long-established and widely accepted part of medical practice. These conferences provide an opportunity for discussing the management and outcome of difficult or interesting cases and act as a forum for sharing knowledge among peers. By these means, the clinico-pathological conference helps to elevate standards of clinical practice and thereby improve the quality of patient care. A recent formal analysis of this review process at the Southampton University Hospitals showed that histological review resulted in an altered diagnosis in 9% of cases, a refined diagnosis in 10% of cases and no diagnostic change in 81%. Over 88% of the diagnostic changes were attributable to the specialist expertise of the reviewing pathologist, and only 4.8% resulted from additional information provided by the clinicians. The amended diagnoses led to major management changes in 3.8%, minor management changes in 2.9% and no change in 93.3%. These findings provided strong support for the long-held contention that clinico-pathological meetings contribute to and improve the clinical management of the patient.

Clinico-pathological conferences may take the form of a meeting with specialised clinical units such as breast, dermatology, ear, nose and throat, oral surgery, gastroenterology, general surgery, urology, nephrology and oncology, or may be hospital Grand Rounds or autopsy demonstrations. In the specialist unit meetings, the pathologist in attendance usually has a special interest in the subspeciality, whereas autopsy demonstrations and hospital Grand Rounds may have input from more junior members such as the trainee pathologist.

At such meetings, the clinicians provide a history for each case, the pathology is reviewed and presented by the pathologist, and the diagnosis and management implications are discussed. These meetings also allow the opportunity of including a more formal audit component which, with a minimum of extra effort and time, would allow assessment of both the diagnostic changes resulting from the pathological review and the effect of these changes on clinical management. While this form of internal audit concentrates largely on diagnostic accuracy, other parameters including turnaround times may also be evaluated. Such conferences, particularly in oncology, provide a mechanism for reaching a consensus on treatment through the empirical process of testing our opinions against one another and by facts.

With the presentation of all views from attending specialists representative of different disciplines, convergence of opinion becomes the accepted course of action.

There are many reasons for participating in tumour conferences. They provide opportunities for pathologists to be in the forefront of cancer education and to be leaders in the field. Pathologists ensure impartiality by serving as arbitrators among surgeons, radiotherapists and medical oncologists, especially in dealing with complex cases. Such clinico-pathological conferences enhance professional ties, foster inter-personal co-operation amongst the medical staff, and furnish a forum for discussion of common problems. They are a visible means for pathologists to affirm their role as educators and also provide a method of continuing medical education as it allows the pathologist to highlight advances in the understanding of the disease and explain the relevance of newer methods and technologies of diagnosis. As neutral participants, pathologists can bring a balance to the conferences, highlighting areas that are often neglected such as staging, literature review, use of tumour registry data, early detection, rehabilitation, tumour classification and even prevention. Scientific interest and even areas of research can be explored through these organ or site-orientated subspeciality conferences.

The attendance at these meeting by outside consultants who provide additional expertise, fosters ties between community hospitals and larger medical centres. They provide a continuing dialogue for review of management principles, methods of follow-up and patient outcome. They are, therefore, an excellent problem-orientated learning resource for students, interns and residents in training. Such meetings allow opportunities to review the process of decision making in medicine, evaluate various approaches to medical education, and improve communication skills. There is no question, to our view, that clinico-pathological conferences fortify knowledge, confirm experience and deepen our sympathy for the human condition.

Attendance at such meetings, whenever the opportunity arises, is an excellent forum for learning for the trainee surgical pathologist. When the opportunity to participate in such meetings presents itself, the trainee should not consider it an onerous task but should view it as an opportunity to fulfil a major part of his/her responsibility and role as a surgical pathologist. It represents an opportunity to participate in patient management as well as to educate fellow clinicians. Teaching is of great benefit to the teacher because the subject must be arranged in his/her own mind so as to be of value to the audience. In doing this, the teacher must first know or learn the subject, and even if he/she thinks he/she knows, gaps in the knowledge will be found that will have to be looked up and clarified. By this process, the teacher's knowledge, insight into and understanding of the subject is, therefore, modified and he/she becomes educated. This happens at even the apparently simplest levels, and, indeed, may be more obvious at simple levels. All types of formal teaching require careful thought and organisation as a mass of facts is considered for the basis of a lesson or talk, and principles have to emerge to make the facts comprehensible to the understanding of the audience. These principles may be new to the teacher, who may not have seen his/her facts in that light before. The facts then become more vivid for the teacher than the learners, because he/she has thought them out for him/herself. Teaching is, therefore, one of the best forms of continuing education.

## Participation at clinico-pathological meetings

The level of technology for visual aids in different institutions will vary but most institutions will have available a microscope with attached television camera linked to a monitor which allows adequate demonstration of microscopic features. Such equipment requires provision of a dedicated seminar room; alternatively, a portable system may be used as it can be moved from room to room. The older direct projection systems often do not provide a sufficiently strong light source for the projection of high magnification views and are cumbersome, so they are now becoming obsolete. When a microscope set-up is not available, the microscopic features of a pathological lesion can be recorded onto a video tape and played back in a video cassette recorder which will be available in most institutions. Macroscopic features can also be recorded and viewed in a similar manner without the necessity of transporting wet specimens. Otherwise, macroscopic images can be viewed on television monitors directly transmitted through video cameras. The use of a microscope and television camera is best suited to a smaller room and smaller audience as adjustments of the microscope and objectives take some time. Video monitors have smaller images than large projection screens, although newer systems also allow the projection of microscope-camera images on to large screen.

The transportation of wet specimens should be done with due consideration to health and safety requirements. Formalin-fixed tissues should not be demonstrated in areas without adequate ventilation facilities unless they are contained in sealed plastic bags. Some specimens, such as necrotic bowel, lose their macroscopic definition

after fixation and are less than ideal for demonstration purposes. In these circumstances, photographs of the fresh specimen projected as slide transparencies would be the best method of demonstration. Similarly, at hospital Grand Rounds, it may be necessary to use projected transparencies to demonstrate the microscopic features as the use of a microscope and television camera is best suited to a smaller room and smaller audience. More formal lectures and presentations are best done using photographic transparencies. Newer electronic technology allows the incorporation and storage of such images together with other scripts and data in a computer disk, to be used with a lap-top computer connected to a video display system or projected onto a large screen for presentation.

### Projection slides

Presentation at meetings is greatly enhanced by the use of overhead projection facilities or photographic transparencies. It is possible, with some thought and planning, to present your information effectively. Even with short notice, neatly typed overhead projection is far more effective than hastily handwritten notes. Such material can be simply made by photocopying typed text and tables onto acetate sheets and colour can be added by passing special acetate sheets through a colour printer. With the ready availability of computerised graphic programs such as PowerPoint (Microsoft) or Aldus Persuasion, attractive overhead transparencies or projection slides can be made, rendering the older dia-diract and diazo techniques obsolete. These software programs are extremely versatile and allow the selection of different colour schemes and patterns for text and background as desired. Standard templates are available in these programs and the colours can be separately selected. Projection transparencies can be produced directly from the computerised software without the need for producing hard copies. The equipment also allows the production of hard copies which can be used as handouts.

With planning, both macroscopic and microscopic images can also be incorporated into these slides and facilities now exist which allow a macroscopic or microscopic image to be stored in the computer and incorporated as desired into a presentation slide. Diagrams and pictures can also be incorporated from other printed sources by using a flat-bed scanner to scan and store the images in a similar way. These images from the computer program can be fed directly into a photographic projection carousel system and, when combined with a lap-top computer, obviates the need for slide projection.

In the preparation of text slides, it is important to give consideration to its contents. Remember, the slides do not stand alone and will be fully elaborated upon by the presenter. Slides are used as prompts for the presenter and they enhance the presentation by allowing the audience to visually focus on the subject or point being discussed. As such, it is important to use bold heading and phrases, avoiding complete formal sentences. It is also important to remember that all too often, far too much information is presented on one slide, making it very difficult to read and comprehend in the relatively short period of time that it is projected. As a guide, no more than nine lines should be placed in any one slide. Complex graphs and tables should be avoided where possible and if they are used, it should be clear that they are only a guide for the presenter and not to be read in detail by the audience. Colour schemes and combi-nations should be carefully selected and the temptation of employing multiple vivid and startling colours should be avoided as they not only distract but can be difficult to read because of poor contrast between fonts and background. Many software programs have standard templates with tested colour combinations and text fonts.

## The art of presentation

With careful thought and practice, it is possible to become a good and effective presenter. The following pointers may be useful.

### Know your audience

Your level of presentation should be geared to the audience and pitched at the average level of knowledge and understanding of the audience. This is especially important when the audience is a mixed group with a wide range of interests and expertise.

It is important to appreciate that an audience of clinicians would have less interest and be less appreciative of detailed descriptions of microscopic features. As such, the number of photomicrographs and electron micrographs should be restricted when speaking to such a group. Use only microscopic illustrations which are essential for the diagnosis or contribute to clinico-pathological correlation. Clinical audiences are more interested in clinico-pathological correlation and prognostication. Much of these features can be illustrated by gross photographs of the specimen to which clinicians are able to relate. With photomi-crographs, it is often useful to clearly identify the tissue and even to point out normal structures to provide a comparison of the microscopic appearances. Line drawings with labels of important land-marks can enhance your presentation.

Always orientate your audience to the photograph, whether it be of gross or microscopic features. With the latter, it can be helpful if a low power photomicrograph be shown first to allow orientation of the pathological changes. High power microscopy is often less useful for the understanding of clinicians with no special interest in the pathology.

## Know your equipment

Before your presentation, familiarise yourself with the equipment you will be using. Know which buttons to press to work the projector – forward, backward and focus.

Know how to turn the microphone on and off, and ensure that it is on before you speak. Microphones fixed to the lectern pick-up extraneous noises transmitted along the surface of the lectern, e.g. from knocking the lectern or placing pointers and glasses with drinking water on the lectern. These microphones are often directional and will only be effective when you speak directly into the microphone. Radiomicrophones carried on the speaker may give rise to interference noise and pick-up and amplify the rustling of clothing and the rattling of necklaces and other ornaments adorning the speaker. Electrical interference can also be very off-putting.

Be familiar with the pointer. Use the pointer on the screen to demonstrate the particular point and turn it off when not in use. Avoid pointing at the audience or having a flickering light roam around the auditorium, both are distressing and distracting to the audience.

Before handing over your slides to the projectionist, ensure that they are clearly marked for sequence as well as for placement into the carousel. Preferably load the carousel yourself and label it with your name, time and venue of presentation.

## Presentation

Good presentation depends on speech delivery as well as audio-visual aids. Endeavour to address the audience rather than the projection screen. Speak slowly, clearly and precisely. Do not mumble or talk too quickly. If you feel that your pronunciation of specific words may not be understood or if the point is too complex, do not hesitate to re-express it in a simpler form. Initially, notes or prompt cards may be required, but it is easy to learn to speak without these aids, using the projected slides of text and morphological images as prompts. Like dictating, avoid extraneous noises and non-contributory sounds such as 'ums' and 'ahs'. Do not fidget or walk around as this can be very distracting. Much may be learnt from listening to oneself on a tape recorder.

It is a useful practice to start your presentation by identifying the problem which you intend to address and to conclude with a very short summary of what you have said. If possible, provide the audience with a 'take home message'. Importantly, pace yourself and keep to the allocated time.

Mastering the art of effective presentation is a very important aspect of a pathologist's training as it allows him/her to fulfil an important component of his/her role, namely that of a teacher and educator, as well as being an integral member of the patient's clinical management team. Effective presentation reinforces and enhances the image of the surgical pathologist and allows a visible means of reaffirming his/her central role in patient management.

## Clinical audits

In addition to pathology audits which form part of peer review and quality assurance programmes, pathologists are also required to participate in clinical audits. This may be part of routine clinical meetings or such audits may fall under the sphere of hospital peer review committees. They may be used to monitor patient management, therapy and follow-up, as well as to assess appropriateness of investigative and biopsy procedures. The role of the surgical pathologist as a neutral and unbiased member of the team allows him/her to contribute to the maintenance of the highest standard of practice and medical care.

# 20 Reference sources

# Introduction

Textbooks and journals are indispensable sources of information for the surgical pathologist. These are numerous and the trainee, with time, will become acquainted with them and will discern which are the most useful for his/her requirements. The choice is a matter of preference, some books being more readable than others while some are better illustrated and serve well as benchtop manuals. This chapter lists a selection of textbooks and journals, some with a brief description of their contents. The list is not intended to be comprehensive.

# Textbooks

## General and systemic pathology

A number of pathology textbooks cover both general and systemic pathology. In most, the opening chapters deal with basic disease processes and mechanisms and contain descriptions of pathology in the separate organ systems. The same books may be used at undergraduate level but they often provide a basis of sound training in anatomical pathology. The most popular of these include:

1   *Muir's Textbook of Pathology*, 13th edition. RNM MacSween & K Whaley (eds). London: Edward Arnold, 1992.
2   *Oxford Textbook of Pathology*. JO'D McGee, PG Isaacson & NA Wright (eds). Oxford: Oxford University Press, 1992.
3   *Robbins' Pathologic Basis of Disease*, 5th edition. RS Cotran, V Kumar & SL Robbins. Philadelphia: WB Saunders, 1994.

## Anatomy and histology

1   *Histology for Pathologists*. SS Sternberg (ed). New York: Raven Press, 1992.

Many trainees starting out in surgical pathology require revision of their knowledge of normal histology. This is an excellent text which places histology in the context of function and pathology.

## Special techniques

### Histotechnology

1   *Theory and Practice of Histological Techniques*, 4th edition. JD Bancroft & A Stevens (eds). Edinburgh: Churchill Livingstone, 1996.

This book is regarded as one of the most comprehensive texts by histotechnologists. While it is not entirely necessary for the trainee to know all the details of staining techniques, an understanding of the principles is essential.

2   *Principles and Practice of Medical Laboratory Science: Basic Histotechnology*. AS-Y Leong. London: Churchill Livingstone, 1996.

This book provides a perspective of the role of the laboratory scientist in the surgical pathology laboratory. It also provides a superficial but comprehensive coverage of the principles and laboratory methods including tissue processing and staining. Both aspects are useful to the trainee pathologist in his/her interaction with technicians and scientists.

3   *AFIP: Laboratory Methods in Histotechnology*. EB Prophet, B Mills, JB Arrington & LH Sobin (eds). Washington DC: American Registry of Pathology, 1992.

## Immunohistochemistry

1  *Applied Immunohistochemistry for the Surgical Pathologist.* AS-Y Leong (ed). London: Edward Arnold, 1993.

This volume provides the background and theory of immunohistochemistry and describes its application in surgical pathology. It is concise and may be used as a text or a reference book. With the multitude of antibodies now available, this book acquaints the trainee with the necessary panels for the diagnosis of various tumours and non-neoplastic disorders.

2  *Immunohistochemistry and Electron Microscopy of Poorly Differentiated and Pleomorphic Tumours.* AS-Y Leong, MR Wick & PE Swanson. New York: Cambridge University Press (to be published in 1996).

This book should be very useful to the surgical pathologist who is frequently confronted with tumours from a variety of anatomical sites which cannot be accurately categorised by the examination of H & E stained sections and require the adjunctive investigations of immunohistochemistry and ultrastructural examination. It presents a practical approach to the diagnostic problem and is amply illustrated with case studies.

## Electron microscopy

1  *Diagnostic Transmission Electron Microscopy of Tumors.* RA Erlandson. New York: Raven Press, 1994.
2  *Ultrastructural Appearances of Tumours*, 2nd edition. DW Henderson, JM Papadimitrou & M Coleman (eds). Edinburgh: Churchill Livingstone, 1986.

3  *Diagnostic Ultrastructure of Non-neoplastic Disease.* JM Papadimitrou, DW Henderson & DV Spagnolo (eds). Edinburgh: Churchill Livingstone, 1992.

## Surgical pathology

1  *Ackerman's Surgical Pathology*, 8th edition. J Rosai. St Louis: Mosby, 1995.

This textbook has become a classic in surgical pathology throughout the world and is a must for trainee pathologists. The latest edition includes chapters on molecular diagnosis in pathology, transplantation pathology, infectious diseases including AIDS, and principles of oncologic practice. Immunohistochemistry has been integrated throughout the book and there is also coverage of flow cytometry with updates on newer monoclonal antibodies and hormone receptors. Computerisation in pathology is also addressed.

2  *Diagnostic Surgical Pathology*, 2nd edition. SS Sternberg. New York: Raven Press, 1994.

This textbook, in two volumes, offers an alternative and is a good benchtop manual for surgical pathologists. It is more difficult to read as there are multiple contributors with their attendant deficiencies and strengths.

## Specialised textbooks

### Bone and joint pathology

1  *Bone Tumors.* JM Mirra (ed). Philadelphia: Lea and Febiger, 1989.
2  *Radiologic and Histologic Pathology of Non-Tumorous Diseases of Bones*

*and Joints*. JW Milgram. Hong Kong: Northbrooke Co Inc, 1990.

Both these books are reference texts.

## Breast pathology

1   *Diagnostic Histopathology of the Breast.* DL Page & TJ Anderson. Edinburgh: Churchill Livingstone, 1987.

This text is now a little dated but is well written and is currently the best text on pre-neoplastic proliferations of ductal epithelium.

2   *Pathology of the Breast.* FA Tavassoli. Connecticut: Appleton and Lange, 1992.

## Cardiovascular pathology

1   *Cardiovascular Pathology*, 2nd edition. MD Silver (ed). Edinburgh: Churchill Livingstone, 1991.

This is a comprehensive reference manual for all aspects of cardiovascular pathology. There are some very good chapters on endomyocardial biopsy interpretation, although much of the content necessarily relates to autopsy pathology and may not be immediately applicable to surgical pathology.

## Cytopathology

1   *Atlas of Diagnostic Cytopathology.* BF Atkinson. Philadelphia: WB Saunders, 1992.

This is an atlas and will complement a textbook of exfoliative cytology.

2   *Comprehensive Cytopathology.* M Bibbo (ed). Philadelphia: WB Saunders, 1991.

This is a large comprehensive textbook of cytopathology and is best used as a reference text.

3   *Manual and Atlas of Fine Needle Aspiration Cytology*, 2nd edition. SR Orell, GF Sterrett, MN-I Walters & DW Whitaker. Edinburgh: Churchill Livingstone, 1992.

## Dermatopathology

1   *Histopathology of the Skin*, 7th edition. WF Lever & G Schaumburg-Lever. Philadelphia: JB Lippincott, 1990.

This is a classic text in dermatopathology. Although many other new textbooks are now available, this remains a very useful and readable text.

2   *Pinkus' Guide to Dermatopathology*, 5th edition. AH Mehregan & K Hashimoto. Connecticut: Prentice-Hall, 1991.

3   *Histologic Diagnosis of Inflammatory Skin Disorders.* AB Ackerman. Philadelphia: Lea and Febiger, 1978.

## Gastrointestinal pathology

1   *Gastrointestinal Pathology. An Atlas and Text.* CM Fenoglio-Preiser, PE Lantz, MB Listrom, M Davis & FO Rilke (eds). New York: Raven Press, 1989.

2   *Pathology of the Gastrointestinal Tract.* S Ming & H Goldman (eds). Philadelphia: WB Saunders, 1992.

## Gynaecological and obstetrical pathology

1   *Blaustein's Pathology of the Female Genital Tract*, 4th edition. RJ Kurman (ed). New York: Springer-Verlag, 1994.

2 *Haines and Taylor: Obstetrical and Gynaecological Pathology*, 4th edition. H Fox & M Wells (eds). Edinburgh: Churchill Livingstone, 1995.

3 *Pathology of the Human Placenta*, 3rd edition. K Bernischke & P Kaufmann. New York: Springer-Verlag, 1995.

## Hepatobiliary pathology

1 *Pathology of the Liver*, 3rd edition. RNM MacSween, PP Anthony, PJ Scheuer, AD Bert & BC Portmann (eds). Edinburgh: Churchill Livingstone, 1994.

2 *Histopathology of the Liver*. G Klatskin & HO Conn. New York: Oxford University Press, 1993.

## Lymphoreticular pathology

1 *Neoplastic Hematopathology*. DM Knowles (ed). Baltimore: Williams & Wilkins, 1992.

2 *Essential Oncology of the Lymphocytes*. IJ Forbes & AS-Y Leong. London: Springer-Verlag, 1987.

## Neuropathology

1 *An Introduction to Neuropathology*. H Adams & DI Graham. London: Churchill Livingstone, 1988.

## Paediatric pathology

1 *Fetal and Neonatal Pathology*, 2nd edition. JW Keeling (ed). London: Springer-Verlag, 1993.

2 *Paediatric Surgical Pathology*, 2nd edition. LP Dehner. Baltimore: Williams & Wilkins, 1987.

## Pulmonary pathology

1 *Pulmonary Pathology*, 2nd edition. DH Dail & SP Hammer (eds). New York: Springer-Verlag, 1993.

This is an excellent and comprehensive textbook which covers many aspects of pulmonary pathology and is particularly strong in the area of pulmonary tumour pathology.

2 *Pathology of Pulmonary Disease*. MJ Saldana (ed). Philadelphia: JB Lippincott, 1994.

3 *Pathology of the Lung*, 2nd edition. WM Thurlbeck & AM Churg (eds). New York: Thieme, 1995.

## Renal pathology

1 *Renal Pathology with Clinical and Functional Correlation*. CC Tisher & BM Brenner (eds). Philadelphia: JB Lippincott, 1989.

This text is one of the foremost reference books in renal pathology.

2 *Pathology of the Kidney*, 4th edition. RH Hepinstall (ed). Boston: Little, Brown & Co, 1991.

This text is a widely used reference source in renal pathology and integrates extensive experimental data. It is produced as a three volume set and is extremely comprehensive.

## Soft tissue pathology

1 *Soft Tissue Tumours*, 3rd edition. FM Enzinger & SW Weiss. St Louis: CV Mosby, 1995.

This is a classic text and an absolute essential for the diagnosis of soft tissue lesions.

## Surgical pathology monograph series

1   AFIP: *Atlas of Tumor Pathology*.
     Washington, DC: Armed Forces
     Institute of Pathology.

These are classic benchtop manuals of
tumour pathology. They represent a series
of fascicles (currently Series III) covering
tumours in a wide range of body sites. The
fascicles are written mostly by American
authors who are internationally acknowledged experts. They contain excellent
illustrations of gross and microscopic
appearances and provide excellent value
for their cost. While almost every body site
has been covered in past fascicles, the
current includes melanocytic and non-
melanocytic tumours of the skin, tumours
of the uterine corpus, gestational trophoblastic diseases, tumours of the cervix,
vagina and vulva, tumours of the thyroid,
parathyroid, mammary gland, bones and
joints, bone marrow, central nervous
system, bladder and kidney, eye and ocular
adnexae and the lower respiratory tract.

2   *Major Problems in Pathology*. Series
     editor: VA LiVolsi. Philadelphia: WB
     Saunders.

This series of monographs was originally
edited by JL Bennington and they currently
cover a wide range of topics representing
problems in surgical pathology. Some of
these monographs are now in their second
edition. The topics covered include the
following:

   *Disorders of the Spleen* (B Wolf & R
      Neiman)
   *Immunomicroscopy* (CR Taylor)
   *Interpretation of Renal Biopsy*, 2nd
      edition (L Striker, J Olsen & G
      Striker)
   *Mucosal Biopsy of the Gastrointestinal
      Tract*, 4th edition (R Whitehead)

*Pathology of the Spinal Cord*, 2nd
   edition (JT Hughes)
*Pathology of the Uterine Cervix, Vagina
   and Vulva* (YS Foo & J Reagan)
*Perinatal Pathology* (JS Wigglesworth)
*Problems in Breast Pathology*, 2nd
   edition (J Azzopardi)
*Surgical Pathology of Bone Marrow* (B
   Wittels)
*Surgical Pathology of Lymph Nodes and
   Related Organs* (ES Jaffe)
*Surgical Pathology of Non-neoplastic
   Lung Disease*, 2nd edition (AA
   Katzenstein & FB Askin)
*Surgical Pathology of the Salivary
   Glands* (GL Ellis, PL Auclair & DR
   Gnepp)
*Surgical Pathology of the Thyroid* (VA
   LiVolsi)
*Thin Needle Aspiration Biopsy* (J Frable)
*Tumours of the Lung* (B MacKay, J
   Lukeman & N Ordonez)

3   *Systemic Pathology*. General Editor:
     WStC Symmers. Edinburgh:
     Churchill Livingstone.

This series started off as a textbook of
systemic pathology but currently, in its
third edition, has been expanded into
separate volumes devoted to specific organ
systems. The series includes the following:

   *Alimentary Tract* (BC Morson)
   *The Breast* (C Elston & IO Ellis)
   *Bone and Bone Marrow* (SN
      Wickramasinghe)
   *Bone, Joints and Soft Tissues* (AJ
      Malcolm, R Reid & M Catto)
   *Cardiovascular System* (MJ Davies, J
      Mann, RH Anderson, WB Robertson
      & N Woolf)
   *Endocrine System* (PD Lewis).
   *Gynaecological and Obstetrical
      Pathology* (MC Anderson)
   *Liver, Biliary Tract and Pancreas* (D
      Wight)

*The Lungs* (B Corrin)
*Male Reproductive System* (ID Ansell)
*Nervous System, Muscle and Eyes* (RO Weller)
*Nose, Throat and Ears* (I Friedmann)
*Skin* (D Weedon)
*Thymus, Lymph Nodes and Spleen* (K Henry & WStC Symmers)
*Urinary System* (KA Porter)

4   *Contemporary Issues in Surgical Pathology.* Series editor: LM Roth. Edinburgh: Churchill Livingstone.

This series currently comprises 10 volumes, each devoted to a specific topic in surgical pathology. They include:

*Liver Pathology* (RL Peters)
*Muscle Pathology* (RR Heffner)
*Pathology of the Colon, Small Intestine and Anus* (HT Norris)
*Pathology of Glomerular Disease* (S Rosen)
*Pathology of the Head and Neck* (DR Gnepp)
*Pathology of the Oesophagus, Stomach and Duodenum* (HD Appleman)
*Pathology of the Placenta* (EVDK Perrin)
*Pathology of the Testis and its Adnexae* (A Talerman & LM Roth)
*Pathology of the Vulva and Vagina* (EJ Wilkinson)
*Tumours and Tumour-like Conditions of the Ovary* (LM Roth & B Czernobilsky)

5   *Biopsy Interpretation Series.* Series Editor: SG Silverberg. New York: Raven Press.

This series of monographs is less extensive than the ones listed above. It currently covers:

*Bladder Biopsies* (PN Braun)
*Breast Biopsies* (D Carter)

*Endometrial Biopsies* (A Blaustein)
*Interpretation of Breast Biopsies* (D Carter)
*Prostate Biopsy Interpretation* (JI Epstein)
*Soft Tissue Sarcomas: Histological Diagnosis* (AD Nash)

6   *International Academy of Pathology Monographs in Pathology.* Series Editor: N Kaufmann. Baltimore: Williams and Wilkins.

These monographs are mainly compilations based on Long Courses presented at the Annual Scientific Meeting of the US and Canadian Divisions of the International Academy of Pathology. Some of these monographs are now dated. They include:

*Adrenal Cortex* (HD Moon & RE Stowell)
*Bones and Joints* (LV Ackerman, HJ Spjut & MR Abell)
*Brain* (OT Bailey & DE Smith)
*Connective Tissue* (BM Wagner & DE Smith)
*Connective Tissue Diseases* (BM Wagner, R Fleischmajer & N Kaufman)
*Current Topics in Inflammation and Infection* (G Majno, RS Cotran & N Kaufman)
*Gastrointestinal Tract* (JH Yardley, BC Mawson & MR Abell)
*Heart* (JE Edwards, M Lev & MR Abell)
*Kidney* (FK Mostofi & DE Smith)
*Kidney Disease: Present Status* (J Churg, BH Spargo, FK Mostofi & MR Abell)
*Liver* (EA Gaul & FK Mostofi)
*Lung* (AA Liebow & DE Smith)
*Lung, Structure, Function and Disease* (WM Thurbeck & MR Abell)
*The Lymphocyte and Lymphocytic Tissue* (JW Rebuck & RE Stowell)

*Ovary* (HG Grady & DE Smith)
*Pancreas* (PJ Fitzgerald & AB
   Morrison)
*Perinatal Diseases* (RL Naeye, JM
   Kissane & N Kaufman)
*Peripheral Blood Vessels* (JL Orbison &
   DE Smith)
*Platelet* (KM Brinkhous, RW Shermer
   & FK Mostofi)
*Reticuloendothelial System* (JW Rebuck,
   CW Berard & MR Abell)
*Skin* (EB Helwig & FK Mostofi)
*Striated Muscle* (CM Pearson & FK
   Mostofi)
*Thyroid* (JB Hazard & DE Smith)
*Uterus* (HJ Norris, AT Hertig & MR
   Abell)

7    *Recent Advances in Histopathology.*
   Edited by PP Anthony & RNM
   MacSween. Edinburgh: Churchill
   Livingstone.

This series is published yearly and is
currently in its 16th volume. It contains
review articles and contemporary topics and
serve as an update of major developments
in histopathology. It provides a useful
source of review for trainees presenting at
College and Board examinations.

8    *Biopsy Pathology Series.* Edited by LS
   Gottlieb, AM Neville & F Walker.
   London: Chapman & Hall.

The series currently includes:

*Bone and Bone Marrow* (B Frisch, SM
   Lewis, R Burkhardt & R Bartt)
*Brain* (JH Adams, DI Graham & D
   Doyle)
*Breast* (J Sloane)
*Bronchi* (EM McDowell & TF Beals)
*Cervix* (DR Coleman & DMD Evans)
*Colon and Rectum* (JC Talbot & AB
   Price)
*Endometrium* (CH Buckley & H Fox)
*Liver* (RS Patrick & J O'D McGee)

*Lymphoreticular System* (DH Wright &
   PG Isaacson)
*Muscle* (M Swash & MS Schwartz)
*Oesophagus, Stomach and Duodenum*
   (DW Day)
*Pathology of the Small Intestine* (FD
   Lee & PG Toner)
*Pulmonary Vasculature* (CA
   Wagenvoort & WJ Mooi)

9    *Pathology Annual.* Edited by PP Rosen
   & RE Fechner. Connecticut:
   Appleton and Lange.

This series is now into volume 29 and is
published yearly, currently as two parts,
devoted to all aspects of diagnostic pathology. Experts throughout the world are
invited to contribute reviews and updates
on subjects of current interest. It is a useful
publication for the trainees, particularly
those presenting for examinations.

## Journals

There are numerous subspeciality journals
but only a few of these will be listed as
they are less likely to be of immediate use
to the trainee. Undoubtedly, the others will
be referred to from time to time and at a
later stage in the trainee's career. Instead,
general and surgical pathology journals are
listed as they are more appropriate to the
trainee who should subscribe to one or two
of these and make a conscious effort to
scan the others for relevant articles and
reviews.

### General medical journals

It is useful for the trainee to subscribe to at
least one general medical journal such as
the *New England Journal of Medicine* or
the *Lancet*. These contain occasional

reviews on aspects of diseases which are useful to the trainee pathologist.

## General clinical pathology

These journals cover all disciplines of clinical pathology and include articles on experimental pathology, microbiology, immunology, haematology, chemical pathology besides autopsy and surgical pathology. While they provide up-to-date information in all these areas, surgical pathology usually occupies no more than one-third of the journals and the trainee can afford to be more selective in the articles to be read.

1   *Journal of Clinical Pathology*
This is the official publication of the Association of Clinical Pathologists of the United Kingdom and it is produced monthly with the aim of publishing original research of relevance to the understanding and practice of clinical pathology.

2   *American Journal of Clinical Pathology*
This is published monthly by Lippincott-Raven for the American Society of Clinical Pathologists.

3   *Pathology*
This is the official publication of the Royal College of Pathologists of Australasia and is published quarterly.

## Anatomical pathology

These journals are aimed more specifically at autopsy and surgical pathology and some deal solely with surgical pathology while others also include experimental pathology and contain review papers.

1   *American Journal of Surgical Pathology*
This journal, published by Raven Press in New York, is sponsored by the Arthur Purdy Stout Society of Surgical Pathology, the Gastrointestinal Pathology Society and the Society for Hematopathology. It probably represents the journal with greatest relevance to surgical pathologists and is essential reading for trainees.

2   *Human Pathology*
This journal aims to provide information of clinical pathological significance in human disease. Its primary goal is the presentation of information drawn from morphological and clinical laboratory studies and more than two-thirds of its pages are concerned with anatomical pathology.

3   *Histopathology*
This is the official publication of the British Division of the International Academy of Pathology. Its purpose is to provide original information on histopathological material which has relevance to the clinical study of human diseases. It is published monthly by Blackwell Science and members of the International Academy of Pathology receive a discounted subscription.

4   *Journal of Pathology*
This is the official publication of the Pathological Society of Great Britain and Ireland with the aim of publishing high quality papers in the fields of pathology and clinicopathological correlation. It is intended for all engaged in the fields of diagnostic and experimental pathology, as well as other workers outside the immediate field of pathology who are interested in disease mechanisms and clinico-pathological correlation.

5   *American Journal of Pathology*
This is the publication of the American Society of Investigative Pathology and published monthly by JB Lippincott. The journal has a strong experimental bias but also provides detailed reviews of the mechanisms of diseases.

6   *Pathology, Research and Practice*
This monthly journal has an international editorial board and represents the official

journal of the European Society of Pathology and is co-sponsored by the American Registry of Pathology. The journal publishes mostly papers related to diagnostic pathology and includes some aspects of experimental pathology and newer techniques in surgical pathology.

### 7   Archives of Pathology and Laboratory Medicine

This monthly journal is published by the American Medical Association and the College of American Pathologists. It covers all aspects of clinical pathology although anatomical pathology comprises a large portion of its pages.

### 8   Advances in Anatomic Pathology

This is a new publication, currently produced bimonthly by Raven Press. It provides major reviews and updates in anatomical pathology and highlights published papers relating to surgical pathology and methodology. It is a useful review journal for trainees as well as the busy surgical pathologist.

### 9   Seminars in Diagnostic Pathology

This is a quarterly publication edited by DJ Santa Cruz and published by WB Saunders Co. Each issue is devoted to a contemporary topic with very informative updates and reviews. It is a very useful journal for trainees.

## Subspeciality journals

### 1   Cytopathology

This is the official journal of the British Society of Clinical Cytology published by Blackwell Science. It is devoted to all aspects of cytology including gynaecological, non-gynaecological and fine needle aspiration cytology and screening.

### 2   Diagnostic Cytopathology

This journal is published monthly by Wiley-Liss. It provides a forum for exchange of information in cytopathology with emphasis on practical and clinical aspects. It is offered as a publication to all members of the Papanicolaou Society of Cytopathology and members of the Academy of Clinical Cytology and Cytopathology.

### 3   Acta Cytologica

This journal is the official publication of the Academy of Clinical Cytology and Cytopathology. It publishes articles on clinical and diagnostic cytology and on applied cell research and methodology.

### 4   Cancer

This is an interdisciplinary journal of the American Cancer Society which aims to integrate scientific information from worldwide sources from all oncological specialities and deals also with cancer prevention, early detection, diagnosis, cure and rehabilitation. A large part of the journal is devoted to these clinical aspects and the trainee should read this journal selectively for these reasons.

### 5   Applied Immunohistochemistry

This is the official publication of the Society for Applied Immunohistochemistry and is one of the few journals devoted entirely to diagnostic immunohistochemistry. It is currently a quarterly publication.

### 6   JCP: Clinical Molecular Pathology

This is a new journal published bimonthly as an edition of the Journal of Clinical Pathology. It is devoted to original research into the molecular aspects of disease and tumours which are relevant to clinical pathology. This journal is the result of the burgeoning information derived from the many new technologies related to the molecular aspects of diseases, information very pertinent to the contemporary surgical pathologist.

7   *International Journal of Gynecological Pathology*

This is published quarterly and represents the official publication of the International Society of Gynecological Pathologists. This is one of the few journals devoted purely to gynaecological pathology.

8   *Ultrastructural Pathology*

This is a bimonthly journal with emphasis on the use of electron microscopy in the study of human disease. It is probably the best journal devoted to diagnostic ultra-structural pathology.

9   *The Breast Journal*

This is a new multidisciplinary journal with an international editorial board devoted to all facets of research, diagnosis and treatment of breast disease.

# 21 Data storage and retrieval

## Introduction

The processing, storage, transmission and retrieval of data is an essential part of the practice of pathology yet uniform standards are lacking. Rapid advances in technology and system affordability have made pathologists increasingly dependent on computerisation in their daily work routines so that pathologists must have an input into this new area of medical informatics as well as the organised management of information technologies, including the evaluation and implementation of computer hardware, software and clinical laboratory automation technologies.

The rising cost of health care has placed pressures on rapid and efficient communication of laboratory results including surgical pathology reports. Computerisation enables storage, organisation, processing and retrieval of vast amounts of information and the potential benefits to pathology laboratories include increased efficiency and quality of services with improved patient care, labour cost savings and enhanced capability for research and teaching. Each laboratory must carefully equate their budget to needs to determine the optimal level of automation. Automation in surgical pathology laboratories, apart from databank systems, has been slow due to the relatively low number of specimens, non-quantitative nature of the data and complexity of interpretation. Technologies now impacting on surgical pathology include Automated Speech-recognition Anatomic Pathology (ASAP) reporting, standardised synoptic gross and microscopic reporting, autofaxing of reports, electronic imaging and telepathology. New electronic technologies also have an impact on pathologist education, not only through computer assisted training and revision programmes such as Intellipath, but also through the use of computers for the storage of reference articles, cases, slides and other data, and its use in the rapid search for relevant references related to subjects of interest.

## Data acquisition

Computerised information systems in surgical pathology became commercially available in the early 1980s with projects such as CoPath developed as a joint venture between Yale University and the Mumps Collaborative, Inc. (Massachussetts, USA). This automated system was founded on the principles that rapid response times were essential, all data needed to be integrated real-time, redundant data entry was to be eliminated, all primary data was to be stored on-line permanently and the system had to be sufficiently flexible to enable modification. Successful systems minimise human intervention in data entry and inquiry, and only those incorporating data in real-time demonstrate cost savings.

All specimens submitted for histological examination must be accompanied by accurate clinical and patient demographic information discussed in detail in Chapter 16. The assignment of a laboratory accession number together with patient demographics, including other data such as name of referring physician, health insurance status, type and nature of specimen and name of accessioning pathologist, is the first point of data acquisition and must be correctly performed.

## Specimen inquiry

Clinicians and pathologists should both be able to make rapid inquiries of pathology case status, even if incomplete, reports, diagnoses and previous pathology tests, not just of histology/cytology but from all clinical laboratories, in a properly organised integrated system. It should be possible to retrieve a given case by identifying the patient's surname, hospital record number, SNOMED diagnosis code or any other variable. On inquiry, the full text of the macroscopic and microscopic description, the diagnosis, with supplementary report if available, the name of the reporting pathologist and the date of completion of each component of the report must be available on screen. Ideally, a user-friendly Windows-based system should be used and there should be access to printing facilities. Draft texts of incomplete reports should not be available.

Ideal systems should be rapid and to be of practical value should have response times of less than a second for standard inquiries and a few seconds for database searches.

## Electronic imaging

Pathology is a morphology-based discipline and the ability to store, retrieve and transmit images with the creation of image databases is a rational complement to text databases already widely in use in pathology laboratories. Imaging system affordability is increasing every day and will soon be routine. Images can be captured with video cameras, still digital cameras and scanners. The transfer of images for consultation (telepathology) is already operational in countries such as Scandinavia.

Images in pathology are derived from a number of sources and include gross specimens, drawings and diagrams, light microscopy, electron microscopy, immuno-fluorescence, molecular diagnostic gels, image analysis data, flow cytometry and tabulated/graphic clinical laboratory data.

PC-based systems with high resolution video cameras connected to frame grabber cards, and in turn a 32-bit ethernet card for communication with a Windows-based CoPath laboratory information system, have been developed. Some advantages of such systems include improved patient care due to the availability of gross images at the time of slide reporting and sign out, comparison of histology with archived images of previous biopsies, capability for instantaneous consultation with other pathologists on the network and improved clinico-pathological conferences.

Libraries of stored video images are an invaluable teaching resource and digitised images of gross specimen diagrams are effective in reducing transfer of possibly soiled paperwork. Video images can be stored on-line, near-line on optical juke boxes, and for older cases and deceased patients, off-line on magnetic tapes or slow optical drives. Just as electronic databases have replaced the need to maintain paper-printed pathology reports, video imaging will replace the current filing systems for macroscopic photographs, drawings and radiographs. Current image database systems are still somewhat slow in operation but better integration with other operating systems and bar code scanning will enhance future use by pathologists.

## SNOP and SNOMED diagnosis coding systems

The development of the SNOP (Standard Nomenclature of Pathology, College of American Pathologists) and SNOMED (Standard Nomenclature of Medicine) coding systems were major developments as they enabled systematic numerical coding of diagnoses to replace free text data entry. This has led to standardisation of diagnostic terminology, and the ability to recover cases by numerical disease category code groupings has enhanced clinico-pathological review and research. Manual entry of SNOMED codes remains one area where errors in data processing are still significant. Automatic SNOMED coding from key words included in the diagnosis is now available and will help overcome this problem.

## Data storage

There are no uniform standards applicable for the duration of storage of pathological specimens and data generated therefrom.

Generally, pathology reports should be stored indefinitely and tissue blocks stored for at least 10 years and as long as possible. The storage of such material is essential for patient care, and the tissues and databases are a vital component of successful clinical-based research.

The guidelines of NATA (National Association of Testing Authorities of Australia) are not clear on wet tissue retention time but histology reports, slides, blocks and 'abnormal' cytology slides must be retained for a minimum of 14 years, whilst 'normal' cytology slides must be kept for a minimum of 2 years. Other agencies recommend retention of blocks, slides and reports and photographs of all positive and significant negative immunofluorescence preparations indefinitely. Practice guidelines will vary in different countries.

In some countries, patients or their next-of-kin appear to retain the legal right of ownership over removed body tissues including blocks and possibly slides, but the pathologist is obliged to examine and sample all tissue specimens. Should wet tissue be handed over to the patient, remove formalin from the container, wash the specimen, place it into 70% alcohol, seal the container and label it with a biohazard sticker. The patient must sign a release form for the specimen. If avoidable, do not release surgical pathology reports, slides or blocks directly to patients but to their physicians.

Pathology information systems should have the potential to hold permanently on-line all case data including clinical and demographic details, the surgical pathology or cytology report (macroscopic, block key, microscopic, conclusion, diagnosis code, comments and special investigations) and billing codes. A section on the report for non-printed comments is helpful to include information such as floaters on the slide or to record intradepartmental consultations and opinions. Database information is also invaluable for administrative tasks such as generating overdue lists and workload recording. It also is essential for cancer registries and, in the case of cervical cancer screening, recall reminders for periodic Pap smears can be computer-generated.

On-line storage of data necessitates construction of system safeguards to avoid loss or corruption of information. Many systems monitor computer terminal log-in, log-out times, incorporate two or more step password protection with user identification, and have refresh screen capabilities to return the monitor screen to a pre-password stage if a user is absent from his/her terminal for any significant length of time. Automatic log-off facilities of non-active terminals of between 5 and 10 minutes is another available safety feature but this can be an annoying feature for pathologists who work with their terminals only intermittently and have to re-log-in each time to access past information or make on-line corrections or edits to a report prior to validation. Data integrity can be maintained by limiting editing only to the accessioning pathologist.

Other precautions to avoid data loss include backing up of data, typically on a daily basis overnight, simultaneously saving all data on two separate storage machines (mirroring) and storage of computer readable data copies (magnetic tapes, microfilm, laser discs) off-site. The introduction of 'virus' into pathology system databases is a real risk and this danger is minimised by the foregoing safety measures. Frequent computer system failures are a major impediment to improving pathology service quality.

## Information access

New biomedical information is currently generated at a tremendous pace and this is so not only in clinical medicine and therapeutics but also in the area of pathology. With the rapid advances and developments in technology, the information accumulated in the realms of diagnostic testing and prognostication is overwhelming and if the pathologist is to continue to serve the vital function of providing the most current and accurate information available, he or she must have effective tools to manage medical informatics. The Internet is one such network which allows immediate access to up-to-date databases. The origin of this network is the Advanced Research Projects Agency Network (ARPANET) which was built by the Department of Defence in the USA in 1969 to link together military computers. With its increasing popularity, many other regional networks were linked to it, including those of many colleges and universities. This expansion resulted into the splitting of ARPANET into two smaller

networks, namely MILNET for the military sites and ARPANET for the non-military sites. Because of the development of faster machines and increasing numbers of machines, ARPANET was replaced in 1990 by the father of the Internet, the NSFNET (National Science Foundation NET), which was much faster and was able to handle the additional load created by the increasing number of workstations. Other countries around the world soon followed this example and built their own smaller networks and in one way or another most of these networks were hooked-up to a US network, thereby linking the computers of the world. This is what is known today as the Internet.

Internet access is often provided free of charge to individual users associated with universities or large research or medical centres. Individuals can be privately connected to Internet via a modem and a standard telephone line or via a modem through one of two types of software packages: Serial Line Internet Protocol (SLIP) or Point-To-Point Protocol (PPP). A number of medical databases are available through Internet, allowing access to sources such as National Institutes of Health (NIH) updates on cancer data for treatment programs and other databases such as MEDLINE, AIDSLINE and CANCERNET, allowing the user to search and retrieve information which is often vital to pathologists who are required to answer questions in relation to consultation, and for access to the most recent information.

Access to Internet also allows the user to send and receive e-mail messages. E-mail has many advantages besides speed and economy. It also allows intradepartmental communication, announcement of departmental news, conferences and scheduled meetings and appointments. The pathologist is also able to communicate with clinicians and laboratory service supervisors who may be difficult to contact by phone. The list of uses is extensive and extends into teaching, research and even day-to-day management of the laboratory.

Mailing lists allow pathologists to join a forum with on-going discussions, questions and announcements about a variety of topics. PATHNET, the Armed Forces Institute of Pathology Mailing List, is a forum for issues related to the study and practice of pathology. PATHO-L, Pathology Discussion Group On-Line, is another forum for any topic related to the science and study of pathology and GRIPE, Group for Research in Pathology Education, is a forum for discussions related to improving pathology education and includes a diverse range of topics from technology to teaching philosophies.

Computers can also be employed in the training of pathologists. Standard textbooks such as the 5th edition of *Robbin's Pathologic Basis of Disease* is available in an electronic version (Pathology TextStack, Keyboard Publishing) inclusive of text with all illustrations and diagrams. Banks of multiple choice questions can be found, such as in QuizBank I and II (Keyboard Publishing) with over 3800 questions, whilst the software of Intellipath (Intelligent Pathology Systems, California) and bar-code-accessed image atlases are marketed by Mosby/Image. Intellipath is an algorithm and image based system intended for both education and case diagnosis and utilises laser disc technology. As of 1994, 14 modules including lymph node pathology with 10 500 images and pigmented lesions of the skin with 2800 images were available and others were being finalised.

Medline data is now readily obtained on CD-ROM or as an inbuilt part of information system networks. CD-ROM databases include Medline Express from the US National Library of Medicine bibliography database, Health ROM from the Australian Government Health Information and DNASIS from Genebank and Serline bibliographic information on biomedical and health science services. These systems provide abstracts of papers published in major health science journals and are also available as on-line databases.

## Personal databases and filing systems

While electronic databases are readily available to the pathologist, it is still often necessary to have photocopies or reprints of relevant articles in personal files for several reasons. Surgical pathology is a morphology-based discipline and it is frequently necessary to have photographic images of the lesion of interest available for comparison to aid in the diagnosis of an uncommon or newly described entity. Furthermore, on-line databases provide only abstracts and full reprints or photocopies may be necessary for discussions with colleagues and for teaching and research. It is thus inevitable that the trainee pathologist will acquire a collection of reprints which will continue to increase with time even after completion of his or her training.

It will be necessary to develop some method of filing these reprints. One of the simplest methods is to file the reprints according to organ systems or by diseases but this soon becomes a cumbersome and unmanageable method when the number of reprints in each file exceeds 100. Furthermore, this method does not allow for cross-referencing, e.g. Hodgkin's disease of the liver will require referencing under 'Hodgkin's disease' as well as 'liver' but can only be physically placed in one file. A more practical method which is not limited by size or number and allows unlimited cross-referencing is to assign consecutive numbers to the reprints as they are acquired and read. Using a card filing system or a personal computer, each reprint can be referenced by as many key words as necessary or by author or authors of the paper, the latter being a less useful way of referencing. The title of the reprint and authors and even abstract of the article can be scanned into the computer and the key words provided in the paper can be used for cross-referencing. This method has several major advantages. It can be done by an assistant, is not limited by size, and reprints are simple to retrieve as they are filed by consecutive numbers and can be separated into manageable groups of 50 or 100. When the collection requires culling, earlier reprints can be discarded without disruption to the system.

Another collection which the trainee pathologist acquires early in his or her training are Kodachromes of macroscopic and microscopic images. A similar method of filing can be employed although the collection of Kodachromes is likely to be much smaller and a simpler method would be to number the Kodachromes consecutively and cross-reference by topography and morphology, e.g. liver: Hodgkin's disease, with referencing under 'liver' and 'Hodgkin's disease'.

It cannot be over-emphasised that a simple method of filing must be adopted as early as possible before one's collection of reprints or Kodachromes becomes too large and filing of the backlog would take too much time.

One problem which the trainee will encounter early in his or her career is the refiling of reprints removed for study and slides removed for lectures and presenta-tion. It is best that these be refiled immediately after use, otherwise they tend to accumulate and never get refiled. While it is often easy to perform this task for reprints, the refiling of Kodachromes that have been used for lectures can be a more tedious process. In particular, if they have been specially selected for a specific topic lecture and periodically reused. In such circumstances, it is best to retain the entire set of Kodachromes in the sequence of their presentation identified either by numbers with colour codes or by drawing a thick oblique line with a marking pen across the side of the stack of Kodachromes arranged in their sequence of use. This will allow identification of the exact placement of each Kodachrome. This entire set of Kodachromes can then be duplicated and the duplicates can be refiled into the main file. The marked set is retained intact for future presentations.

## Further reading

Di Giorgio CJ, Richert CA, Klatt E, Becich MJ 1994 E-mail, the Internet and information access technology in pathology. Seminars in Diagnostic Pathology 11: 294–304

Langford LA 1995 Electronic imaging: a guide for anatomic pathologists. Advances in Anatomic Pathology 2: 141–152

Schubert E, Gross W, Becich MJ 1994 Computer-assisted instruction in pathology residency training: design and implementation of integrated productivity and education work stations. Seminars in Diagnostic Pathology 11: 282–293

# 22 Professional examinations, subspecialisation and research

It would be inappropriate to conclude this compendium without a short discussion on professional examinations, subspecialisation and research. These subjects are not of immediate concern to the pathologist starting his or her training but are of obvious relevance for the future.

## Professional examinations

### Examination and training requirements

Without a higher degree or qualification in pathology, you are unlikely to be licensed to practise as a specialist or consultant pathologist. While the regulations for licensing differ in different countries, in most, it will be necessary to complete a prescribed period of training and to pass a written and perhaps also practical examination set by a professional body representing pathologists in your country. Most examinations will attempt to establish whether a candidate has achieved a satisfactory level of competence during his/her training, which will enable him/her to function as a consultant pathologist.

Pathology training is essentially an apprenticeship, and it is necessary to ensure that you obtain the best training possible by working in a department which allows access and exposure to most aspects of pathology including specialised areas of surgical pathology such as neuropathology, cytopathology, renal gynaecological pathology and paediatric pathology. It may be necessary to rotate through different institutions to obtain the required breadth of training.

### Study and preparation

Before approaching the written examination it is necessary for the candidate to

have developed a system of learning. The principles of learning are simple, though it is hard to put into effect. Training in surgical pathology is a 'hands-on' process but it requires constant reinforcement by theoretical consideration of the practical work. This can be done by discussion, formal teaching sessions, by reading and by auditing the work. In surgical pathology, the frequent and constant exposure to the same disease or pathology in the form of diagnostic cases at routine cut-up and reporting, at slide seminars and daily slide review sessions provide an excellent opportunity for reinforcement. In every encounter between two or more people, whether spoken or written, there is potential for learning. Most of the learning is done on the job but you will need to think about how to reinforce this. It can be done by personal effort and study and may be helped by attending lectures and seminars. In essence, successful learning is attained only through personal effort, even though it may be directed and helped along by your seniors and supervisors. Learning must be planned and made effective personally as no one else can do it for you.

In your approach to the professional examination, it is important to realise that the examination is very much a 'game situation', often with limited relevance to the way in which surgical pathology is actually practised. The exam is an artificial situation designed in an attempt to assess your level of competency, your knowledge, and your ability to apply it in a practical manner. Like all games, it has rules, subtleties and refinements, but it is necessary to win as the price of losing is expensive, if nothing else. It is, therefore, important to know the rules of the examination or 'game'. These rules should be available through the bodies conducting the examination and it would be of immense help to obtain copies of past examination questions. This will provide you with an insight into the breadth and depth of the examination. It will also allow you the opportunity of practising answers for the exam.

The surgical pathologist has access to a wide range of books and journals and during the period of his/her training, it is important to assimilate new information as it appears in these journals as well as to read review articles which are often timely and relate to subjects of contemporary interest and importance. In this respect, it is important to develop a correct reading habit. Reading is a technique that may be learned so that it can be effective for the purposes at hand. While many systems of reading have been described, it is necessary for you to decide at the onset whether an article should be skipped, skimmed, read or studied. A great deal of reading material, even in learned journals, may be skipped entirely as being of no relevance to you and your requirement at the time. Do not waste your time on idle browsing unless that is your conscious intent, as it might be with a glossy magazine. But, if it is your intention to read for a purpose, then be selective in what you read and most material can be skipped entirely. Skim when you want to have an outline of what is written without taking too much notice of it and when you do not wish to read anything in detail. Skimming is ideal for reading large volumes of committee minutes, with which we are inundated from time to time. In these, headings alone are enough to tell you whether to skip or skim. In longer, continuous prose, a glance at the first and last sentences in each paragraph might be sufficient to tell you all that you wish to know, provided the author has done his/her job well. If the author has not, then do not waste your time. If his/her prose is

unclear, so probably is his/her thinking, and you have no time for slovenliness.

Skimming may be used for most pathology journals. You want a clue as to what the article is about without extreme detail, the title of the article may be enough for you or may put you off entirely. Summaries may or may not be useful but are enough to indicate whether to skip, skim, read or, rarely, study.

Reading means paying careful attention to what has been written so as to understand it but not necessarily reproduce it in detail later. Reading falls short of the attention needed to study. You should be interested in the subject and reading is meant to satisfy that interest. It is a technique that you might use with a novel and the pace of reading is important since you are doing it for leisure. You can savour the style, the content and the plot slowly, or you can simply get on and enjoy the story. A journal article demands greater attention than this, but it is up to you to decide.

Studying, in essence, consists of reading, recalling and reviewing. The key word is 'reinforcement', driving the material that you have read into your memory for recall when needed, in examinations, in diagnostic or clinical situations, or teaching sessions. You should first look over the summary so that you can see what the paper is about, then you read the work completely. Next you 'recall' it by going over it in your mind to see that you remember and understand the contents. Alternatively, you might write notes or talk to someone else about what you have learnt. This allows you to identify the gaps in your learning and you can correct these by turning back and going over the piece again. At the next learning session, you review the work done before and quickly recall it to yourself to check that you know it. You can then move on to the next section and read, recall and review. Taking notes may help to reinforce this memory process. This is the core of the learning process. Surgical pathology is a morphology-based discipline and pathology articles are invariably well illustrated. Pay careful attention to the photographs and read the legends as they provide another opportunity of imprinting the image in your memory. Examining a tissue section with the lesion or pathology provides yet another opportunity of recalling and revising.

Few people give the technique of reading any thought, having learnt to do it in childhood. One may think that reading is ingrained and it is to be used always in roughly the same way. But by thinking of the varying purposes of reading gives flexibility so that you know why you are doing it. Often, rather than mechanically wading through a number of articles in one reading session, it may be useful to make short notes or paragraph summaries of the more important sections of the article. Subsequent informal discussion with colleagues or in the context of a journal club will aid in hammering the knowledge in so that it is relevant and will stay in our mind. At all cost, avoid reading books or journals as a chore as it is a certain way to become disillusioned and disheartened with the task in hand!

## Examination techniques

Examinations seem to be an integral part of a career in medicine and yet examination technique is not taught as part of the medical curriculum. Doctors have to take so many exams that they are experts in the subject; yet some fail because of lack of technique. Failure, for whatever cause or reason, is destructive of self-confidence, making it harder to pass a failed exam

subsequently. Do not take an examination unless you have really done the work for it. Be sure to go through the curriculum before commencing your preparation. While some professional boards and colleges still conduct the written examination in the form of essay-type questions, multiple choice questions are also commonplace. If the latter is so, in preparation for the exam, you must practise answering multiple choice questions. The examining body will not let you have any of their questions because they belong to their secret bank of questions; however, there are dozens of books for practice. There are many forms of multiple choice questions and it will serve you well to find out from your examining body, from a recent candidate, or from an examiner just what kind of multiple choice question paper is set and be prepared to know the technique you need. With a large number of questions to be answered in a restricted time, it is probably best to go through them all, entering the answers to those you are sure of. Then go back and work through those you have left out first time around. You must try to be systematic. If wrong answers are definitely penalised by deduction of marks, do not guess the answers and be sure you know how to erase wrong answers that you wish to correct. As with all examinations, read the instructions very carefully before you start to be sure that you know exactly what is expected of you.

The short answer question is a common component of the written examination. Adhere rigidly to the instructions as you get no credit for straying and interpreting them in the manner you wish. If 10 lines of script are asked for, do not write 20. Examiners give considerable thought to the form and format of the examination and how they should be marked so that it annoys them if candidates do not stick to the rules.

The essay-type question allows you a freer hand but these often have specific intent which is stated in the question, so ensure that your answer is relevant and do not stray as it will not earn you marks. It is useful to construct an essay plan, using headings and key words to represent contents of a sentence or paragraph. You must develop the ability to translate a plan into an essay and this can be done with regular practice, starting with a plan from which the essay is written within a reasonable time limit. Generally, 45 minutes is allowed per question and the plan can be done within 5 minutes at the beginning. Write this plan into the answer script, clearly deleting this plan when you have completed your answer. This has several advantages. Firstly, it allows you to formulate your thoughts and organise your answer rather than commencing writing freestyle immediately which very often results in distorted answers, with over-detailed description at the beginning and gradual deterioration towards the end as time begins to run out. Also, facts are often recalled out of sequence or in a random fashion and these can be more readily slotted into an essay plan but it is much more difficult to modify free prose-style answers to accommodate these variations. The outline may also have another benefit in that although not part of the formal answer, it is clearly visible to the examiner and it will allow an immediate overview of the general organisation. In the event that the answer cannot be completed, it will also show that you have considered all the major points in your plan and will indicate the direction of the answer and what was intended. The plan should be laid out neatly, with enough gaps to add in infor-mation which comes to mind during the course of writing the answer.

It is important to estimate how much time to allocate for each question and subsection and to adhere to it. Ensure that your hand writing is legible. Few examiners read every word of an answer but skim through it looking for the facts asked for, the development of an argument, logic and perhaps also watching for the use of English. Use headings when appropriate. Each paragraph should start with a sentence that states what the paragraph is about, and any new thought, fact or statement needs a new paragraph. You must do everything in your power to make the reading of your answer easy for the examiner who must not have to work hard to find out what you know. He/she might become impatient if you make him/her struggle either with your handwriting or with your style. If these are good, they may even help to gloss over deficiencies in your knowledge.

## Subspecialisation

The surgical pathologist is the last of the true generalists. All disciplines of medicine have undergone subspecialisation with internist physicians and surgeons subspe-cialised as nephrologists and urologists, cardiologists and cardiothoracic surgeons, endocrinologists and endocrine surgeons, hepatologists and hepatobiliary surgeons, etc. Each of these subspecialities demands equally specialised knowledge from the pathologist. It is difficult, if not impossible, to provide this expertise without some degree of subspecialisation by the surgical pathologist.

Clinical subspeciality training requires attachment to the appropriate subspeciality unit as the clinical trainee requires exposure to clinical material. However, in the case of surgical pathology, we have the distinct advantage in that much of the training can be done on archival material in the form of microscopic slides, tissue blocks, electron micrographs and detailed pathology reports without the requirement for patients. Aided by the extensive literature available on the subject, slide seminars, conducted courses and workshops, the pathologist is able to do most of his/her basic training in a subspeciality without attachment to a subspeciality pathology unit or a pathologist with the appropriate special interest, although, in most cases, this latter process successfully completes the training. Thus, it is advisable for the trainee to choose at least two to three areas in which to develop a subspeciality interest. Of course, it is possible to change these selections as you progress in your training or even later in your career. In contrast, it is extremely difficult for a cardiologist to switch interest to another area such as endocrinology or neurology.

## Research

Research as an educational tool is often misunderstood. Few people are destined to be Nobel Prize Laureates or will make a major, lasting contribution to the sum of medical knowledge. However, it should be evident by now that the surgical pathologist has an integral role which encompasses diagnosis, patient care, education and, inevitably, research. All doctors, in particular pathologists, should be alert, inquiring and show special interest in some subject. Research is not done solely so that it will look good on your curriculum vitae. It is done because it is fun to find new things out and it heightens critical faculties and enthusiasm for what you are doing. What

you find out may not be new to others who know about the subject, but research is also a voyage of discovery of things for oneself. Until you become a recognised expert in the field, your research is most likely to benefit you the most. It adds mainly to your private knowledge and development, and with luck, to public scientific knowledge. Quite apart from any obvious importance of your work, you will have contributed to the thinking and teaching about your subject in your immediate circle. Progress in medical knowledge generally comes from the glacial process of addressing a series of very small questions related to a given problem and not the galvanic process of discovering a single generic solution to the problem! In everything, there is a point at which knowledge runs out and is inadequate. There are always new ways of looking at pieces of knowledge and correlating them in ways different from previously so that new insights emerge. If you perform research, this will certainly happen to you personally, giving a little glow of satisfaction, and the insights may be illuminating to others also. Even old problems can bear looking at again and they come up fresh again because someone has recently thought about them in a slightly different way than before. You can do it too, and you should.

It has been said that 'inspiration comes from work and not work from inspiration'. Too many pathologists wait for inspiration when what is needed is work. Furthermore, when you begin critical questioning, it carries over into all your diagnostic work. There is no necessity for research to be separated from everyday practice. Research is an attitude of mind linked to intellectual and practical energy. The everyday workload is often used as an excuse to avoid the much harder work of thinking, and the research that flows from it.

Publication is the proper endpoint of research as it marks the completion of a piece of work and makes the author review what he/she has done and appraise it. It concentrates the mind, it may add to public knowledge, and the work is submitted to a wider critical audience. The object of writing up a piece of research is to make you appraise just what it is that you have done. Until you write, your ideas will be nebulous and undisciplined. Writing refines your ideas and makes you discard some and develop others. It is a voyage of self-exploration, and the polishing of a piece that you have personally wrought. Whether or not it impresses anyone else is of less consequence, as it is yours and you have done it. If it is, in fact, published, then your pleasure will be greater. Even worse than the ignorance is the dismissal of research effort as being trivial. The lazy and complacent are often heard to say that most of what is published is a waste of time, paper and trees, and that the authors would have been better employed getting on with their diagnostic work and not having to produce papers. This entirely misconceives the purpose of research which is a form of advanced education for the researcher. It is a form of thought and way of life above the humdrum. Formal education lifts the educated above the ruck, but research and publication carries on the process of education so that it is continuing, and enlivens day-to-day work. Once it has been tasted it transforms, and the change in the pathologist is visible in all he/she does. Of course, most research is trivial if it is compared and measured only by its contribution to public useable knowledge, but research is also to be measured by what it does to those who perform it. It is evidence of a striving, lively mind engaged in the highest intellectual activity of which it is capable. Research completes and binds the component roles and function of the surgical pathologist as a diagnostician, clinician and teacher.